Memory Improvement

Douglas J. Herrmann / Herbert Weingartner
Alan Searleman / Cathy McEvoy
Editors

Memory Improvement

Implications for Memory Theory

Springer-Verlag
New York Berlin Heidelberg London Paris
Tokyo Hong Kong Barcelona Budapest

Douglas Herrmann
National Center for Health Statistics
Hyattsville, MD 20782, USA

Herbert Weingartner
NIMH
Bethesda, MD 20892, USA

Alan Searleman
Department of Psychology
St. Lawrence University
Canton, NY 13617, USA

Cathy McEvoy
Department of Aging and Mental Health
University of South Florida
13301 Bruce B. Downs Blvd.
Tampa, FL 33612-3899, USA

With 4 Illustrations

Library of Congress Cataloging-in-Publication Data
Memory improvement : implications for memory theory / edited by
Douglas Herrmann ... [et al.].
p. cm.—
Includes bibliographical references and indexes.
ISBN-13: 978-1-4612-7656-2 e-ISBN-13: 978-1-4612-2760-1
DOI: 10.1007/978-1-4612-2760-1
1. Memory—Congresses. 2. Mnemonics—Congresses. I. Herrmann, Douglas J.
[DNLM: 1.Memory—congresses. BF 371 M5326]
BF371.M4515 1992
153.1'2—dc20
DNLM/DLC 92-2169
for Library of Congress

Printed on acid-free paper.

Softcover reprint of the hardcover 1st edition 1992

Production managed by Christin Ciresi; manufacturing supervised by Vincent Scelta.
Camera-ready copy prepared by the editors using Wordperfect.

9 8 7 6 5 4 3 2 1

ISBN-13: 978-1-4612-7656-2

For Our Spouses

Donna Herrmann	*Liz Weingartner*
Janice Searleman	*Douglas Nelson*

Preface

This text contains the lectures presented at a conference titled "Memory Improvement: Implications for Memory Theory" which was held at Union College in October of 1990. We thank Union College, the Teabod Spencer Fund, and the Pew Foundation for their support of this conference. We are especially appreciative of Seth Greenberg and Hugh Foley for their efforts in making this conference possible.

Individually and collectively, the four of us had been thinking of convening a conference to examine the most recent findings about memory improvement and to demonstrate the relevance of the new approach to memory improvement for a scientific understanding of human memory. Much to our good fortune, Dave Burrows of Skidmore College directed us to Seth and Hugh because he knew they were considering holding a conference concerned with everyday memory. After a discussion, it was agreed that the conference would assume the focus found in this text.

It is important to note that this conference departs from the traditional specialist conference. Such conferences typically involve specialists presenting and defending their research of recent years on a particular topic. All papers (except the first two and final two) review the major findings that illustrate how a certain psychological factor (psychopharmacology, emotional state, metamemory, strategies, practice, external aids, social interaction, context, and attention) may be influenced to produce memory improvement. The authors of chapters who have done research pertinent to a review include it, but with the same emphasis as would be given to other comparable findings. As a result, this text presents the latest and the most thorough examination of the methods and findings of memory improvement ever published. Moreover, the second chapter presents a new historical analysis of memory theories as they bear on memory improvement. Finally, the last two chapters of the text (by McEvoy and by Zacks and Hasher) present the first comprehensive attempt to relate memory improvement phenomena to the theories of memory improvement and to memory theory in general.

DOUGLAS HERRMANN
HERBERT WEINGARTNER
ALAN SEARLEMAN
CATHY MCEVOY

Contents

Contributors

DEBORAH L. BEST Department of Psychology, Wake Forest University, Winston-Salem, North Carolina 27109, USA

STEPHEN J. CECI Department of Human Development and Family Studies, Cornell University, Ithaca, New York 14853, USA

MICHELLE DESIMONE Department of Human Development and Family Studies, Cornell University, Ithaca, New York 14853, USA

PAMELA BEARD EL-DINARY Department of Human Development, University of Maryland, College Park, Maryland 20742, USA

MICHAEL M. GRUNEBERG University College of Swansea, Swansea, Wales, United Kingdom

LYNN HASHER Department of Psychology, Duke University, Durham, North Carolina 27706, USA

DOUGLAS J. HERRMANN National Center for Health Statistics, Hyattsville, MD 20782, USA

PAULA T. HERTEL Department of Psychology, Trinity University, San Antonio, Texas 78284, USA

CHRISTOPHER HERTZOG School of Psychology, Georgia Institute of Technology, Atlanta, Georgia 30332, USA

MARGARET JEAN INTONS-PETERSON Department of Psychology, Indiana University, Bloomington, Indiana 47405, USA

SARAH JOHNSON Department of Human Development and Family Studies, Cornell University, Ithaca, New York 14853, USA

CATHY L. MCEVOY Department of Aging and Mental Health, University of South Florida, Tampa, Florida 33612 , USA

GEORGE L. NEWSOME, III Department of Psychology, Indiana University, Bloomington, Indiana 47405, USA

DAVID G. PAYNE Department of Psychology, State University of New York at Binghamton, Binghamton, New York 13901, USA

DANA J. PLUDE Department of Psychology, University of Maryland, College Park, Maryland 20742, USA

MICHAEL PRESSLEY Department of Human Development, University of Maryland, College Park, Maryland 20742, USA

ALAN SEARLEMAN Department of Psychology, St. Lawrence University, Canton, New York 13617, USA

HERBERT WEINGARTNER National Institute of Mental Health, Bethesda, Maryland 20892, USA

MICHAEL J. WENGER Department of Psychology, State University of New York at Binghamton, Binghamton, New York 13901, USA

ROSE T. ZACKS Department of Psychology, Michigan State University, East Lansing, Michigan 48824, USA

The New Approach to Memory Improvement: Problems and Prospects

Michael M. Gruneberg

It is of course an honor to be asked to make an introduction to a conference in the area of one's particular interest; all the more so when the conference is on a topic that, until recently, I for one despaired of being taken seriously by academic psychologists. I think it fair to say that this conference is further evidence, if any were needed, that such despair was misplaced, and that, notwithstanding the attack on practical applications by such as Banaji and Crowder (1989), the application of memory studies to real-life problems is moving toward center stage.

The change in climate that allows the serious scrutiny of practical application has a number of important implications, not all of which have been taken on board by academic psychologists. First and foremost, it allows the serious treatment of whole areas that had previously been regarded as marginal. Memory improvement is undoubtedly one of these areas. Partly, I think this marginal view of memory improvement was because the area seemed to have little to offer that was new. Since the time of the Greeks, memory improvement has been associated with mnemonic systems, which could be demonstrated to work efficiently, indeed dramatically, but which didn't actually seem to be of much use in real life. Herrmann and Searleman (1990), for example, note the failure of memory improvement courses to have any effect on behavior in follow-up evaluations: hence Park, Smith, and Cavanaugh's (1990) recent approving quote of Bacon that mnemonic aids were "a barren thing for human uses" (p. 326). Partly, however, the lack of interest may have reflected an embarrassment that academic psychologists have at getting their hands "dirty" in practical, nontheoretical areas. I believe this conference shows that both these reasons are invalid.

In the first place, the work of Herrmann and Searleman (1990) in particular, with their multimodal approach to memory improvement shows, as do the multiplicity of approaches at this conference, that many new ways of improving memory are emerging including the importance of physical states, mental states, and the knowledge that individuals have about the range of effective strategies. Herrmann and Searleman's thesis, that these factors need to be integrated with task specific repertoires of behavior, surely opens up enormous possibilities for advances in the practical advice and help that academic psychologists can give to the man in the street. My only minor difference with them is a matter of emphasis on the value of traditional mnemonic strategies. In my view, some repertoires would benefit from the adaptation of some traditional mnemonic strategies--that in order to herald in the new it may be worth trying to recycle at least bits of the baby, if not the bathwater!

The other possible worry of academic psychologists, that there is little of theoretical value in investigating memory improvement, has also been shown to be unfounded by the contents of this conference. It always had to be a dubious argument. In the first place, practical problems are surely the testbed of theoretical ideas. The strongest argument against Banaji and Crowder's wish to confine the study of memory to the controlled condition of the laboratory is that this would prevent any real test of theories in the real world. It is as if a plane designer is not interested in whether the plane actually flies, as long as it flies on paper. To confine work on memory to the laboratory is to miss possible complex interactions that occur in real life and that materially affect memory performance. An example we gave in our reply to Banaji and Crowder (1989) is of the correlation between knowledge base and memory (e.g. Gruneberg, Morris, & Sykes, 1991). Under "real-life" conditions, when subjects heard real football scores, the correlation between knowledge of football and retention of new scores was .82. When subjects knew that the scores were made up, the correlation dropped to .36 (Morris, Tweedy, & Gruneberg, 1985). Presumably the real-life nature of the experience affected willingness to process incoming information. If the relationship had not been tested in a real-life situation, the extent of the underlying relationship between knowledge base and retention would not have been demonstrated. To be fair to Banaji and Crowder, it must be noted that they are concerned to ensure scientific rigor and control and as a scientific aim this cannot be faulted. The problem is, in an imperfect world, we sometimes have to settle for less than perfection if we are to gain insights into important phenomena. Indeed, it has often been noted when dealing with any new phenomena, even in the laboratory, that we often at first fail to control important variables until further research reveals their significance.

It is not only as a test bed of theoretical ideas in the laboratory, however, that practical application to the real world is important. Is it not self-evident that many questions in science start in the real world and become refined and controlled in the laboratory? This leads to hypothesis testing and ultimately model building and theory construction in order to account for the phenomena investigated. One of the excitements of memory research in general and the area of memory improvement in particular is that many of the approaches are so new that their theoretical implications can, at present, only be guessed at. Theorizing is only fruitful when there is a body of data, and the change that is making theory building possible is the change in the climate of the last 20 or so years that has led to the accumulation of a significant body of empirical data. As we all know, data and theory are equally necessary if research is to become guided by a coherent framework to advance both practical application and understanding of the underlying mechanisms of memory.

The aim of this conference is, of course, to examine the theoretical implications of the new approach to memory improvement. It is held against the background of the paper published last year by Banaji and Crowder (1989) who questioned whether anything of theoretical interest had emerged as a result of all the activity on practical application and the study of everyday memory. Well, of course it depends on what is meant by worthwhile in this context, but already the multimodal approach to memory improvement put forward by Herrmann and Searleman (1990) has focussed on the considerable complexity of understanding memory performance over and above the complexity involved in understanding the classical, if you like, structural memory problems of encoding, storage, and retrieval. It is clear that memory performance cannot be understood without taking account of phýsical conditions such as time of day; mental conditions such as motivation, mood and depression; attitudes such as feeling confident of success; or social context conditions such as those involving control of social flow of information.

Yet even psychologists approaching memory from a different perspective, such as Weinert (1988) note that merely looking at structural aspects of memory itself is too simplistic if one is to understand memory performance. Weinert notes three other factors which must be taken into account: first, the strategies employed on a memory task; second, the knowledge that an individual has about these strategies (metamemory); and third, the knowledge base to which new information is related. How these factors interact with encoding, storage, retrieval, and context factors such as physical and mental condition is what determines memory performance.

When it comes to proposing theories of memory improvement, therefore, a great deal of the groundwork has already been done. Without some kind of theoretical framework, work on memory improvement and indeed any aspect of memory performance, will be fragmented, as some critics have already indicated. On the other hand, my own view is that exactly what theory of memory improvement is put forward is less important than that a framework for research is put into place. An analogy might be with Herzberg's theories in organizational psychology. Few organizational psychologists would now accept that Herzberg's two-factor theory was supported by empirical evidence, yet Herzberg's influence on organizational psychology is of the greatest importance. Why? The reason is that the framework he proposed for conceptualizing factors involved in job satisfaction still guides our thinking. It is still useful to distinguish between context and content factors and to divide these further into distinct but related aspects of job satisfaction differing in their importance to overall satisfaction and dissatisfaction in various ways. Of course, theories are never right or wrong; they are the best guides available and change with challenge and new evidence. The point I am making is that we need not be too concerned that present theories might in some respects be inadequate in order to provide what is necessary and useful now--a conceptual and theoretical framework to give coherence to otherwise disparate and unrelated aspects of the area.

Apart from providing a framework for a theory of memory improvement, it is clear that different aspects of memory improvement investigation can feed back into a better understanding of the basic mechanisms of memory. Indeed, the arguments of Banaji and Crowder, that little of theoretical value can emerge from the study of practical application could only have been written by those who have never tried to solve practical problems.

My own interest in metamemory for example, started as a result of investigating the first-letter mnemonic aid--Richard of York Gave Battle In Vain to remember the colors of the rainbow, for example. The question posed was the extent to which first-letter cueing might be of value in overcoming memory blocks. To investigate this, we had to produce memory blocks, but of course, the question arises--what is a block; is it something you are certain you know, pretty sure you know, think you know, and so on. It became necessary to investigate the relationship between cued first-letter recall and degree of underlying memory block as measured by a self-rated feeling of knowing. Results showed that where feeling of knowing (Gruneberg & Monks, 1974) was certain, cued recall of unrecalled capitals of countries was .53; where subjects did not know, cued recall probability was .16. This, of course, merely confirms previous findings such as those of Hart (1965) of a relationship between degree of feeling of knowing and evidence of later retention. However, obviously matters could not be left there--what exactly was it that subjects know they know? The study led inevitably to trying to gain a greater understanding of the mechanism of feeling of knowing. Since then, the concept of metamemory has undergone a considerable transformation as the paper by Hertzog at this conference makes clear. I am not, of course, suggesting that my work on first-letter cueing led to important insights into metamemory. What I would argue is that it illustrates that tackling practical problems cannot be easily divorced from the need to inform our theoretical understanding. To suggest that pursuing practical application is somehow harmful to our advancing theoretical knowledge, as suggested by Banaji and Crowder (1989), is surely as far from reality as it is possible to be.

Earlier I suggested that some of the implications of the new interest in applying memory research had not fully been taken on board by academic psychologists, and I think it worth spending a few minutes discussing these. Most psychologists interested in memory improvement are, of course, interested in furthering our basic understanding of memory processes, but most, too, probably would like to think that theoretical insights would also feed back into practical application. As I indicated at the 1988 Practical Aspects of Memory Conference (Gruneberg, 1988), I feel that one problem is that psychologists are still too reluctant to go from the laboratory or the field study to the sustained effort that is required in implementing changes in the real world.

The second nettle that must be grasped is that of making one's findings and knowledge available. Academics by-and-large don't like publicity, don't like their colleagues to have publicity, and certainly don't like their colleagues to see any financial gain from their efforts, unless, of course, they are joint authors, or partners in the consulting firm! It is not an entirely flippant point. If we want theoretical insights to feed back into something that will benefit the man and woman in the street with his or her memory problems, one major way of doing this is through publicity and publication or both. It cannot be done by osmosis, nor can it be done well by leaving it to others less expert than the developers, because they will often fail to understand what it is they are dealing with. In any case, there is no army of technocrats out there waiting to take up our ideas. There is no choice but to publish or publicize memory research ourselves in a way that is intelligible to the recipient. Elizabeth Loftus has done this with her court appearances on eyewitness evidence. Herrmann (1990) has done this in relation to new memory improvement methods through the publication of a book written and promoted with the general public in mind. Geiselman and his colleagues (e.g., Fisher & Geiselman, 1988) have done this in relation to the cognitive interview, and Pressley and El-Dinary have extended strategic learning to the class situation (this volume). I must declare an interest in that I have been involved in publishing language courses that use mnemonic strategies (Gruneberg, 1985, 1987). There are, of course, a number of other such attempts, but I think it fair to claim that such attempts by academic psychologists are few and far between. Of course, not everyone, but certainly more academic psychologists interested in memory improvement should involve themselves in publicizing their findings and in presenting their work in such a way that others can readily find it and use it. For unless more academic psychologists interpret as well as further our current knowledge for the benefit of those outside psychology, we are in danger of being regarded as self-indulgent and unproductive.

It has to be said that the whole question of making material available in the form that nonprofessionals can use is fraught with difficulties. The difficulty of dealing with the press is well known--they are interested in stories, not detailed accuracy. The greater problem is perhaps dealing with other professionals--teachers in education, for example, where even the notion of memory improvement is sometimes highly suspect. Higbee (1978, 1988) has frequently written about misconceptions of teachers and others over mnemonic aids, but the problem goes much deeper. Any attempt by an "outsider" to improve ways of teaching a specialist subject area, for example, can be seen as threatening competence and of undermining the current theory of teaching in that area. In particular, memory problems are often seen as low level problems, and memory improvement strategies are therefore seen as low level strategies. Many teachers would, I suspect, agree with Howe (1970) when he states, "If something is worth learning there is almost always a meaningful way of learning it." That Howe is a psychologist just shows how deep-seated the problem is of looking at memory improvement in the context of education. Yet, such a view as Howe's is, in my view, hopelessly idealistic. It is, after all, hardly a matter of dispute that the majority of our children are left lost and confused by conventional teaching methods in a host of subjects from maths to foreign languages to science. There are, of course, meaningful ways of learning aspects of these--our children clearly need help in seeing this but also need help with their problems in remembering what they are taught. My main point, however, is that despite difficulties in regard to the application of memory improvement strategies, academic psychologists in the area of memory improvement must face these problems if we are going to use our theoretical insights to help those whom we feel could benefit.

I should like to finish, however, by stating the obvious. Of course, there are problems, but surely in the history of memory research, there never has been a time when so many advances in our understanding have been made, when so many topics have been seriously investigated by so many prominent academic psychologists, and when the potential to apply our knowledge has been so great. Our problems are more the problems of success than of failure, as the holding of this conference so clearly demonstrates.

References

Banaji, M.R., & Crowder, R.G. (1989). The bankruptcy of everyday memory. *American Psychologist*, *44*, 1185-1193.

Fisher, R.P., & Geiselman, R.E. (1988). Enhancing eyewitness memory with the cognitive interview. In M.M. Gruneberg, P.E. Morris, & R.N. Sykes (Eds.), *Practical aspects of memory: Current research and issues* (Vol. 1, pp. 34-39). Chichester: Wiley.

Gruneberg, M.M. (1985). *Computer linkword: French, German, Spanish, Italian, Greek, Russian, Dutch, Portuguese, Hebrew*. Penfield, NY: U.S.A. Artworx.

Gruneberg, M.M. (1987). *Linkword French, German, Spanish, Italian*. London: Corgi Books.

Gruneberg, M.M. (1988). Practical problems in the practical application of memory. In M.M. Gruneberg, P.E. Morris, & R.N. Sykes (Eds.), *Practical aspects of memory: Current research and issues* (Vol. 1, pp. 555-557). Chichester: Wiley.

Gruneberg, M.M., & Monks, J. (1974). Feeling of knowing and cued recall. *Acta Psychologica*, *38*, 257-265.

Gruneberg, M.M., Morris, P.E., & Sykes, R.N. (1991). The obituary on everyday memory and its practical application is premature. *American Psychologist*, *46*, 74-76.

Hart, J.T. (1965). Memory and the feeling of knowing experience. *Journal of Educational Psychology*, *56*, 208-216.

Herrmann, D.J. (1990). *Supermemory*. Emmaus, PA: Penn-Rodale.

Herrmann, D.J., & Searleman, A. (1990). The new multimodal approach to memory improvement. In G.H. Bower (Ed.), *Advances in learning and motivation* (Vol. 26, pp. 175-205). New York: Academic Press.

Higbee, K. (1978). Some pseudo limitations of mnemonics. In M.M. Gruneberg, P.E. Morris, & R.N. Sykes (Eds.), *Practical aspects of memory: Current research and issues* (Vol. 1, pp. 147-154). Chichester: Wiley.

Higbee, K. (1988). *Your memory*. Englewood Cliffs, NJ: Prentice Hall.

Howe, M.J.A. (1970). *Introduction to human memory*. New York: Harper & Row.

Morris, P.E., Tweedy, M., & Gruneberg, M.M. (1985). Interest, knowledge and the memory of soccer scores. *British Journal of Psychology*, *76*, 416-425.

Park, D.C., Smith, A.D., & Cavanaugh, J.C. (1990). Metamemories of memory researchers. *Memory & Cognition*, *18*, 321-327.

Weinert, F.E. (1988). Epilogue. In F.E. Weinert, & M. Perlmutter (Eds.), *Memory development* (pp. 381-396). Hillsdale, NJ: Erlbaum.

Memory Improvement and Memory Theory in Historical Perspective

Douglas Herrmann and Alan Searleman

For over 2000 years, scholars have advanced various explanations for memory phenomena (Herrmann & Chaffin, 1988). Until this century, most of these explanations relied almost exclusively on either traditional memory variables (such as duration of study, amount of rehearsal, presence or absence of appropriate retrieval cues) or the capacities and limitations of the memory system itself (i.e., the processes of registration, retention, and remembering). During the past two decades, however, there's been increasing evidence that memory performance is also influenced by variables identified with other *modes* of psychological processing. In other words, converging evidence suggests that human memory is also directly or indirectly influenced by an individual's physical, emotional, and attitudinal states.

With an ever increasing number of links being identified between these other modes of psychological processing and memory performance, it is now reasonable to attempt to develop broader theories of memory that can account for all modes of processing that affect memory. This offers the promise of providing a more complete account of memory capabilities, which in turn, should prove useful for conducting future human memory research and for the aiding of people who suffer from various clinical memory disorders (and for improving memory in nonclinical populations as well). A major goal of this conference is to provide an opportunity for evaluating the practical and theoretical importance that these other modes of psychological processing have on memory performance in general and in particular, how they can be utilized to optimize memory skills and ability.

Since the advent of modern memory research by Ebbinghaus (1885/1964), research on memory improvement has typically (and regrettably) had a relatively low priority. For reasons that are not completely clear, the optimization of memory performance has often been viewed as being primarily only an applied issue. Whereas other sciences routinely considered ideal states (e.g., a frictionless machine, processes that occur in a vacuum, processes that occur in a sterile environment), the optimization of memory skills was evidently too close to the applied world for the new science of memory (Hoffman & Senter, 1978).

The purpose of this chapter is to discuss the various approaches taken to memory improvement in the past and present. We will not provide a chronology of the development of memory theories (for such a chronology see Herrmann & Chaffin, 1988; Hoffman & Senter, 1978; Mitchell, 1911; Wilson, 1987; Yates, 1966). Instead, we will outline how different types of memory theories have dealt with the phenomena of memory improvement. Finally, we will conclude with a brief overview of the conference.

A Review of Memory Theories

Although literally hundreds of memory theories have been advanced both before and since Ebbinghaus (1885/1964), they may be regarded as expressions of a much smaller number of fundamental theoretical alternatives. To simplify consideration of past theories, we propose that essentially eight types of memory theories have been advanced over the past 2000 years. We fully recognize that it is certainly possible to classify memory theories in other plausible ways. However, we chose the particular taxonomy of theories that appears in Table 2.1, largely because it allows us to discuss how various memory theories have or have not considered the problem of improving memory ability. The eight types of theories are summarized in Table 2.1, and their implications for how memory aptitude may be improved are discussed as follows. The first 2 theories date back to antiquity; the remaining theories were primarily inventions of the late 19th and 20th centuries.

Biological Theory

Memory is ultimately a biologically based process. Many studies have shown that the administration of a certain treatment (such as the intake of certain chemicals, medicines, or vitamins or the introduction of electrical stimulation) may alter memory physiology (such as consolidation processes) so as to either improve or retard acquisition and retrieval of information (Baltes & Kliegel, 1986; Chorover & Schiller, 1965; Hebb, 1949; Lynch, 1986; McGaugh, 1989; Rosenzweig, 1984; Squire, 1987; Weingartner & Parker, 1984).

The memory mechanisms assumed by a biological theory have differed across time and researchers, ranging from *RNA* and protein codes, to reverberating neuronal circuits, to synaptic changes caused by long-term potentiation, to the particular importance of some central nervous system structures and circuits (e.g., the medial temporal and the diencephalic regions of the brain). Regardless of the particular mechanism(s) supposedly involved, it has traditionally been assumed that any biological intervention affects either all of the memory system or a system component that is involved in all memory tasks (such as short-term memory).

Table 2.1. Taxonomy of General Theories of Memory

Theory	*Mechanisms involved in Acquisition and Retrieval*
Biological	Physiological structures and brain chemistry
Classical	Mnemonics, changing ways of learning with images and associations
Behaviorist	A response conditioned to a stimulus, or two stimuli associated with each other in a memory task, or to characteristics common to similar tasks
Motivational	A behavior is learned to manage anxiety associated with memory tasks
Educational	A learning set, changing from repeated attempts to learn a domain of knowledge
Information Processing	Routine ways (strategies) for processing information, presumably inferred from prior experience
Cognitive	Levels of processing, presumably changing through normal development and task/domain specific strategies acquired through repeated task/domain experience
Multimodal	Manipulations of memory performance through all psychological systems

Classical Theory

The oldest theory of memory, except for perhaps the biological theory, was formulated in ancient Greece (Yates, 1966). This theory assumes that memory phenomena involve the use of *mnemonics*, which are previously memorized procedures that guide rehearsal of to-be-learned information. The first recorded mnemonic technique, invented in the 3rd century BC by the poet Simonides, required that items be registered in memory by imagining them in the "loci" of a familiar place. Later, when attempting to remember the material, the loci are imagined and thereby provide a "mental structure" with which to retrieve each item.

Behaviorist Theory

The behaviorist theory grew out of an associative tradition going back to antiquity (Warren, 1921), but its primary methodology comes from the 20th century (Skinner, 1938; Watson, 1913, 1925). There are two major ways that memory occurs according to a behaviorist model. Both ways require the classical or operant conditioning of a response to a memory task. First, a person's response to a stimulus in a particular memory task can be conditioned so that when that stimulus is later presented, memory of the appropriate response to make will occur. Second, a person's response to a class of two or more memory tasks may be conditioned so that a certain stimulus will elicit a memory process. Thus, an encoding response (like paying attention) might be conditioned to occur to certain learning tasks. Given sufficient motivation to respond, behaviorist theory assumes that memory improvement depends upon increasing the strength of the association between stimuli or between a stimulus and a response.

A modern variant of the behaviorist theory is the PDP (parallel distributed processing) model, or "connectionist" model. This model assumes that patterns of stimulation devoid of reinforcement lead to the registration of memories and that reinstatement of these patterns leads to the later retrieval of those memories (McCelland & Rumelhart, 1985). Memory is improved by conditioning a person to have the appropriate encoding or retrieval responses.

Motivational Theory

Freud (1901) proposed that unconscious and conscious motivations were responsible for much of the forgetting that people manifest in everyday life. While psychoanalysis has never been regarded as a way for people to improve their memory, this approach to memory problems paved the way to more recent attempts for improving memory performance by means of teaching people to cope with anxiety. Such attempts have been applied to the teaching of study skills (Spielberger, Gonzales, & Fletcher, 1979) and in helping the elderly deal with everyday memory problems (Yesavage, Sheikh, & Lapp, 1989).

Educational Theory

While educational theory also has its roots in antiquity (Mann, 1979), modern variants of this theory find most of their roots in the neobehaviorist learning theories. Educational theory assumes that learning is rewarding in its own right and that registration in memory of a particular association is dependent on whether or not a person has already learned the set of associations that are conceptually necessary to learn the new association, in other words, learning sets (Gagne & Paradise, 1961; Harlow, 1949). Like behaviorism, the educational theory assumes that memory phenomena are associative in nature, but unlike behaviorism, educational theory assumes that a learning set can change without conditioning.

Information-Processing Theory

These theories, inspired by computer technology, assume that memory registration and retrieval are affected by the degree to which information is processed in a memory task. Like many computers, the memory system is governed by a central processor. The central processor controls the distribution of attention to information that is to be registered in long-term memory or to produce the retrieval of other information held in long-term memory (Atkinson & Shiffrin, 1968). The distribution of attention is voluntarily regulated by a previously learned program, called a "routine" or "strategy." For example, a routine for rehearsal might voluntarily dispose a person to read an item, then repeat the item to oneself, and finally say the item aloud (Underwood, 1971, 1978). In this regard, information-processing theories suggest that memory improvement critically depends upon the amount of attention that is voluntarily devoted to a memory task.

Cognitive Theory

Modern cognitive psychology began by adopting the information-processing framework (Neisser, 1967, 1976). However, whereas the information-processing model assumed that the central processor governed the amount of processing given to a piece of information, the new cognitive model assumed that the central processor controlled qualitative (rather than quantitative) aspects of processing, sometimes called "levels" of processing. For example, one level involves paying attention to sensory properties of a stimulus whereas another level involves paying attention to the semantic aspects of a stimulus (Craik & Lockhart, 1973). Subsequent research has suggested that processing is probably not best characterized in terms of levels but, instead, according to the types of tasks and domains of information encountered (Baddeley, 1982, 1986; Chase & Ericsson, 1982; Ericsson, 1985; Herrmann, Buschke, & Gall, 1986; Morris, Bransford, & Franks, 1977). In addition, it soon was recognized that besides depending on the kind of task, processing also varied with a person's experience with a type of task--novel tasks had to be processed in a very deliberate fashion while well learned tasks could be processed more automatically (Anderson, 1981; Hasher & Zacks, 1979; Shiffrin & Schneider, 1977).

Multimodal Theory

Memory improvement, as just seen, has been conceived by the foregoing theories in several fundamental ways. Each theory assumes different kinds of memory processing and different mechanisms that carry out the processing. Despite these differences, they share one notable similarity--they all assume that memory phenomena are manifestations of just the memory system, either in terms of the physiology of memory or learned memory processes. In the 1970s researchers from several different theoretical backgrounds (especially gerontology, neuroscience, and clinical neuropsychology) proposed that memory should not be conceived so simply.

The impetus for a new approach came about partly because the classical methods of memory improvement (method of loci, peg-word, and others) often had not produced an adequate improvement in performance. For example, research has repeatedly shown that these methods are not useful for all tasks. They are less readily applied to more complex material (such as learning a poem, a document, or a story) than they are to simpler material (such as learning a shopping list). In addition, the classical methods are not applicable to some situations at all. Try using the method of loci to mentally encode a person's face or a peg-word system to remember the exact shades of eight different color chips of blue paint. You would no doubt find that these tasks would be very difficult to perform. Finally, and perhaps most damning of all, even in situations that are best suited for the use of the classical methods of memory improvement (i.e., list learning), most people who are explicitly trained in their use (including memory researchers themselves) usually choose not to use them once they are beyond the period of memory training because the classical methods are so taxing for most people to use (Bellezza, 1983; Higbee, in press; Lapp, 1983; Park, Smith, & Cavanaugh, 1990).

Because the classical methods were often found to be inadequate, many researchers and practitioners developed new methods for memory improvement (Backman, 1989; Druckman & Swets, 1988; Herrmann, 1990; Herrmann, Rea, & Andrzejewski, 1988; Herrmann & Searleman, 1990; Khan, 1986; Labouvie-Vief & Gonda, 1976; McEvoy & Moon, 1988; Poon, 1980; Pressley, Borkowski, & Schneider, 1987; Pressley, Forrest-Pressley, Elliott-Faust, & Miller, 1985; Wilson & Moffat, 1984; Yesavage, 1985; Yesavage et al., 1989). The new memory improvement methods not only included novel ways to mentally manipulate information but, of probably even greater significance, examined ways to improve memory performance by optimizing the psychological and physiological systems in which the memory system itself is embedded. Memory improvement depends on influencing all psychological modes of processing. Specifically, these other psychological modes of processing involve a person's physiological condition, emotional state, attitudes, social behaviors, and sensory/perceptual interactions with the environment.

It is important to point out that the proposal that memory is influenced by other psychological modes is not really a new idea. Not only in modern times (e.g., Herrmann & Searleman, 1990; Jenkins, 1974; Perlmutter, 1988) but even over a hundred years ago, similar notions were being put forth (Feinaigle, 1812; Middleton, 1888), so the new approach, instead of being truly new, more properly should be considered a modern reexamination of the interdependence of the memory system and other modes. The multimodal approach may be seen as a synthesis of the approaches that preceded it (Herrmann & Searleman, 1990).

Figure 2.1 illustrates where and when other modes might have their influence on the functioning of the memory system. As illustrated, mental manipulations directly affect the memory processes of registration, retention, and remembering, while physical and social manipulations influence these same memory processes but in a more indirect way by means of the sensory and response systems. Such manipulations could affect what the sensory system pays attention to by orienting receptors to stimuli relevant to certain memory tasks. For example, a physical manipulation might involve the positioning of one's gaze to better see a person's face to aid the registration process. A social manipulation can affect what is expressed by the response system. For instance, during conversations with others, we all make verbal or gestural responses to others to make it clear that we remember shared past events (or at least to give the impression that we remember when, in fact, we may not). Manipulations of one's physical condition, emotional state, and attitude also affect the registration, retention, and remembering components, as well as the sensory and response systems but in a more delayed and passive manner (represented by a dotted line).

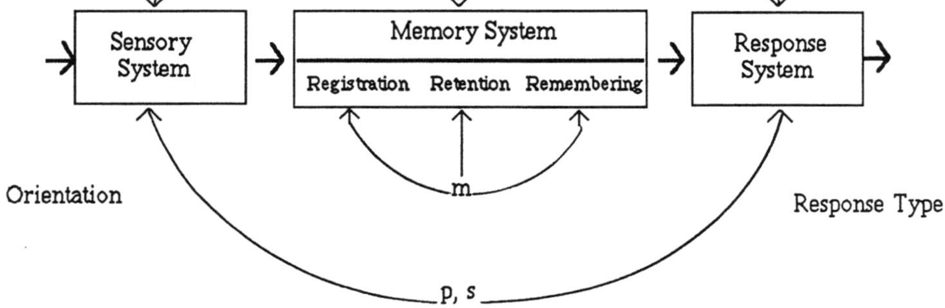

Figure 2.1. A Multimodal View of Memory (c - condition, e - emotion, a - attitude, m - mental manipulations, p - physical manipulations, s - social manipulations)

Discussion

Just as each of the aforementioned classes of theories has implications for how memory might be improved, the reverse is also true: The facts of how memory may be improved have implications for what is the most appropriate theory of memory. The purpose of this conference is to examine recent findings about memory improvement and to demonstrate the relevance of these findings to memory theory. These findings pertain not only to new ways to mentally manipulate information in memory tasks but also to how to make use of techniques that can facilitate memory performance by optimizing physical, emotional, and attitudinal states. Because new memory improvement methods have been developing so rapidly, there has not been sufficient opportunity for the research community to consider the effects of these methods or their implications for how general memory theories might be revised to best account for memory performance. This conference provides an opportunity to consider the theoretical importance of the new approach to memory improvement for a scientific understanding of human memory.

The conference consisted of lectures that described how different psychological modes of processing can affect memory performance: psychopharmacology (Weingartner & Herrmann), emotional state (Hertel), metamemory (Hertzog), strategies (Pressley & El-Dinary), practice (Payne & Wenger), external aids (Intons-Peterson & Newsome), social interaction (Best), context (Ceci, DeSimone, & Johnson), and attention (Plude). After a review of the latest innovations in memory improvement, the conference concluded with an examination of the implications of these findings for a theory of memory improvement (McEvoy) and for memory theory in general (Zacks & Hasher).

The findings presented extend our understanding of memory and challenge our conception of how independently the memory system functions with respect to the rest of the psychological system. The evidence that the participants presented also demonstrated that control over memory performance can be exerted in a much more diverse fashion and over a much wider time interval than previously believed. For example, manipulations that affect memory performance through the control of physical condition must occur before task performance (such as by watching what one eats, ensuring a series of nights with sound sleep before an important memory task, or by carrying out relaxation techniques).

The research reviewed at this conference also indicates that the notion of the memory task deserves reexamination and possibly redefinition. The memory task has been as immensely useful construct in elucidating stimulus and task variables that affect basic processes or that interact with content manipulations in memory performance. However, because this construct precludes consideration of relevant variables of the other modes of psychological processing, it's appropriate to propose that the object of memory research be expanded to also include any relevant variables of the memory "situation," that is, ones that precede, attend, or are part of a memory task (Bruce, 1985; Cohen, 1989; Goethals & Solomon, 1989; Greeno, 1989; Kelly & Stephens, 1989; Lave, 1988; Neisser, 1982, 1985; Perlmutter, 1988; Rabbitt, 1988; Schacter, 1984; Wilson, 1987). The results of this conference also indicate the need to improve methodology in memory research. In particular, the multimodal influences suggest that more controls be used in research and that subject characteristics need to be assessed more fully (Buschke, 1987; Poon et al., 1986). A careful examination of how memory can be improved will not only lead to better ways to remedy memory problems but will also result in more sophisticated research methodology and theorizing about how memory functions.

References

Anderson, J.R. (Ed.). (1981). *Cognitive skills and their acquisition*. Hillsdale, NJ: Erlbaum.

Atkinson, R.C., & Shiffrin, R.M. (1968). Human memory: A proposed system and its control processes. In K.W. Spence & J.T. Spence (Eds.), *The psychology of learning and motivation* (Vol. 2, pp. 90-95). New York: Academic Press.

Backman, L. (1989). Varieties of memory compensation of older adults in episodic remembering. In L. Poon, D. Rubin, & B. Wilson (Eds.), *Everyday cognition in adulthood and late life* (pp. 509-544). New York: Cambridge University Press.

Baddeley, A.D. (1982). Domains of recollection. *Psychological Review, 89*, 708-729.

Baddeley, A.D. (1986). *Working memory*. New York: Basic Books.

Baltes, P.B., & Kliegel, R. (1986). On the dynamics between growth and decline in the aging of intelligence and memory. In K. Poeck (Ed.), *Proceedings of the thirteenth world conference on neurology* (pp. 1-7). Heidelberg, Germany: Springer-Verlag.

Bellezza, F.S (1983). Mnemonic-device instruction with adults. In M. Pressley & J.R. Levin (Eds.), *Cognitive strategy research* (pp. 51-73). New York: Springer-Verlag.

Bruce, D. (1985). The how and why of ecological memory. *Journal of Experimental Psychology: General, 114*, 78-90.

Buschke, H. (1987). Criteria for the identification of memory deficits: Implications for the design of memory tests. In D.S. Gorfein & R.R. Hoffman (Eds.), *Memory and learning* (pp. 331-347). Hillsdale, NJ: Erlbaum.

Chase, W.G., & Ericsson, K.A. (1982). Skill and working memory. In G.H. Bower (Ed.), *The psychology of learning and motivation* (Vol. 16, pp. 2-58). New York: Academic Press.

Chorover, S.L., & Schiller, P.H. (1965). Short-term retrograde amnesia in rats. *Journal of Comparative and Physiological Psychology*, *59*, 73-78.

Cohen, G. (1989). *Memory in the real world*. Hillsdale, NJ: Erlbaum.

Craik, F.I.M., & Lockhart, R.S. (1973). Levels of processing: A framework for memory research. *Journal of Verbal Learning and Verbal Behavior*, *11*, 671-684.

Druckman, D., & Swets, J.A. (1988). *Enhancing human performance*. Washington, DC: National Academy Press.

Ebbinghaus, H. (1964). *Memory*. Trans. A. Ruger & C.E. Bussenius. New York: Dover. (Original work published 1885.)

Ericsson, K.A. (1985). Memory skill. *Canadian Journal of Psychology*, *39*, 188-231.

Feinaigle, M.G. von (1812). *The new art of memory*. London: Sherwood, Neely & Jones.

Freud, S. (1901). *The psychopathology of everyday life*. Harmondsworth: Penguin.

Gagne, R.M., & Paradise, N.E. (1961). Abilities and learning sets in knowledge acquisition. *Psychological Monographs, 75, (14 Whole No. 518*, 308).

Goethals, G.R., & Solomon, P.R. (1989). Interdisciplinary perspectives on the study of memory. In P.R. Solomon, G.R. Goethals, C.M. Kelley, & B.R. Stephens (Eds.), *Memory: Interdisciplinary approaches* (pp. 1-13). New York: Springer-Verlag.

Greeno, J.G. (1989). A perspective on thinking. *American Psychologist*, *44*, 134-141.

Harlow, H.F. (1949). The formation of learning sets. *Psychological Review*, *56*, 51-65.

Hasher, L., & Zacks, R.T. (1979). Automatic and effortful processes in memory. *Journal of Experimental Psychology: General*, *108*, 356-388.

Hebb, D.O. (1949). *The organization of behavior*. New York: Wiley-Interscience.

Herrmann, D. (1990). *Supermemory*. Emmaus, PA: Rodale.

Herrmann, D.J., Buschke, H., & Gall, M. (1986). Improving retrieval. *Applied Cognitive Psychology*, *9*, 27-33.

Herrmann, D.J., & Chaffin, R. (1988). *Memory in historical perspective*. New York: Springer-Verlag.

Herrmann, D.J., Rea, A., & Andrzejewski, S. (1988). The need for a new approach to memory training. In M.M. Gruneberg, P.E. Morris, & R.N. Sykes (Eds.), *Practical aspects of memory* (Vol. 2, pp. 415-420). Chichester: Wiley.

Herrmann, D.J., & Searleman, A. (1990). The new multimodal approach to memory improvement. In G.H. Bower (Ed.), *Advances in learning and motivation* (Vol. 26, pp. 175-205). New York: Academic Press.

Higbee, K.L. (in press). What do college students get from a memory improvement course? *Reading Improvement*.

Hoffman, R., & Senter, R.J. (1978). Recent history of psychology: Mnemonic techniques and the psycholinguistic revolution. *Psychological Record, 28*, 3-15.

Jenkins, J.J. (1974). Remember that old theory of memory? Well, forget it! *American Psychologist, 29*, 785-795.

Kelly, C.M., & Stephens, B.R. (1989). Thoughts on interdisciplinary approaches to memory. In P.R. Soloman, G.R. Goethals, C.M. Kelly, & B.R. Stephens (Eds.), *Memory: Interdisciplinary approaches*. New York: Springer-Verlag.

Khan, A.U. (1986). *Clinical disorders of memory*. New York: Plenum.

Labouvie-Vief, G., & Gonda, J.N. (1976). Cognitive strategy training and intellectual competence in the elderly. *Journal of Gerontology, 31*, 327-332.

Lapp, D. (1983). Commitment: Essential ingredient in memory training. *Clinical Gerontologist, 2*, 58-60.

Lave, J. (1988). *Cognition in practice*. Cambridge, England: Cambridge University Press.

Lynch, G. (1986). *Synapses, circuits, and the beginnings of memory*. Cambridge, MA: A Bradford Book, The MIT Press.

Mann, L. (1979). *On the trail of process: A historical perspective on cognitive processes and their training*. New York: Grune & Stratton.

McClelland, J.L., & Rumelhart, D.E. (1985). Distributed memory and the representation of general and specific information. *Journal of Experimental Psychology: General, 114*, 159-188.

McEvoy, C.L., & Moon, J.R. (1988). Assessment and treatment of everyday memory problems in the elderly. In M.M. Gruneberg, P.E. Morris, & R.N. Sykes (Eds.), *Practical aspects of memory* (Vol. 2, pp. 155-160). Chichester: Wiley.

McGaugh, J.L. (1989). Modulation of memory processes. In P.R. Solomon, G.R. Goethals, C.M. Kelley, & B.R. Stephens (Eds.), *Memory: Interdisciplinary approaches* (pp. 33-64). New York: Springer-Verlag.

Middleton, A.E. (1888). *Memory systems: New and old*. New York: G.S. Fellows.

Mitchell, J.M. (1911). Mnemonics. In *The Encyclopedia Britannica*/ (Vol. 18). Cambridge: Cambridge University Press.

Morris, C.D., Bransford, J.D., & Franks, J.J. (1977). Levels of processing versus transfer appropriate processing. *Journal of Verbal Learning and Verbal Behavior, 16*, 519-534.

Neisser, U. (1967). *Cognitive psychology*. New York: Appleton, Century, Crofts.

Neisser, U. (1976). *Cognition and reality*. San Francisco: Freeman.

Neisser, U. (1982). *Memory observed*. New York: W.H. Freeman.

Neisser, U. (1985). The role of theory in the ecological study of memory: Comment on Bruce. *Journal of Experimental Psychology: General, 114*, 272-276.

Park, D.C., Smith, A.D., & Cavanaugh, J.C. (1990). Metamemories of memory researchers. *Memory & Cognition*, *18*, 321-327.

Perlmutter, M. (1988). Research on memory and its development: Past, present, and future. In F.E. Weinert & M. Perlmutter (Eds.), *Memory development: Universal changes and individual differences* (pp. 353-380). Hillsdale, NJ: Erlbaum.

Poon, L.W. (1980). A systems approach for the assessment and treatment of memory problems. In J.M. Ferguson & C.B. Taylor (Eds.), *The comprehensive handbook of behavior medicine* (Vol. 1, pp. 191-212). New York: Spectrum.

Poon, L.W., Gurland, B.J., Eisdorfer, C., Crook, T., Thompson, L.W., Kasniak, A.W., & Davis, K.L. (1986). Integration of experimental and clinical precepts in memory assessment: A tribute to George Talland. In L.W. Poon (Ed.), *Clinical memory assessment of older adults* (pp. 3-10). Washington, DC: American Psychological Association.

Pressley, M., Borkowski, J.G., & Schneider, W. (1987). Good strategy users coordinate metacognition, strategy use and knowledge. In R. Vasta & G. Whitehurst (Eds.), *Annals of child development* (Vol. 4, pp. 89-129). Greenwich, CT: JAI Press.

Pressley, M., Forrest-Pressley, D.L., Elliott-Faust, D., & Miller, G. (1985). Children's use of cognitive strategies: How to teach strategies, and what to do if they can't be taught. In M. Pressley & C.J. Brainerd (Eds.), *Cognitive learning and memory in children* (pp. 1-47). New York: Springer-Verlag.

Rabbitt, P. (1988). Does fast last? Is speed a basic factor determining individual differences in memory? In M.M. Gruneberg, P.E. Morris, & R.N. Sykes (Eds.), *Practical aspects of memory* (Vol. 2, pp. 161-168). Chichester: Wiley.

Rosenzweig, M.R. (1984). Experience, memory, and the brain. *American Psychologist*, *39*, 365-376.

Schacter, D.L. (1984). Toward the multidisciplinary study of memory: Ontogeny, phylogeny, and pathology of memory systems. In L.R. Squire & N. Butters (Eds.), *Neuropsychology of memory* (pp. 13-24). New York: Guilford.

Shiffrin, R., & Schneider, W. (1977). Controlled and automatic human information processing II. Perceptual learning, automatic attending, and a general theory. *Psychological Review*, *84*, 127-190.

Skinner, B.F. (1938). *The behavior of organisms*. New York: Appleton, Century, Crofts.

Spielberger, C.D., Gonzales, H.P., & Fletcher, T. (1979). Test anxiety reduction, learning strategies, and academic performance. In H.F. O'Neill & C.D. Spielberger (Eds.), *Cognitive and affective learning strategies* (pp. 111-131). New York: Academic Press.

Squire, L. (1987). *Memory*. New York: Oxford University Press.

Underwood, B.J. (1971). Recognition memory. In H.H. Kendler & J.T. Spence (Eds.), *Essays in neobehaviorism: A memorial volume to K.W.*

Spence. New York: Appleton, Century, Crofts.
Underwood, G. (1978). *Strategies of information processing*. London: Academic Press.
Warren, R.C. (1921). *A history of the association psychology*. New York: Scribners.
Watson, J.B. (1913). Psychology as a behaviorist views it. *Psychological Review*, *20*, 158-177.
Watson, J.B. (1925). *Behaviorism*. London: Kegan Paul, Trench, Trulner.
Weingartner, H., & Parker, E.S. (1984). *Memory consolidation: Psychobiology of cognition*. Hillsdale, NJ: Erlbaum.
Wilson, B. (1987). *Rehabilitation of memory*. New York: Guilford.
Wilson, B., & Moffat, N. (1984). *Clinical management of memory problems*. Rockville, MD: Aspen Systems.
Yates, F. (1966). *The arts of memory*. Chicago: Chicago University Press.
Yesavage, J.A. (1985). Nonpharmacologic treatments for memory losses with normal aging. *American Journal of Psychiatry*, *142*, 600-605.
Yesavage, J.A., Sheikh, J.I., & Lapp, D. (1989). Mnemonics as modified for use by the elderly. In L. Poon, D. Rubin, & B. Wilson (Eds.), *Everyday cognition in adulthood and late life* (pp. 598-611). New York: Cambridge University Press.

Clinical and Pharmacological Perspectives for Treating Memory Failures

Herbert Weingartner and Douglas Herrmann

In this chapter, we provide a brief review of some of the current schemes, or models, that are available for defining the structures and processes that are involved in memory functions from both a psychological and biological perspective. This perspective is relevant for considering strategies for improving memory since the techniques that prove useful would be logically based upon what we know about the structures and processes that together operate to establish and maintain memory. We provide an overview of some of the prototypic types of memory failures associated with prevalent neuropsychiatric disorders. We discuss some pharmacological strategies that have been developed on the basis of what we know about the psychobiology of normal and impaired memory functions. In discussing these issues we first consider some of the methodological issues that must be taken into account in using drugs to alter memory functions. We review findings from studies demonstrating the highly selective memory response to drug treatments in normal controls and memory-impaired Alzheimer's disease patients.

The efficacy of methods that allow us to repair systems that are not functioning normally has been built upon an understanding of the mechanisms and determinants that govern the normal operation of those systems. It is appropriate that this conference considers the complex issue of how memory functions might be improved through a detailed analysis of what we know about the mechanisms of normal memory functions and an equally detailed understanding of how memory can fail. The application of memory theory at several levels of analysis is clearly relevant to improving memory functions and knowledge gained from applying theory is then also useful in testing and elaborating features of memory theories.

Psychobiological View of Different Types of Memory

One of the debates that continues unabated in the psychology literature has to do with how many different memory systems can be identified (Tulving, 1985). The distinction between episodic, or recent context and sequence dependent memories (*episodic memory*), as opposed to memories that represent our knowledge base, particularly in terms of semantic representations (*semantic memory*) has long been considered a valid dichotomy. We know that memory processes that require conscious awareness, that is those processes that are *explicit*, appear to be determined by somewhat different neural systems for memory functions than are processes that are *implicit* and outside of awareness (Graf, Squire, & Mandler, 1984; Jacoby & Witherspoon, 1982; Perruchet & Baveux, 1989; Schacter, 1987). Another distinction between different memories that has been emphasized, particularly by neuropsychologists, is the memory for information that varies with respect to *modality* such as verbal in contrast to pattern information (lateralization of memory functions for different types of to-be-remembered information). Mechanisms and determinants of memory processes that can be performed *automatically*, without intention or sustained concentration, as opposed to memory functions that require *effort*, sustained and directed cognitive processing, also appear to be different (Hasher & Zacks, 1979; Hirst & Volpe, 1984; Kahneman, 1973; Schneider & Shiffrin, 1977; Shiffrin & Schneider, 1977). Whether or not someone does remember some event, processes involved in either judging the accuracy of memory performance or predicting memory performance (i.e., self-monitoring cognitive operations that are associated with memory) can also be altered by factors that are independent of those that might influence the actual accuracy and completeness of memory performance. These *metacognitive memory* functions have only recently been of renewed interest to cognitive psychologists and clearly have been seen as important in the study of impairments of memory.

Simple associative learning and memory (performance) has been generally ignored by most cognitive psychologists interested in human information processing. However simple Stimulus-Response (S-R) conditioning accounts for a good deal of learning and memory of important behaviors such as tastes, interests, and aversions. Furthermore, the psychobiological basis of S-R conditioning has been well defined, and changes in that system have also been described in memory-impaired mammals other than man (Thompson, 1986). The circuitry that determines simple conditioning such as the eyeblink involves neurobiological systems that are substantially different from those necessary for explicit memory. In addition, it should be pointed out that a cascade of serial and parallel processes are engaged when we are presented with information that may or may not be memorable at a later point in time. These component processes are determined by some unique psychobiological features and have been characterized in several generations of information-processing models. Functions such as sensory processing and integration, attentional processes, decision processes, stages in memory acquisition, memory consolidation (emphasized most frequently in studies of memory in lower animals), and retrieval processes are just a few of the many processes that can be altered in highly specific ways in both normal and memory-impaired subjects. Any one of these cognitive memory functions can be altered by some treatment, while other domains of cognitive functioning are left unaffected. Likewise, clinical states like those described in the next section can be expressed in the form of highly selective alterations in cognition with some functions spared while others are markedly impaired.

How Does Memory Fail? Clinical Examples of Different Forms of Memory Impairments

Remediation of disturbance in memory should logically be based upon an understanding of the mechanisms of memory failures. In this section, we consider some typical examples of disturbances in memory.

There are many forms of memory failure. Some are the direct result of impairments in biological hardware systems, defined in terms of both neuroanatomy and neurochemistry of those brain systems that are involved in establishing long-term memory traces of experience. For example, lesions of the hippocampus are associated with impairments in memory. Likewise, treatments that disrupt the cholinergic nervous system also lead to failures in memory, and this system is seen as being directly involved in some memory consolidation functions (part of the extrinsic, mediating system that supports memory trace formation). Other forms of memory impairment may be the result of impairments in systems that, although not directly involved in the formation of memory, play an important extrinsic, modulatory, cognitive role in memory (Herrmann & Searleman, this volume; Lister & Weingartner, 1987; Tariot & Weingartner, 1986). For example, alterations in attention or motivation have powerful effects on information processing and therefore affect memory.

Both behaviorally defined and biologically driven conditions can produce impaired memory functions. The most common conditions that produce disorders of memory include head trauma, infections such as encephalitis, vascular diseases such as strokes, and degenerative central nervous diseases such as Alzheimer's and Korsakoff's disease. The features of the memory impairments in these last two disorders, summarized below, typify the highly specific ways that memory may fail. Many behavioral conditions and psychiatric disorders also result in impaired memory functions. For example, conditions that alter arousal, anxiety, and stress that might occur in nominally normal individuals, as well as changes in mental functions seen in syndromes such as hyperactive attention deficit disorders, dissociative disorders, or states of depression can result in highly specific deficits in memory. Below we summarize in some detail the types of memory changes that are apparent in one of these prototypic psychiatric disorders, namely depression.

Cognitive Failures in Depression: Failures in Effort-Demanding Cognitive Processes

Depression is not a unitary diagnostic entity. There are several subgroups of depressed patients. For example, psychobiological factors differentiate patients with unipolar and bipolar affective disorder (the latter would include patients with a history of mania along with a history of depression); patients who, unlike normals, do not respond to some provocative drug treatment such as dexamethasone, which ordinarily would suppress corticosteroids; patients with agitated, in contrast to, retarded forms of depression; and patients with or without a positive family history of depression. However, despite subtle differences in cognitive symptoms that distinguish these subpopulations of depressed patients, they also share a good deal in common in terms of the nature of the cognitive impairment that is linked to their depression. The severity of these cognitive symptoms is directly related to the severity of the depression that is present.

Several aspects, or domains, of cognitive functioning appear to be selectively impaired while other cognitive functions are spared in depressed patients (Cohen, Weingartner, Smallberg, Pickar, & Murphy, 1982; Roy-Byrne, Weingartner, Bierer, Thompson, & Post, 1986; Weingartner, Cohen, Martello, & Gerdt, 1981). In general, when depressed patients attempt memory tasks that do not have a time limit or when information is presented in a highly structured fashion, performance is unimpaired. Depressed patients are also effective in accessing their previously acquired knowledge in long-term memory. In addition, depressed patients are unimpaired when asked to process information automatically. Attentional processes are near normal unless patients are confronted with so much information that it exceeds normal processing capacity.

However, depressed patients tend to over-organize or overgeneralize the use of some scheme that would integrate their experiences. Both implicit and explicit cognitive functions are impaired or spared as a function of the degree to which they require effort and concentration for successful performance to take place. In fact, effort-demanding implicit cognitive operations are particularly likely to be disrupted in depression.

Retrieval of information and memory representations of experience are also altered in depression. Mood states, such as depression, serve as a context that biases what can be retrieved from memory. Mood states, such as depression or elation, influence the types of retrieval strategies that are generated for searching what is in memory. Therefore, under altered mood state conditions, a depressed patient may not recall some past experience that may be available for recall but may be temporarily inaccessible in the depressed mood. This profile of cognitive changes, as well as others that have been cited in studies of depression, are depicted in Table 3.1.

Table 3.1. Types of Cognitive Functions that are Altered in Amnestic Disorders, Depression, and Dementia (Alzheimer's Disease).

Type of process	*Disorder*		
	Amnesia	*Depression*	*Dementia*
Explicit memory	↓↓	↓↓	↓↓
Meta-cognition	↓↓	–	–
Encoding processes	↓	↓	↓↓
Automatic cognitive processes	↓↓	–	↓↓
Effort-driven memory processes	↓↓	↓↓	↓↓
Access to knowledge memory	–	–	↓↓
S-R conditioning	–	?	?
Implicit memory processes	–	↓ * *	↓↓
Decision processes	?	– ?	– ?

? Functioning in this domain has not been adequately studied
– Spared functions
↓ Impaired and very impaired ↓↓ functions
** * Recently reported findings*

Dementia of an Alzheimer's Type (DAT): Failures in Attention, Memory, and Other Cognitive Functions Including Impairments in Accessing Information from Long-Term Memory

Alzheimer's disease is the most common and disabling disease that compromises cognitive functioning in the elderly. The cognitive changes associated with DAT are obvious, particularly as the disease progresses. In DAT, the cognitive changes begin in a mild form, often indistinguishable from the cognitive changes that might be apparent in depression, as secondary to stress, as a side effect of various medications, or as changes that have been associated with normal aging. In fact, during the early stages of the disease, the diagnosis of DAT may be quite difficult and is largely established by excluding other neurological and neuropsychiatric diseases. As DAT progresses, one can note dramatic changes in many cognitive functions, particularly those components of memory that are ordinarily spared in other neuropsychiatric disorders, such as depression or amnesia. Not only is recent explicit episodic memory altered, but in addition, progressive impairments are seen in implicit memory functions, access to information that is part of a knowledge base in long-term memory, procedural memory, language functions, and learning of procedures. Unlike the cognitive changes that are apparent in depression, the memory changes that are seen in DAT are even more dramatic for those cognitive functions that ordinarily can be accomplished automatically. Furthermore, unlike depression or the memory failure that is apparent in amnestic syndromes (see Table 3.1) the DAT patient often fails to remember because of basic, intrinsic difficulties in encoding and decoding events. This is directly attributable to impairments in rapidly accessing knowledge memory, making it difficult for these patients to organize and bring meaning to their ongoing experiences and thereby compromising memory (Grafman, Thompson, Weingartner, Lawlor, & Sunderland, in press; Weingartner, Grafman, Boutelle, Kaye, & Martin, 1983).

In the past decade, we have learned a great deal about the neuropathology of DAT that may be related to the cognitive changes that are expressed in the disease. This knowledge base has served to provide the rational for the development of experimental treatment strategies. Some of these pathognomonic changes in the brains of DAT patients include alterations in brain cells such as the appearance of neurofibrillary tangles, neuritic plaques, granulovacular degeneration, and an actual loss of neurons. In addition, it also appears that even for surviving neurons, one can note a loss of the number of synapses per neuron and a restriction in the synaptic active zones (Buell & Coleman, 1979, 1981; Davies, Mann, Sumpter, & Yates, 1987; Hamos, DeGennaro, & Drachman, 1989). Cholinergic neurons, particularly in the basal forebrain are particularly likely to be lost in DAT. The resulting cholinergic deficit in DAT occurs even in the early stages of the disease, even before its cognitive expression is clear. The extent to which cholinergic central nervous system involvement is present is positively correlated with the cognitive (particularly memory) symptoms that are present (Whitehouse et al., 1982). The finding of the *cholinergic deficit* in DAT has been the driving theme for the development of therapies that might potentially reverse or at least slow down the course of the disease. Many studies have been completed or are still being proposed to test the efficacy of treating DAT patients with cholinergic precursors, such as choline; with drugs that would effect the enzyme that degrades acetylcholine, such as physostigmine or an oral form of that drug (THA); or through the use of drugs that might directly stimulate the postsynaptic cholinergic neuron, such as with the use of arecoline. It should be pointed out that aside from the cholinergic nervous system, many other neurochemical systems have been shown to be involved in DAT. For example, there appears to be abnormal catecholaminergic functioning in DAT patients, which has prompted several groups to attempt to stimulate this system alone or in combination with cholinergic drugs.

In evaluating the effectiveness of any of these pharmacological treatments, it is important to appreciate how cognitive functions fail in DAT. The ideal target drug response in these patients would be one in which positive changes in recent memory occur because these patients more effectively access and make use of their previously acquired knowledge and skill base that is part of their long-term memory. Table 3.1 attempts to summarize the features of the memory changes that are apparent in DAT.

Amnesia: A Failure in Recent Explicit Memory with a Sparing of Implicit and Knowledge Memory

Amnestic syndromes are associated with a wide variety of neurological conditions including Korsakoff's disease, some focal head injuries, and some strokes. These patients typically have difficulty remembering recently acquired experiences. However, their recent memory difficulties can be discriminated from those seen in depression or in DAT patients. What differentiates an amnestic disorder from some of the memory impairments evident in other neuropsychiatric disorders is the sharply defined islands of spared memory functions. The typical amnestic patient maintains many of the cognitive, memory skills that are often impaired in DAT. For example, previously acquired semantic knowledge and skills that are part of long-term memory are unaltered in the amnestic syndrome. Language function is typically normal. In fact, it is this normal access to both semantic information and knowledge memory that is the basis upon which the amnestic patient confabulates, or fills in the blanks of recent memory. Some memories of recent experiences are also quite spared. For example, all kinds of associative conditioning can be retained in these patients, just like in normal subjects. Furthermore, these patients can be taught rules and procedures and will then retain those skills and perform them even after a long delay between training and performance (Cohen & Squire, 1980). Many other aspects of experience are believed to persist in memory, based on the fact that performance on some tasks is influenced by previous training. However, when amnestic patients are asked to identify the source of their experience with some task or stimulus, they frequently cannot explicitly identify how this knowledge was acquired. That is, these patients show dramatic failures in memory when we ask them to explicitly recall some experience. For example, we can teach an amnestic patient to solve a problem and later demonstrate that the solution has been retained, implicitly, in memory. However, the patient is unaware of the circumstances in which that experience got into memory, the context in which that experience was acquired, or the events that led up to or followed that experience, functions that would be associated with episodic memory. It is, in fact, the dramatic dissociation between what amnestic subjects can and cannot remember that has served as the primary data base for distinguishing between implicit and explicit memory functions.

Some features of the memory impairment in amnesia are also similar to those seen in DAT patients. For example, both amnestic and DAT patients are equally impaired in explicit recall of both information that is processed automatically as well as for experience that requires concentration and effort. This feature of the amnestic memory impairment is similar to that seen in DAT patients (Strauss, Weingartner, & Thompson, 1985) but very different from the features of memory impairment seen in depression (Weingartner et al., 1981). Another similarity may exist between the cognitive-memory dysfunctions in DAT and in amnestic Korsakoff's disease involving impairments that have been identified with frontal lobe functioning. Recent research has suggested that at least some of the determinants of the memory impairments seen in amnestic patients with histories of alcoholism, as well as DAT patients, may be attributable to frontal lobe pathology (Janowsky, Shimamura, Kritchevsky, & Squire, 1989). Studies have shown that cognitive test performance in Korsakoff's disease patients resembles the performance of patients with frontal lobe lesions. Cognitive behavior that requires initiating and planning strategies are presumed to reflect frontal lobe pathology, which may then also be reflected in memory performance. Perhaps frontal lobe damage can explain some of the memory deficits that are observed in patients with Korsakoff's syndrome.

Heterogeneity of Impaired and Unimpaired Functions in Memory Disorder Patients

Perhaps the most important point to be stressed is the extensive neuropathological heterogeneity for groups of patients that are defined clinically as having amnesia, Korsakoff's amnestic disorder, DAT, or suffering from depression. In some patients, this may mean that the lesions that produce impaired memory are limited to only those structures that are involved in memory, while in other patients lesions may also include systems that can alter motivation, mood, emotion, activation, planning, and so forth. We know that in many patients that we define as suffering from an amnestic disorder, not only are memory functions altered, but other behavioral systems can also be seen as dysfunctional, systems that also have an impact on cognitive memory performance. For example, the ability of these patients to make accurate judgments about their own memory performance (alterations in metamemory), their apathy, and their inability to release from proactive interference, may not necessarily reflect changes in memory per se that are attributable to the disease but may also reflect changes that have to do with other aspects of the disorder (e.g., damaged frontal lobes), which may be present in some of these patients and not others.

Table 3.1 summarizes the features of spared and impaired memory functioning in the typical amnestic individual in contrast to the pattern of cognitive memory dysfunctions seen in the typical depressed and DAT patient. It should, however, be pointed out that it is rare to see pure amnestic patients (or for that matter DAT or depressed patients) in the clinic. An enormous amount of heterogeneity appears both in the clinical and neuropathological presentation of each of the clusters of syndromes that are summarized here. In fact, the prototypic patient is rare (Bowden, 1990).

Developing Drugs that May Improve Memory Functions: Some Research Considerations

The development of treatments of memory impairments in some neuropsychiatric disorders is based upon what we know about the neuropathology of that disease along with basic research knowledge about the neurobiological determinants of memory. For many disorders, this is defined by neuroanatomical variables, neurochemical deficits, or both, along with knowledge of neuroanatomical and neurochemical systems that play either a modulatory or mediating role in memory.

One common approach to the problem of testing the efficacy of memory treatments involves the use of various types of animal models of cognitive dysfunctions that may appear in humans. The approach is to create some lesion and then study whether some treatment might attenuate the cognitive deficits produced by that lesion. If that lesion involves compromising some neurochemical system, then one approach to treatment is a direct replacement of that neurotransmitter, or a drug strategy that can affect the postsynaptic neuron, or by using a drug that alters the rate at which a neurotransmitter might be metabolized. Another approach, one that is illustrated in some detail below, involves inducing, in a reversible fashion in normal controls, the deficit state that might be present in some clinical population. For example, it is possible to use drugs as tools for simulating amnesia (with benzodiazepines), dementia (using anticholinergic agents), or depression (with the use of drugs that depress catecholamine activity) in healthy, normal volunteers. One could then investigate whether some potentially useful treatment can acutely reverse the cognitive deficit produced by some drug.

The logic of the drug treatments that have been used to treat Parkinson's disease has also guided the search for treatments for the cognitive deficit in DAT. Parkinson's disease is a disease that involves the dopamine system. Therefore, some treatment that would elevate levels of brain dopamine would be viewed as therapeutic in treating Parkinson's disease patients. This is the same type of logic that has led to the development of several strategies for treating the memory impairment of DAT with drugs that would affect the cholinergic nervous system either directly or indirectly. We know that DAT is associated with a cholinergic dysfunction (although many other systems are also involved), so drugs that would improve cholinergic functioning should be helpful in these patients. Consequently, investigators have studied the effects of drugs that singly or in combination would be expected to affect either activity at the presynaptic neuron, receptors on the postsynaptic neuron, or activity at cholinergic synapses, such as altering the activity of enzymes that degrade the neurotransmitter acetylcholine. However, we also know that in DAT, catecholaminergic activity is also compromised, which has led to the use of drugs that would have an impact on that system. One example of how catecholaminergic drugs might be helpful in improving memory functions in DAT is provided in the summary of a study that was designed to explore how a monamine oxidase inhibitor might be clinically useful. This is presented in the concluding section of this paper. Some clinical researchers have attempted to alter both cholinergic and catecholaminergic functioning in DAT with a combination of drug treatments as a means of improving memory functioning.

Another type of direct intervention for correcting what is wrong with the brain is through the use of brain transplants. In fact, a long history of research in lower animals has shown such an approach to be effective in reversing behavioral deficits resulting from brain lesions in rodents. Some, albeit limited, use of transplant methods has begun in treating clinical populations such as Parkinson's disease patients. Yet another technique for directly treating what is wrong with the brains of cognitively impaired neuropsychiatric patients is through the use of treatments that might serve to promote the repair or regeneration of damaged or lost neurons with the use of substances that might stimulate nerve growth factor. Transplant and regeneration procedures are still in the early stages of development in terms of application in humans and have yet to be used to remedy memory deficits. However, such methods are likely to be tested in the relatively near future.

Another approach to treating cognitive impairments in DAT is through the use of drugs that alter central nervous system functions in selected brain systems in either nominally unaffected subjects that are at risk for some disease or in patients who are in the early stages of that disease. The strategy here is to either prevent the occurrence of the disease or to perhaps retard the onset or rapidity of the progression of the disease.

Even a cursory review of the scientific-clinical literature on drug manipulations of memory functions in neuropsychiatric patients shows how difficult it is to do carefully controlled studies in this area. The methodological hurdles and difficulties make reliable and effective development of drug treatment of memory functions proceed slowly and often in directions that prove not to be useful. In the section below, we consider some of the more obvious methodological issues that must be thought through in evaluating pharmacological treatments of memory impairments. The concluding section provides a summary of findings that emerge from the use of two of the approaches discussed in reversing the types of memory deficit that are expressed in DAT and in drug treated normals that temporarily demonstrate a DAT like memory impairment.

Methodological Issues

Even when there is good reason to believe that a particular drug is theoretically appropriate for treating a memory impairment, the effectiveness of drugs is often limited by various aspects of how the treatments are administered. There are several classes of methodological considerations that might influence the effect of a drug on memory.

Peripheral in Contrast to Central Factors

It has often been taken for granted that a drug must enter the central nervous system to affect memory. Recently, more attention is being paid to the role of peripheral mechanisms in cognitive processes. A growing body of evidence supports such a role, especially for the catecholamine, opiates, and pituitary-adrenal hormones. This may occur in several ways. For example, peripheral agents to which the blood-brain barrier is relatively impermeable may cross the blood-brain barrier in minute quantities or may have metabolic by-products that cross. Alternatively, a substance may affect areas of the brain that are poorly protected by the blood-brain barrier or may indirectly affect the brain via peripheral autonomic afferents. Within the context of the models developed above, such peripheral influences are an aspect of the "extrinsic" modulatory system.

Subjects

One of the common observations in studies of alterations in memory function in either normal subjects or in patient populations is that of variability of response to some treatment. Reports of drug effects on memory often simply report effects in terms of overall difference in mean memory performance in contrast to differences in how specific subject or patient characteristics may modulate how a drug alters brain functioning. For example, the baseline level of arousal may dramatically alter the potential memory-enhancing effects of some drug. Drug-induced augmentation of arousal can shift individuals beyond the optimal range of the inverted U-shaped curve of arousal into over-aroused deterioration. Restoring performance that has been impaired from fatigue or other drugs or retarding performance decline from "time-on-task" effects is easier.

Dose-Effect Relationships

Another important methodological consideration in the study of drugs that might be considered for improving memory is that under the same conditions, different doses of the same drug may exert different pharmacological effects.

Simple assumptions that larger doses will exert more of a given effect and smaller doses less of an effect can be erroneous. For example, certain doses of the cholinesterase inhibitor, physostigmine, can exert small positive effects on memory performance, but both higher and lower doses in the same people can impair performance on the same tasks. These inverted U-shaped patterns of performance illustrate the importance of using multiple drug doses. A "best dose," or the dose of drug at which performance is measured to be maximal, can best be determined by administering different doses of the drug, each for a standardized period of time. This requires the use of repeated measures design with the capability of repeating equivalent forms of a battery of memory tests that would be useful in assessing a set of well characterized and relevant cognitive functions.

Task Sensitivity

Although obvious, many studies that would examine the potential memory-enhancing effects of some drug treatment ignore issues of appropriateness of both the memory target response and the level of difficulty of some evaluative procedure for a given patient group. Appropriate drug sensitivity means there is empirical evidence that the task quantitatively measures the specific effects of the study drug through a range of doses. A task is disease or deficit sensitive when it quantitatively measures the particular range of deficits associated with the clinical entity under study. For example, an appropriate task for measuring the effects of a cholinergic agonist on memory in patients with DAT would be one with established sensitivity to cholinergic agents as well as sensitivity to the cognitive deficits of Alzheimer's disease. Ideally, the task would also have some clinical relevance for the patients being studied, so it is useful to report the magnitude of a change in memory performance in addition to whether it is statistically significant. An important dimension of task sensitivity is the difficulty of the task for each individual subject. In many drug trials, the subjects show a wide range of cognitive deficits. With tasks that the more impaired subjects can handle, the less impaired individuals may become bored or quickly reach a ceiling, so significant improvement cannot be measured. Conversely, a task that an unimpaired subject finds an interesting challenge may excessively frustrate an impaired individual and precipitate a catastrophic emotional reaction that negatively influences subsequent testing.

Task Specificity

It is clear that just as different forms of neuropsychiatric disorders produce specific and somewhat unique forms of spared and impaired patterns of memory dysfunctions, so to do drugs that alter memory functions. This is the case both for drugs that disrupt memory and agents that might improve memory functions (see the example of L-Deprenyl effects on memory in DAT that is presented below). It is precisely for that reason that it is important to evaluate drug effects on memory using batteries of cognitive tests made up of interrelated and contrasting tasks with different specificities for the cognitive domains they are designed to assess. The aim would be to identify and quantify islands of spared versus impaired cognitive functions that result from some drug manipulation. In this way, it may be possible to appreciate how different drug interventions alter different cognitive functions and that different patient populations present with different forms of cognitive impairments, requiring different forms of treatment.

Two Illustrations of How Drug Strategies Can Be Used to Treat Memory Impairments in DAT

This final section provides a summary sketch of the types of findings that have been obtained in studies that have explored various types of drug treatments in DAT patients. It should be immediately pointed out that at this point in time, there is no treatment for DAT. Thus, no drug treatment has reliably returned the DAT patient to a normal functioning state. On the other hand, a good deal of progress has been made in this area of research, and a number of treatments are available that can potentially alter some of the cognitive symptoms and clinical expression of this progressive disease. Most of this research progress has been directly built upon our knowledge of the neuropathology of DAT (Bartus, Dean, Beer, & Lippa, 1982; Coyle, Price, & DeLong, 1983; Gottfries, 1985; McGeer, McGeer, Suzuki, Dolman, & Nagai, 1984; Weingartner, Sitaram, & Gillin, 1979). Furthermore, some trials are currently underway that are examining whether some of these drugs, when administered early, can slow the course of the disease. In somewhat more detail, we then summarize findings from two different types of studies that were designed to explore the potential cognitive-enhancing effects of two types of drugs. In one study, DAT patients were treated with a drug that would enhance catecholamine activity. In the other study, normal controls were first administered a cholinergic antagonist that produced a dementia-like memory impairment along with either a placebo pretreatment or a peptide that was hypothesized to attenuate the drug-induced dementia.

The drugs that have been studied have consisted of four types. The most commonly tested drugs are those whose target response is the cholinergic nervous system. Some of these drugs act at the presynaptic neuron, others alter the activity of the enzyme that typically degrades the neurotransmitter acetylcholine (e.g., physostigmine or tacrine), and others act on the postsynaptic receptor (e.g., arecoline). A second class of drugs alter catecholamine activity either presynaptically, in terms of altering the degradation rate of catecholamine, or postsynaptically. A third group of drugs have been labeled nootropics, and their action in altering memory functioning remains ill defined. The frequently tested drug, hydergine, belongs to this class of drugs. Finally, neuropeptides and drugs that might alter brain peptides have also been tested in DAT patients. In general, none of these classes of drugs have been excluded as possible treatments of the memory impairments associated with DAT. However, although some positive results have been obtained, effects have been small, highly dose dependent (where dosing is often tailored to individual patients), and frequently only subsamples of patients demonstrate a positive response. This is perhaps not surprising given the enormous heterogeneity in the expression and course of the disease that is commonly noted in studies of DAT.

The use of cholinergic agonists, such as physostigmine and tacrine, as tools for altering memory in DAT patients has had a long history (Beller, Overall, & Swann, 1985; Christie, Shering, Ferguson, & Glen, 1981; Davis & Mohs, 1982; Kaye et al., 1982; Sitaram, Weingartner, & Gillin, 1978; Tariot et al., 1988). Other cholinergic drugs have also been studied extensively in DAT patients. For example, previous research using the cholinergic agonist, arecoline (Christie et al., 1981), has demonstrated some improvement in memory (for pictures) in DAT patients. In our hands, this cholinergic drug had no reliable acute effect on any of a number of types of cognitive memory functions. Neither access to knowledge memory as assessed by a category retrieval test, nor free recall of verbal material, nor recognition memory for pictures was improved following drug administration. This was the case despite the fact that a clear and robust drug effect was evident, including activation with increased motor behavior, tachycardia, and increased blood pressure. It may in fact be that the dysphoric aspects of the activating effect of the drug actually blocked the possibility of demonstrating a positive effect on memory functions (Tariot et al., 1988 for details of findings). Our laboratory, as well as many other groups, continue to explore the potential value of direct cholinergic agonists.

Treating DAT Patients with a Catecholamine-Enhancing Drug: An Example of Drug-Induced Alteration in Effort-Demanding Memory Functions

Based on the fact that the catecholamines play a role in memory and cognition and that central monamine systems are disturbed in many DAT patients, we attempted to stimulate this system using L-Deprenyl, a centrally active monamine-enhancing drug. This drug does not have a significant negative effect on cholinergic functioning, which is already compromised in DAT, and acts as a monamine oxidase inhibitor thereby enhancing catecholaminergic activity. We studied the memory effects of L-Deprenyl in 17 well characterized middle stage DAT patients (who met DSM III and NINCDS-ADRDA workshop DAT criteria). These patients were first treated with a placebo for 7 days, then 10 mg of L-Deprenyl per day for 28 days, followed by 40 mg of L-Deprenyl for 35 days, followed by placebo for 14 days. Throughout the study, and during each study phase of the design, a number of biological measures were assessed, such as cerebrospinal fluid monamine metabolites and sympathetic nervous system activity, along with clinical status and several types of memory functions. A detailed presentation of methods used and observed clinical findings is presented elsewhere (Tariot et al., 1988). Here we summarize the key conclusion that can be drawn from the considerable body of data obtained from that study. Many of these conclusions underscore the importance of the methodological issues that must be considered in designing studies of how drugs might alter memory functions.

The patients studied were evaluated several times during each phase of this study. Physiological and other behavioral effects, such as mood and activation, were evaluated at regular intervals throughout the study phase of the experiment. In addition, three previously validated sets of methods were used to assess attention, access to semantic memory (a domain that is compromised in DAT and is likely to play a role in determining impairments in other memory domains), and effort-demanding episodic memory functions.

Subjects were presented with standardized lists of 12 unrelated common nouns. Each list of words was read at a 3 second per word rate. The subject was then asked to remember as many of the words as possible. The words not remembered were repeated, and again the subjects were asked to try to remember all of the words on the original list--the words remembered on the previous trial as well as the words that were prompted because the subject did not remember them on the previous trial. This procedure was repeated for six trials or until all of the words had been successfully remembered. In the second cognitive procedure that was administered, subjects were read, at a 2 second rate, 12 words that were typical examples of members of a category such as parts of the body, vegetables, fruit, or four-legged animals. The items chosen for presentation represented the full and systematic range of frequencies of occurrence that represent category membership. Six of the 12 words were read once, and 6 of the words were read twice. After hearing each word, the subject was asked to identify whether the word was presented before (within the last few seconds). Immediately after completing this phase of the procedure, subjects were presented with another category name and were asked to generate as many category exemplars as possible. Subjects did this for 90 seconds. This procedure was used as a means of assessing semantic memory, as well as preventing rehearsal of the words that had just been presented. Subjects were also asked to complete several mood-rating scales. Following this and 15 minutes after having heard the list of words that contained six singly and six doubly presented items from some category, the subject was asked to remember several types of things. First, subjects were asked to recall the words on that particular list, followed by a recognition-memory test in which they were asked to identify whether a presented word had been presented as a stimulus or was a new word, a distractor. If a word was judged as *old*, then the subject was also asked to estimate how often that word had been presented at the time the list of words were first read to the subject. Finally, the subject was asked to estimate the judged certainty of being correct in recognition-memory word responses.

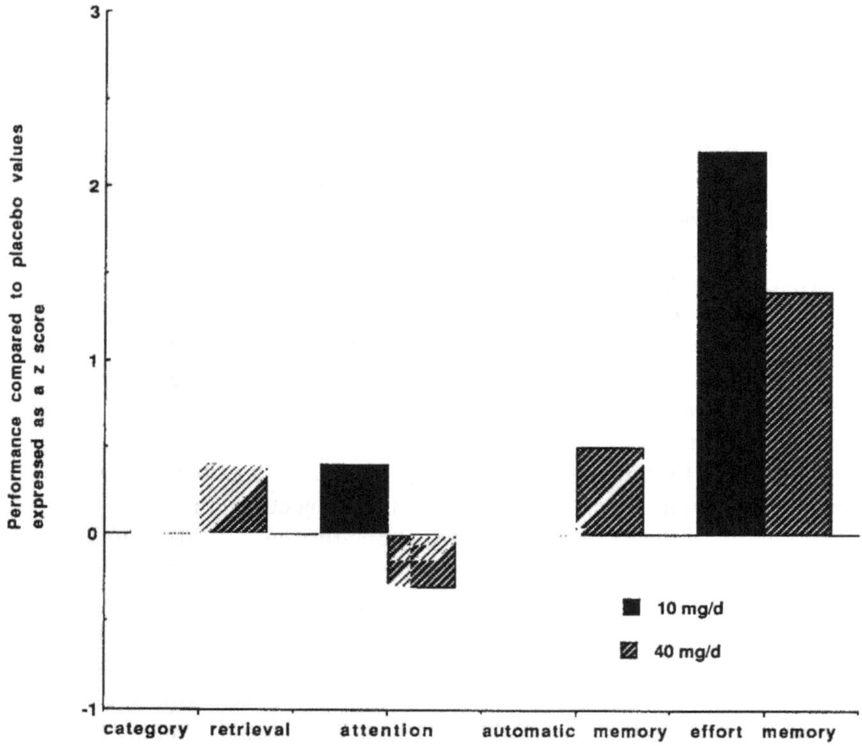

Figure 3.1. L-Deprenyl effects on psychobiologically distinct components of cognitive functioning.

Some changes in the moods of patients were noted, including appearing less anxious while on the active drug. The patients also appeared to be more sociable on the drug. These broadly defined behavioral changes that were evident were statistically reliable but more evident while subjects were treated with the lower of the two doses of L-Deprenyl. Reliable improvements in cognitive functioning were clear during the active drug phase of the study, and the positive effects disappeared when placebo treatment was reactivated during the last phase of the study. However, the pattern of cognitive changes produced by L-Deprenyl were consistent with what might be expected of an antidepressant type cognitive response rather than an antidementia type response. That is, changes in memory that appeared following L-Deprenyl treatment, particularly at the 10 rather than 40-mg dose per day, were limited to changes in effort-demanding memory performance, which is what would occur if depressed patients were treated with a drug that lifts depressive symptoms. What was not altered were other types of memory functions such as the ability to access semantic memory. These findings are summarized in Figure 3.1. One might characterize the memory-improving effects as clinically useful despite the fact that the response was not considered to be mediated by those mechanisms that are more central to the determinants of memory failure in DAT patients, which makes it difficult for these patients to appreciate and encode experiences. The treatment allowed these patients to persist, to persevere, in accomplishing a difficult cognitive task through a mechanism in which MAO inhibition leads to increased catecholamine activity that in turn activates subjects. Perhaps a treatment that can alter both catecholaminergic as well as cholinergic functioning would further enhance memory functions in DAT patients by improving both effort-demanding and semantic-memory functions. This hypothesis is currently being tested in our clinical laboratory.

Creating a Drug-Induced Dementia in Normal Controls and then Reversing that Cognitive Impairment with Another Drug

In another recently completed set of studies, we have tested whether various drugs, such as amphetamine or the brain tripeptide thyrotropin-releasing hormone (TRH) might reverse the memory- impairing effects of scopolamine (Molchan et al., 1990). In a series of studies, we have been able to demonstrate that the cholinergic antagonists, such as scopolamine, can produce in both normal young controls as well as in normal elderly subjects the type of memory deficit that is so readily apparent in untreated DAT patients. Those effects are dose dependent and involve alterations in attention, working memory, effort-demanding as well as automatic cognitive operations, and access to knowledge in semantic memory. Furthermore, these very same effects are also observed superimposed on the DAT clinical picture when DAT patients are treated with cholinergic antagonists such as scopolamine. It therefore appears that cholinergic antagonist-treated subjects model the memory impairment of DAT.

In a recently completed experiment, we tested whether the brain tripeptide TRH might reverse all or part of the scopolamine-induced memory impairment using cognitive methods just like those described above. Memory was impaired in normal subjects treated with scopolamine in doses that would produce a memory impairment equivalent to that seen in middle stage DAT patients. In some conditions, subjects were pretreated with placebo. In another condition, the same subjects were pretreated with TRH before being administered TRH. Given what we know about the sites of action of TRH we could predict that TRH would reverse the memory-impairing effects of scopolamine. If that were to prove to be the case, then it would also suggest that this might be yet another potential useful strategy for treating the memory impairment that is present in DAT. Some components of impaired memory, particularly effort-demanding explicit memory functions, were attenuated by TRH treatment. In addition, some aspects of the scopolamine-induced impairment in accessing semantic memory were also attenuated following TRH treatment.

These results were not surprising since TRH receptors are concentrated in the limbic system, and more specifically in the hippocampus and the amygdala, structures known to play a crucial role in memory. Furthermore, these are the structures that we know are involved in DAT. We also know that TRH interacts with several neurotransmitter systems including the cholinergic system. These findings are therefore important, because they point to a possible neuromodulatory role of TRH on the cholinergic nervous system, suggesting that TRH might be useful in facilitating human memory. These studies also illustrate a research strategy that can be useful in developing neuropharmacological tools for improving memory in which we begin by inducing a memory failure and then study how we might reverse that failure.

Some Conclusions and Prospects for Improving Memory in Clinical Populations

Diseases that disrupt central nervous system functioning can produce highly specific changes in memory functioning. An understanding of how cognitive functions, such as memory, are altered is key in the programmatic development of treatment or remediation strategies that would prove helpful in the remediation of those impairments. The types of findings that will prove useful for understanding the nature of the varieties of memory failures include: systematic quantitative clinical studies contrasting different populations of memory-impaired patients, animal modeling of those impairments that have been characterized in humans, behavioral modeling that might define the mechanisms of different types of memory operations in nominally unimpaired subjects, quantitative analysis of the neurobiology of memory systems in lower animals and in even very simple systems (at the level of aggregates of small numbers of neurons), and pharmacological studies of memory functions in both humans and other animal preparations. The latter types of studies have taught us that psychoactive drugs often produce highly specific rather than general changes in memory.

In considering drug treatments for improving memory, it must be understood that any observed change in memory functions can also be highly specific to one domain but not another, often in narrowly defined dose ranges, and in some subjects but not others. For example, in the treatment of DAT patients, one often notes that it is the less impaired patient that benefits from some treatment. Furthermore, one patient might respond positively to one dose of a drug and negatively to another dose, which might improve memory performance in some other patient. In many ways, the types of findings that are obtained in studies of drug manipulations of memory parallel those seen in studies of behavioral manipulations and training strategies that would improve memory. Here, too, we generally observe effects that, when apparent, are highly task specific (see Herrmann & Searleman, 1990). After all, behavioral manipulations and drugs, if they act to alter memory, both do so by altering how the brain processes information.

What are the prospects for the development of memory-enhancing drugs? Clearly, the likelihood of success is linked to the thoroughness of our understanding of the neurobiology of normal and impaired memory functions. Certainly our appreciation of the anatomy and neurochemistry of many brain systems has grown dramatically during the last 2 decades. Based on this knowledge base, it should be possible to develop drug treatments that can have at least a modest effect on cognitive functions in nominally normal individuals and not only impaired patient populations such as early stage DAT patients. The changes in normal cognitive functioning would likely be in those areas where some modest deficit state exists. This would be the case in normal elderly or in subjects with conditions such as stress, information overload, or impaired arousal (e.g., sleep deprivation) that can disrupt normal cognitive functioning. Likewise, as is apparent at this conference, our understanding of the psychology of memory functions has also grown during this same period. The real challenge for researchers interested in developing tools that would improve memory is to bring into the same laboratory the knowledge and skills of contemporary neuroscience with the sophisticated and subtle understanding of the differentiated picture of memory that is provided by cognitive science.

Endnote 1

Herbert Weingartner is most grateful for continued support from The Upjohn Corporation that allows us to develop the tools for assessing changes in cognitive functions in response to drug treatments of memory-impaired subjects. Harry Bowen and Joseph Fleishaker of The Upjohn Corporation have been particularly active in support of this research.

References

Bartus, R.T., Dean, R.L., Beer, B., & Lippa, A.S. (1982). The cholinergic hypothesis of geriatric memory dysfunction. *Science*, *217*, 408-417.

Beller, S.A., Overall, J.E., & Swann, A.C. (1985). Efficacy of oral physostigmine in primary degenerative dementia. *Psychopharmacology, 87*, 147-151.

Bowden, S.C. (1990). Separating cognitive impairment in neurologically asymptomatic alcoholism from Wernicke-Korsakoff syndrome: Is the neuropsychological distinction justified? *Psychological Bulletin, 107*, 355-366.

Buell, S.J., & Coleman, P.D. (1979). Dendritic growth in the aged human brain and failure of growth in senile dementia. *Science, 206*, 854-856.

Buell, S.J., & Coleman, P.D. (1981). Quantitative evidence for selective dendritic growth in normal human aging but not in senile dementia. *Brain Research, 214*, 23-41.

Christie, J.E., Shering, A., Ferguson, J., & Glen, A.I.M. (1981). Physostigmine and arecoline: Effects of intravenous infusions in Alzheimer presenile dementia. *British Journal of Psychiatry, 138*, 46-50.

Cohen, N.J., & Squire, L.R. (1980). Preserved learning and retention of pattern-analyzing skill in amnesia: Dissociation of knowing how and knowing that. *Science, 210*, 207-210.

Cohen, R.M., Weingartner, H., Smallberg, S.A., Pickar, D., & Murphy, D.L. (1982). Effort and cognition in depression. *Archives of General Psychiatry, 39*, 593-597.

Coyle, J.T., Price, D.L., & DeLong, M.R. (1983). Alzheimer's disease: A disorder of cortical cholinergic innervation. *Science, 219*, 1184-1190.

Davies, C.A., Mann, D.M.A., Sumpter, P.Q., & Yates, P.O. (1987). A quantitative morphometric analysis of neuronal and synaptic content of the frontal and temporal cortex in patients with Alzheimer's disease. *Journal of Neurological Science, 78*, 151-164.

Davis, K.L., & Mohs, R.C. (1982). Enhancement of memory processes in Alzheimer's disease with multiple-dose intravenous physostigmine. *American Journal of Psychiatry, 139*, 1421-1424.

Gottfries, C.G. (1985). Alzheimer's disease and senile dementia: Biochemical characteristics and aspects of treatment. *Psychopharmacology, 86*, 245-252.

Graf, P., Squire, L.R., & Mandler, G. (1984). The information that amnesic patients do not forget. *Journal of Experimental Psychology: Learning, Memory, and Cognition, 10*, 164-178.

Grafman, J., Thompson, K., Weingartner, H., Lawlor, B.A., & Sunderland, T. (in press). Script generation as an indicator of knowledge representation in patients with Alzheimer's disease. *Neurology.*

Hamos, J.E., DeGennaro, L.J., & Drachman, D.A. (1989). Synaptic loss in Alzheimer's disease and other dementias. *Neurology, 39*, 355-361.

Hasher, L., & Zacks, R.T. (1979). Automatic and effortful processing in memory. *Journal of Experimental Psychology: General, 108*, 356-388.

Herrmann, D.J., & Searleman, A. (1990). The new multimodal approach to memory improvement. In G.H. Bower (Ed.), *Advances in learning and motivation* (Vol. 26, pp. 175-205). New York: Academic Press.

Hirst, W., & Volpe, B.T. (1984). Automatic and effortful encoding in amnesia.

In M.S. Gazzaniga (Ed.), *Handbook of cognitive neuroscience* (pp. 369-386). New York: Plenum.

Jacoby, L.L., & Witherspoon, D. (1982). Remembering without awareness. *Canadian Journal of Psychology, 36*, 300-324.

Janowsky, J.S., Shimamura, A.P., Kritchevsky, M., & Squire, L.R. (1989). Cognitive impairment following frontal lobe damage and its relevance to human amnesia. *Behavioral Neuroscience, 103*, 548-560.

Kahneman, D. (1973). *Attention and effort*. Englewood Cliffs, NJ: Prentice-Hall.

Kaye, W., Sitaram, N., Weingartner, H., Ebert, M., Gillin, J.C., & Smallberg, S.A. (1982). Modest facilitation of memory in dementia with combined lecithin and anticholinesterase treatment. *Biological Psychiatry, 17*, 275-280.

Lister, R.G., & Weingartner, H.J. (1987). Neuropharmacological strategies for understanding psychobiological determinants of cognition. *Human Neurobiology, 6*, 119-127.

McGeer, P.L., McGeer, E.G., Suzuki, J., Dolman, C.E., & Nagai, T. (1984). Aging, Alzheimer's disease, and the cholinergic system of the basal forebrain. *Neurology, 34*, 741-745.

Molchan, S.E., Mellow, A.M., Lawlor, B.A., Weingartner, H.J., Cohen, R.M., Cohen, M.R., & Sunderland, T. (1990). TRH attenuates scopolamine-induced memory impairment in humans. *Psychopharmacology, 100*, 84-89.

Perruchet, P., & Baveux, P. (1989). Correlational analyses of explicit and implicit memory performance. *Memory & Cognition, 17*, 77-86.

Roy-Byrne, P., Weingartner, H., Bierer, L., Thompson, K., & Post, R. (1986). Effortful and automatic cognitive processes in depression. *Archives of General Psychiatry, 43*, 265-267.

Schacter, D.L. (1987). Implicit memory: History and current status. *Journal of Experimental Psychology: Learning, Memory, and Cognition, 13*, 501-518.

Schneider, W., & Shiffrin, R.M. (1977). Controlled and automatic human information processing: I. Direction, search, and attention. *Psychological Review, 84*, 1-66.

Shiffrin, R.M., & Schneider, W. (1977). Controlled and automatic human information processing: II. Perceptual learning, automatic attending, and a general theory. *Psychological Review, 84*, 127-190.

Sitaram, N., Weingartner, H., & Gillin, J.C. (1978). Human serial learning: Enhancement with arecoline and choline and impairment with scopolamine. *Science, 201*, 274-276.

Strauss, M.E., Weingartner, H., & Thompson, K. (1985). Remembering words and how often they occurred in memory-impaired patients. *Memory & Cognition, 13*, 507-510.

Tariot, P.N., Cohen, R.M., Welkowitz, J.A., Sunderland, T., Newhouse, P.A., Murphy, D.L., & Weingartner, H. (1988). Multiple dose arecoline infusions in Alzheimer's disease. *Archives of General Psychiatry, 45*, 901-905.

Tariot, P.N., & Weingartner, H. (1986). A psychobiologic analysis of cognitive failures. *Archives of General Psychiatry, 43*, 1183-1188.

Thompson, R.F. (1986). The neurobiology of learning and memory. *Science, 233*, 941-947.

Tulving, E. (1985). How many memory systems are there? *American Psychologist, 40*, 385-398.

Weingartner, H., Cohen, R.M., Martello, J.D.I., & Gerdt, C. (1981). Cognitive processes in depression. *Archives of General Psychiatry, 38*, 42-47.

Weingartner, H., Grafman, J., Boutelle, W., Kaye, W., & Martin, P. (1983). Forms of memory failure. *Science, 221*, 380-382.

Weingartner, H., Sitaram, N., & Gillin, J.C. (1979). The role of the cholinergic nervous system in memory consolidation. *Bulletin of the Psychonomic Society, 13*, 9-11.

Whitehouse, P.J., Price, D.L., Struble, R.G., Clark, A.W., Coyle, J.T., & DeLong, M.R. (1982). Alzheimer's disease and senile dementia: Loss of neurons in the basal forebrain. *Science, 215*, 1237-1239.

Improving Memory and Mood Through Automatic and Controlled Procedures of Mind

Paula T. Hertel

Memory procedures and emotional states function together. Affective tone permeates episodes of memory functioning. Memory functions centrally in episodes of emotional disturbance, serving to feed the episode with fuel from past events or to repress those events when one hopes to escape or avoid the episode. When cognitive procedures are impaired by emotional states such as depression and anxiety, people do not perform the tasks and achieve the goals that could help to repair their moods. In the context of these considerations, then, we must view the improvement of memory as not merely a possible outcome of change in emotional states, but as a factor in effecting such change. Memory improvement and mood improvement function together.

In this chapter, I examine the relationship between memory functions and the negatively valenced emotional states of anxiety and depression. Isen (1984), Bower (1981), and others have discussed the relation of positively valenced states to memory, showing that a positive mood improves intentional memory for positive and sometimes neutral events. However, in a very practical sense, knowing that one can sometimes remember better in a good mood is trivial to the goal of memory improvement; the problem becomes one of trying to attain the good mood. Also, people in elated states don't care very much about possible memory difficulties that arise from extreme arousal or from attempts to recall negative events. In contrast, people care a great deal about impaired functions associated with depression and anxiety (Beck, Rush, Shaw, & Emery, 1979; Poon, 1980). Furthermore, our knowledge of *angry* memory is limited, and it would seem to be a transitory phenomenon unless anger is accompanied by depression. These are the reasons for restricting my topic to depressive and anxiety-related phenomena in memory. The central goals in improving the memory functions of depressed and anxious people are restoration to *normal* levels and eventual mood repair.

This chapter is organized according to the considerations noted at the outset. The first section briefly reviews the major findings in the literature on memory impairment associated with depression and anxiety. The emphasis is placed on findings that offer interesting implications for memory improvement. The second section pertains to memory improvement during mood impairment. Improving one's memory provides a reduction in the number of things one must feel depressed or anxious about. It also helps to achieve more important goals that might eventually assist in mood repair. The third section takes up the bidirectional relation of memory functioning and disturbed mood. In this section, I review the literature on cognitive biases associated with depression and anxiety, with an eye toward their alleviation. The third section is based on the assumptions that the best way to improve memory functioning is to repair the disturbed mood and that such repair involves important adjustments in memory procedures.

The literatures on mood-related effects in memory are guided by various theoretical perspectives (e.g., schema theory, network theory). Following the lead of others (e.g., Clark & Isen, 1982; Eysenck, 1982; Hasher & Zacks, 1979), I appeal to the theoretical distinction between automatic and controlled processes in order to establish a framework for this review. In the manner outlined by Kahneman (1973), I refer to procedures that can occur without attention or conscious awareness as automatic processes. Controlled processes are those that require attention or the use of resources that are essentially limited by a relatively fixed capacity for conscious thought. An emphasis on specific cognitive procedures holds the greatest promise for research on memory improvement (see Herrmann & Searleman, 1990).

Memory Impairment in Depressed and Anxious States

Many reviews of mood and memory emphasize research on the association of mood with the emotional meaning of the materials or events to be remembered (i.e., mood congruence; e.g., Blaney, 1986; Ingram, 1984; Isen, 1984; Johnson & Magaro, 1987). I briefly address issues related to mood congruence below, where I take up the interrelation between mood and memory improvement. Here I review research on memory impairment when depressed or anxious subjects encounter relatively neutral information. Relatively neutral materials probably constitute a large portion of what one encounters in occupational or educational settings.

Although symptoms of depression and anxiety correlate highly in some populations, there are potentially important differences in their effects on memory functions (Ingram, Kendall, Smith, Donnell, & Ronan, 1987). Unfortunately, few researchers have taken measures of both types of affect, so the similarities and differences in the findings on depression and anxiety should be viewed with caution (see Greenberg & Beck, 1989). Furthermore, the findings I review are gathered from different types of depressive populations (experimental inductions, dysphoric college students, outpatients with depressive symptoms and syndromes, and hospitalized depressives with and without other nosologies) and different types of anxious populations (students with test, state, or trait anxiety; phobics; and patients and students with other anxiety-related disorders). In my discussions of depressive and anxiety-related phenomena, I ignore possible differences associated with the type of population unless those differences have contributed to a reliable taxonomy of corresponding effects on memory functioning. For the most part, this has not been the case (cf., Ingram & Kendall, 1987; Williams, Watts, MacLeod, & Mathews, 1988).

Depressive Deficits

A number of reviews of depressive deficits in memory conclude that depression is associated with a reduction in effortful or controlled processing within a limited capacity system (e.g., Ellis, & Ashbrook, 1988; Williams et al., 1988). According to this view, depression depletes the resources needed to perform more difficult processing tasks. Depletion occurs through physiological limitations on processing capacity or through the allocation of attention to irrelevant features of self or context (Beck, 1967; Ellis & Ashbrook, 1988). Depressed subjects in memory experiments, then, presumably have limited ability to employ controlled processes such as organization and elaboration--processes that require attention within the limited capacity system (see Hasher & Zacks, 1979) and benefit subsequent attempts to remember.

Within this general framework of depressive deficits in controlled processing, some research has emphasized the organization (or the structure) of the materials to be remembered. Williams et al. (1988) and Ellis and Ashbrook (1988) have suggested that well structured or organized materials make fewer processing demands. Recall of clearly structured prose passages like those used by Hasher, Rose, Zacks, Sanft, and Doren (1985) does not reflect depressive deficits, whereas recall of more obtuse text does (see Watts & Cooper, 1989). As early as 1976, Russell and Beekhuis showed that the ability to sort nouns into obvious categories during the learning task was not impaired by psychotic depression. Depressed patients in studies by Weingartner, Cohen, Murphy, Martello, and Gerdt (1981) showed recall deficits with unstructured word lists but not when the lists were clearly categorized. So in the sense of inherent structure of materials to be remembered, depressive deficits occur with poorly structured materials. Accounts of depressive deficits that emphasize depletions in resources tend to maintain that depressed subjects lack the resources to detect or to impose the structure that will benefit later recall.

Other specifications of impaired processing point to deficits in elaborative processing. Roy-Byrne, Weingartner, Bierer, Thompson, and Post (1986) found depressive deficits in recalling elaborated materials from a semantic orienting task but no deficit in frequency judgments, which are often not affected by elaborative processing.

Ellis, Thomas, and Rodriguez (1984, Experiment 1) showed that college students who were experimentally induced to feel depressed did not recall words that were each studied in elaborated sentences as well as did neutral subjects; perhaps they failed to expend the resources needed to fully process the elaborated contexts or to use them at the time of recall (see Ellis, Thomas, McFarland, & Lane, 1985). In another experiment that employed induction procedures, Ellis et al. (1984, Experiment 3) showed a depressive deficit in recall of words placed in contextually difficult (less obvious) sentences but not in recall of words from sentences that were highly related to the words. Hertel and Rude (1991b) failed to replicate these findings with naturally depressed college students. (Also see Hasher et al., 1985; Ingram, 1989; Isen, 1984; for discussions of possible differences in memory effects associated with naturally occurring versus experimentally induced depression.) Recently, however, we have replicated the findings of Ellis et al. (1984, Experiment 3) with clinically depressed outpatients. The results of this experiment suggest modifications to previous speculations about the nature of depressive deficits in controlled processing.

In the incidental learning phase of an experiment by Hertel and Rude (1991a), outpatients exhibiting symptoms of unipolar depression, recovered outpatients, and nonpsychiatric controls judged the semantic fit of words into easy or difficult sentence frames. One learning condition was similar to the procedure of Ellis et al. (1984, Experiment 3): The word and the frame were displayed concomitantly, and subjects judged the fit whenever they chose to do so during the duration of the trial. Another condition restricted the display of the word to 1 second at the beginning of the trial; subjects were required to repeat the word and make the judgment at the end of the trial. In this second condition, then, the subjects' attention was focused on the task, in that they were required to rehearse the words and possibly encouraged to process them more elaboratively in the context of the sentence, whereas in the unfocused condition, subjects' attention was less constrained to focus on the task. The unfocused condition produced a depressive deficit in the subsequent free recall of words from the difficult contexts. In contrast, depressed subjects in the focused learning condition recalled those words as well as did both control groups.

Clearly, these results suggest that depression does not limit the ability to allocate sufficient resources to a more difficult task. Yet an emphasis on controlled processes is still quite appropriate: When the task was unfocused, depressed subjects might have paid less attention to the materials; perhaps they allocated attention to task irrelevant processing. However, under focused learning conditions that were at least as demanding, depressed subjects performed as capably as nondepressed subjects. Hertel and Hardin (1990) describe deficits of the type that was demonstrated in the unfocused condition as depressive deficits in initiative. Unlike subjects in a neutral mood, depressed subjects fail to spontaneously initiate controlled processes that would benefit intentional remembering. When procedures are guided by instructions or when tests of memory bypass the advantage of uninstructed procedures employed spontaneously by nondepressed subjects, initiative ceases to be the issue and depressed subjects do not show memory impairments.

Deficits in initiative might be understood as difficulties in detecting the optimal strategy. Experiments by Leight and Ellis (1981), conducted with experimental inductions of depressive and neutral moods, have shown depressive impairments in the discovery of higher order structure for letter strings. In the varied-input condition, the learning task encouraged but did not instruct for the discovery of higher order meaning. In the constant-input condition, such discovery was made more difficult. Following the learning phase, subjects were transferred to a similar task with new letter strings, under either varied or constant conditions. The important result for the present purposes was that nondepressed subjects who received varied input on the learning task detected the higher order meaning and transferred that strategy to the second task, regardless of their mood or the conditions of input during the second task. A depressed mood prevented the detection of the optimal strategy, but once it had been discovered under neutral conditions, depressed subjects used the strategy effectively.

Depressive deficits in initiative might also be understood as motivational disturbances. Experimentally depressed subjects tend to report less curiosity and are less motivated to read about psychology experiments (Rodrigue, Olson, & Markley, 1987). Riskind (1989) suggested that reduced interest in external events might even cause a reduction in the allocation of resources to cognitive tasks. Along these lines, Cohen, Weingartner, Smallberg, Pickar, and Murphy (1982) obtained a high correlation between sustained motor effort and recall at longer delays in a short-term memory task (for depressed subjects only). Because these tasks share few elements, the authors suggested that they are related through a central motivational state. Such a central mechanism could also determine the tendency to initiate strategies beyond the requirements of the task.

Retarded initiation of voluntary action is emphasized by Coyne and Gotlib's (1983) review of depression research. Similarly, Rehm (1982) related loss of initiative to deficits in self-monitoring and self-control. Retarded initiative, however, does not imply that depressed subjects simply suffer from low levels of arousal or lack incentives. Several investigators provide evidence that depressed people are ultimately very cooperative (Coyne & Gotlib, 1983), that simple manipulations of incentive do not affect depressed subjects more than others (Richards & Ruff, 1989), and that CNS arousal characterizes depression (e.g., Kuhl & Helle, 1986). Clearly, the relation between depression and specific motivational constructs has not been well delineated.

Kuhl and Helle (1986) have developed an interesting approach to understanding the cooccurrence of central arousal and behavioral passivity in depression. They proposed that chronic depression is maintained by unfulfillable (degenerated) intentions. Intentions to achieve essentially unattainable goals use resources needed to enact new intentions. Thus, to the extent that they are "on one's mind," they induce arousal while ensuring passivity in ongoing tasks. One test of this account established a very minor unfulfillable goal (cleaning up a messy table) that, for depressed subjects only, seemed to remain active during subsequent tests of prospective memory (remembering to number pages) and memory span for words. Kuhl and Helle's work is compatible with the notion that ruminations occupy the cognitive capacity needed for ongoing tasks, but the ruminations are not necessarily self-related, and they interfere with the initiation of new tasks as well as with routine processing demands.

Finally, Watts, MacLeod, and Morris (1988b) suggest that the depressive mind is not always actively engaged in task irrelevant thoughts when deficits are observed in memory tasks. Mind wandering seems to occur during prose processing or retrieval, but when depressed subjects are engaged in planning during problem solving (e.g., the Tower of Hanoi) the mind "goes blank." Going blank seems to reflect difficulties in thinking about what to do next.

Anxiety-Related Deficits

In reviewing research on anxiety-related deficits in memory functions, Eysenck (1982) and Wine (1980) offered interpretations that emphasized attentional capacity. As in the hypothesis with depressive deficits, capacity is presumably occupied by extra-task processing. Unlike accounts of depressive deficits, however, Eysenck proposed that anxious subjects attempt to compensate with increased effort; they do better at easy tasks, while still showing the deficit in difficult tasks. Thus, anxiety reduces the reserve of resources for controlled processing, with arousal mediating the effects related to task difficulty. Moreover, arousal seems to have consequences for cue utilization (Easterbrook, 1959). Task irrelevant cues are eliminated by moderate levels of arousal, but higher levels seem also to eliminate more central, relevant cues (see Geen, 1980, for a review of cue utilization in test anxiety).

A particularly good summary of evidence of anxiety-related deficits in memory is provided by Williams et al. (1988, Ch. 3). Such deficits involve impaired elaboration, referred to by Williams et al. as biases toward surface level processing. Anxiety also seems to reduce the use of organizational processes, but such reduction sometimes is compensated for by other means. For example, Mueller (1976) has shown evidence of less clustering by anxious students without an overall deficit in free recall.

In general, anxiety-related deficits occur under conditions that are widely similar to those in which depressive deficits arise. Impaired elaborative and organizational processes are associated with susceptibility to sources of distraction that use resources within a limited capacity system. Ingram and

Kendall (1987) suggested that anxious subjects' task irrelevant focus is less self-oriented than what seems to be the case with depressives, but when the overlap between depression and anxiety is eliminated, so is the evidence for differences in self-focus (Ingram, 1990). Some anxious subjects, however, do show signs of excessive preoccupation with stressful situations and misperceive their demands (Ingram et al., 1987). They sometimes compensate by increasing their efforts on aspects of the task that are under their control (easier tasks that benefit from high levels of arousal).

Finally, it might be important to consider that almost all demonstrations of mood-related impairments have used tests of intentional remembering (see Jacoby & Kelley, 1987). As has been found by Hertel and Hardin (1990), with depressed college students, mood impairments may not occur on tests where remembering is not the focus of attention but, instead, may occur in the course of performing other tasks. (Mood congruency, however, has been demonstrated in such tasks; these effects are described below.) Moreover, unintentional uses of memory clearly outdistance intentional uses of memory in their frequency and importance of occurrence. The irony of this observation lies in the realization that mood-impaired people are not aware that unintentional uses of memory may be unimpaired. They notice failures to remember when they are trying to remember. An important step in future research on memory impairment and complaints should be taken in the direction of exploring unintentional uses of memory by depressed and anxious people.

Memory Improvement During Mood Impairment

In their multimodal approach to suggestions for memory improvement, Herrmann and Searleman (1990) made distinctions between "content" manipulations, such as standard mnemonic techniques, and "process" manipulations, such as changes in emotional states. According to their view, process manipulations in the realm of depressive and anxiety-related deficits are somewhat synonymous with mood improvement (addressed in the next major section of this chapter). Evidence of mood dependent memory, also taken up briefly by Herrmann and Searleman, is mixed in the realm of depression and anxiety. Some researchers see mood dependent memory as a special case of mood congruency (e.g., Blaney, 1986); others doubt its existence or stress that it occurs only when other contextual cues are weak (e.g., Bower & Mayer, 1989). Even if mood dependent memory turns out eventually to be a reliable phenomenon, we might wonder what it offers in the way of memory improvement techniques, beyond instructions to make one's mood during study comparable to one's mood during testing, or vice versa. In this section, then, I restrict my review to research on memory improvement in the realm of content and strategy manipulations used with depressed and anxious subjects. The aim is to find ways of improving memory performance to be used by people experiencing ongoing impaired moods.

The major question that arises in considering memory improvement techniques for depressed and anxious people is whether such improvement indeed is possible without mood repair. For example, after reviewing the evidence for depressive deficits in cognitive capacity, Williams et al. (1988, Chapter 3) wondered if depressed subjects are able to process "deeply;" some clinical studies have shown that depressives benefitted less than normals from inherent structure (i.e., the approximation of word lists to text). The implication is that depressed and anxious people should be resigned to function on low capacity as best they can. However, research that has focused on structuring not the materials but the task itself, through instructions and design, holds more promise for believing that people with impaired moods can engage the procedures that lead to good performance on memory tests. The advice that emerges from this research, described next, is to understand componentially the requirements of tasks to be completed by mood-impaired people, to construct methods for engaging the necessary procedures, and above all, not to abandon them to the weaknesses of their own initiative or to their irrelevant thoughts.

Specific Procedures for Memory Improvement

Because disturbances in the focus of attention characterize both types of mood impairments, it makes sense that there have been several successful attempts to improve memory by mobilizing the attention of depressed and anxious subjects for task appropriate processing. The evidence described above regarding the elimination of depressive deficits in recall by requiring attention to the target words during incidental learning (Hertel & Rude, 1991a) is one example of such an attempt. Instructions to image during initial exposure to materials is yet another way. If subjects cooperate, imagery improves memory by way of both elaborative and organizational procedures. According to Watts, MacLeod, and Morris (1988a), imagery instructions improved severely depressed subjects' memory for prose, even though they still reported losses of concentration. Edmunson and Nelson (1976) showed that imagery instructions helped highly anxious students (as well as nonanxious students). In general, reviews of attempts to improve the performance of test anxious students on memory tasks (e.g., Geen, 1980) emphasize the importance of directing attention to task relevant features and away from sources of distraction.

Directing attention away from sources of distraction experienced by depressed people can be achieved by increasing task demands. Krames and MacDonald (1985) obtained this result in a dual-processing task with varying degrees of cognitive load. Nondepressed subjects recalled more words from the beginning of lists under low loads than under high loads, but the reverse was true for the depressed outpatients, who showed a "distraction effect" under low loads and recalled at higher levels as load increased. Ruminations apparently can be overridden by attention-demanding tasks.

Attention-demanding tasks, of course, do not necessarily mobilize attention in ways that benefit memory performance. Many tasks are susceptible to the use of special strategies that are not specified by instructions. Hertel and Hardin (1990), for example, emphasized the importance of guiding depressed subjects in their use of controlled strategies for recognition. In these experiments, experimentally depressed, naturally depressed, and nondepressed college students completed two different tests of memory for homophones whose less frequent meanings (e.g., pear instead of pair) had been biased in an incidental study phase. In the first test of memory (spelling), the number of homophones spelled in line with the studied bias indexed the unintentional use of memory and did not show a depressive deficit. Tests of unintentional uses of memory typically do not show effects of elaborative learning or invite strategic procedures during testing, and so nondepressed subjects should not show the advantage of initiating unrequired procedures. Tests of intentional remembering, such as recognition, are susceptible to uninstructed procedures, and on the following test of recognizing homophones from the study phase, depressive deficits were revealed. Specifically, nondepressed subjects tended to use strategies for recognition that employed the intervening spelling test, whereas recognition and spelling were stochastically independent for depressed subjects. Most important for research on memory improvement were the results from attempts to provide all subjects with strategies that might have been employed spontaneously by nondepressed subjects. When they were directed to recall the study phase as they spelled (Experiment 2) or to use their performance on the spelling test as a bridge to the study phase during recognition (Experiment 3), the recognition performance of depressed subjects improved.

The investigation of impairments in strategic processing has been the focus of research on problem solving in depression. Silberman, Weingartner, and Post (1983) found that depressed subjects focused less on a single hypothesis than did nondepressed subjects and solved fewer problems. Yet, when they were required to list their hypotheses while solving, depressed subjects improved. Similarly, Abramson, Alloy, and Rosoff (1981) discovered that when depressed subjects were provided with hypotheses for problem solving, they performed as well as normals.

In summary, we might conclude that depressed people can be helped to perform well on tests of intentional remembering if they are required to attend to task relevant features and guided to employ appropriate strategies. Although anxious people probably do not suffer from the lack of initiative, they nevertheless need help in focusing on the relevant features of the task. One might surmise from the comments of Ingram and Kendall (1987) and Wine (1980) that anxious people would also profit from specifications of strategies for unstructured situations. Yet, what can be done more generally in memory-training programs to encourage depressed and anxious people to develop skills for use beyond the task at hand?

Memory Training

According to Williams et al. (1988, Ch. 3), there have been few, if any, demonstrations of long-term instructional effects for depression and anxiety. Poon (1980) outlined a multifaceted program that includes specific suggestions for practicing learning strategies and for developing retrieval plans. Yet, as Watts et al. (1988a) aptly comment, "the main challenge is likely to be getting [depressed people] to actually use the strategies" (p. 187). No one (depressed, anxious, or "normal" people alike) likes to use the effortful, controlled procedures that typify memory improvement techniques. Indeed, Poon's program includes many motivational components to encourage practice.

Long-term improvement in the real world also depends heavily on what one might call "prospective metamemory." Practiced and skilled we may be, but we still must consciously remember to use the techniques, at least until they become automatic or habitual. Prospective metamemory might be best achieved if training and practice take place in a variety of settings and tasks so that cues to use the procedures are linked to the situations in which they are needed.

Finally, it seems likely that a stable of mnemonic and search techniques might not be the thing to emphasize in training programs with depressed and anxious people. What seems to be particularly necessary is practice at staying on task, perhaps assisted by external aids. Training in breaking down the components of cognitive tasks might help to override depressive deficits in initiative and planning. In this regard, main-line research on memory might do well to emphasize specific procedures of mind (Kolers & Roediger, 1984). Functional approaches, such as the description of relations among classes of cues (Watkins, 1990), offer direct application to memory training.

Any program designed to improve memory functions in the long run must also consider factors beyond training in specific skills and strategies (Poon, 1980). For example, a reduced sense of self-efficacy in cognitive tasks is associated with depressed moods (Bower, 1983) and test anxiety (Wine, 1980). Self-efficacy determines what one attempts to do and how well one persists in doing it (Bandura, 1977). Therefore, training in self-efficacy--through experience in structured tasks--might help to improve performance on unstructured memory tasks (also see Hertzog, this volume). In addition, Kuhl and Helle (1986) advised that we teach depressed people strategies for disregarding intentions unrelated to the task at hand.

Improvement in Mood and Memory

Improvement in memory functioning of mood-impaired people seems best achieved by repairing the disturbed moods. Does mood repair actually help? Our assumption that it does relies on evidence that mood-impaired subjects do not perform as well as others. Most of these studies are correlational; even in the ones that employ experimental inductions, some other phenomenon associated with the induced mood may actually cause the deficit (see Riskind, 1989). What is needed is research in which mood-impaired subjects are randomly assigned to treatments for mood repair or to wait lists, with a demonstration of pretreatment deficits and posttreatment recovery.

If mood repair does improve memory performance, the method of treatment seems to be critical. For example, remediation of memory difficulties associated with test anxiety has not been achieved reliably by treating the emotional component of anxiety through relaxation techniques (see Williams et al., 1988, Ch. 3; Wine, 1980). Furthermore, one cannot repair mood disturbances without involving memory functions. The success of attempts at mood repair is clearly affected by ongoing memory procedures such as mood congruent attention and retrieval.

Selective attention to mood congruent aspects of current experience and selective remembering of mood congruent aspects of events from the past constitute ubiquitous findings in the literature on mood and memory (see reviews by Blaney, 1986; Bower, 1981; Isen, 1984; Johnson & Magaro, 1987). However, the selectivity of these procedures is commonly thought to be an automatic aspect of feeling state, with controlled processes operating on the material that is automatically selected for attention (Clark & Isen, 1982; but see the superb critique by Blaney, 1986). Mood is presumably maintained by automatic selection and repaired by controlled processes. Sometimes controlled processes such as active rehearsal of mood-related materials are thought to operate in such a way as to reconcile their meaning and achieve self-control (e.g., Rehm, 1982); sometimes controlled processes direct attention away from further processing and toward more neutral material. Next, I describe a few examples of mood congruent effects that illustrate these proposed phenomena.

In the realm of automatic selection, several studies (reviewed by Williams et al., 1988, Ch. 10) have shown selective attention to threat-related words by anxious subjects. Also, Eysenck, MacLeod, and Mathews (1987), for example, showed that trait anxious subjects spelled homophones in the direction of threat-related meaning (e.g., die vs. dye). Similar effects have been found in depression; for example, a depressed mood has been associated with lowered thresholds for detecting failure-related words (Postman & Brown, 1952) and emotional words in general (Small & Robins, 1988). Yet, according to Williams et al., depressive effects in automatic selection have not been demonstrated when anxiety is controlled.

Automatic retrieval processes, to the extent to which they characterize procedures in tests of unintentional memory, also are implicated in anxiety. Subjects in a study by Mathews, Mogg, May, and Eysenck (1989) were asked to imagine scenes for threatening and nonthreatening words and to judge their pleasantness. Later they were provided with three-letter stems for old and new words and told to complete them with the first word that came to mind. Subjects with generalized anxiety disorders completed the stems of old threatening words more often than other types and more often than did controls. In the controlled-processing test of cued recall, however, anxiety-related differences were not obtained. Furthermore, others cited by Mathews et al. have found that anxious subjects actually recall fewer threatening than nonthreatening words. Perhaps controlled processes operate to avoid further processing of threatening materials.

Illustrations of mood congruent effects on intentional recall abound. Symmetries with respect to depression and anxiety are most often found when materials have been processed self-referentially (e.g., Greenberg & Beck, 1989; Ingram et al., 1987). Such symmetries led Ingram and Kendall (1987) to suggest that anxious and depressed subjects engage similar procedures, with the products of the procedures exhibiting differences associated with the type of mood. Others might point out that controlled procedures operate to different ends, as a consequence of motivational factors such as avoidance (in anxiety) or mood repair (in depression). We can reasonably assume that controlled procedures would be involved in attempts at mood control. Such attempts would not always be important in typical experimental contexts (and therefore symmetries between depression and anxiety can be demonstrated), but they would more likely arise in natural contexts for retrieving personal memories (see Costanzo & Hasher, 1989).

A framework for reconciling the sometimes disparate findings on mood congruency has been offered by Williams et al. (1988, Chapter 10). Their model holds that depression and anxiety involve different types of biases in specific procedures that are either passive (automatic) or awareness based (controlled). Anxiety operates like automatic priming in moving resources toward threatening materials. Later, awareness-based procedures direct resources away from threatening materials, thereby inhibiting the development of cues for recall. In contrast, depression biases the products of controlled processes by deploying resources to the recruitment of depression-related information. The model provides links to certain notions of adaptation: Anxiety helps people to avoid danger, so automatic aspects of information processing are sensitive to anxiety; one function of depression is to come to terms with loss, so controlled procedures are sensitive to depression.

Based on their model, Williams et al. (1988) provide some suggestions for remediation of impaired mood. Treatments that emphasize positive aspects of experience can, through rehearsal, make them more likely to be automatically selected. Furthermore, treatment may help mood-impaired people to become aware of the ways that automatic processes contribute to their mood states.

Such awareness might not directly modify the state, but it could provide opportunities for the counterconditioning of emotional processes. For example, if threatening stimuli are not avoided, reactions other than fear can be conditioned and erroneous ideas about threat can be challenged (see Foa & Kozak, 1986). A similar point is made by Beck et al. (1979): By concentrating attention on "automatic" negatively valenced thoughts, depressed people could then redirect resources to more productive focal points and those procedures might become more automatic with practice.

More generally, cognitive therapies have been shown to be effective in the treatment of depression (e.g., Teasdale, Fennell, Hibbert, & Amies, 1984) and the "worry" component of anxiety (Wine, 1980). Cognitive therapies include techniques of cognitive restructuring of depressive or worrisome thoughts. Teasdale (1983) tells us that cognitive therapy helps the client to gain access to more realistic thoughts; such access can be attained through the guidance of thoughts or the improvement of mood, which provides automatic access to positive thoughts. The processes involved in restructuring might well involve redirecting resources to more productive thoughts in both conscious and unconscious ways (Williams et al., 1988, Chapter 10).

Conclusions

In reviewing what we have learned to date about memory improvement, Herrmann and Searleman (1990) reached three conclusions. First, people will not continue to use very effortful techniques. According to some formulations, the use of such techniques by depressed and anxious people is inherently limited by their moods. Alternatively, my review has led to the conclusion that the attention of depressed and anxious people can be mustered for effortful processing by structuring the requirements of the task. This capability, however, does not obviate the problems associated with long-term improvement in intentional remembering. Some remediation might be achieved through training in prospective metamemory, which would require a clearer understanding of functional aspects of memory.

Functional analyses emphasize specific aspects of the task under consideration. Similarly, Herrmann and Searleman's (1990) second conclusion was that memory training should focus on skills that are specific to the materials and task at hand. The notion of specificity should also be extended to the domain of mood-related impairments, such as difficulties in planning and in attending to task-related cues.

Third, the focus of memory training should be "multimodal." One of the modes addressed by Herrmann and Searleman (1990) is the emotional state of the rememberer. The authors suggest that various modes operate in ways that are both central and peripheral to the memory system. This observation clearly holds for depressive and anxious memory. Impaired moods perhaps function peripherally to affect motivations associated with planning and task initiation. Impaired moods function centrally to channel the focus of attention, sometimes away from the task and sometimes toward mood-related aspects of experience. The distribution of resources to mood-related material may function to maintain the mood and associated memory problems, but it can be used therapeutically to repair the mood by summoning controlled processes in situations where automatic processes typically hold sway.

Gaining control seems to be what memory training is all about. In contrast, losing control by practicing to make effortful procedures automatic (Klatzky, 1984) or by using memory unconsciously (Jacoby & Kelley, 1987) might turn out to be better advice to give depressed and anxious people. Because we rarely consider the unconscious effects of past experience, memory complaints surely are based on failures to intentionally remember. Who knows what deleterious effects are exerted by beliefs about impaired memory and the concomitant resolution to try harder? Unless the depressed or anxious person understands specifically how to improve memory, trying harder to remember may merely exacerbate the impairment by providing more salient examples of failure that increase anxiety and depression.

Endnote 1

The writing of this chapter was supported by Grant #RO3 MH44044 from the National Institute of Mental Health.

References

Abramson, L.Y., Alloy, L., & Rosoff, R. (1981). Depression and the generation of complex hypotheses in the judgment of contingency. *Behavior Therapy and Research*, *19*, 35-45.

Bandura, A. (1977). Self-efficacy: Toward a unifying theory of behavior change. *Psychological Review*, *84*, 191-215.

Beck, A.T. (1967). *The diagnosis and management of depression*. Philadelphia: University of Pennsylvania Press.

Beck, A.T., Rush, A.J., Shaw, B.F., & Emery, G. (1979). *Cognitive therapy of depression*. New York: Wiley.

Blaney, P.H. (1986). Affect and memory: A review. *Psychological Bulletin*, *99*, 229-246.

Bower, G.H. (1981). Mood and memory. *American Psychologist*, *36*, 129-148.

Bower, G.H. (1983). Affect and cognition. *Philosophical Transactions of the Royal Society of London*, *B302*, 387-402.

Bower, G.H., & Mayer, J.D. (1989). In search of mood-dependent retrieval. In D. Kuiken (Ed.), Mood and memory: Theory, research, and applications [Special Issue]. *Journal of Social Behavior and Personality*, *4*, 121-156.

Clark, M.S., & Isen, A.M. (1982). Toward understanding the relationship between feeling states and social behavior. In A.H. Hastorf & A.M. Isen (Eds.), *Cognitive social psychology* (pp. 73-108). New York: Elsevier.

Cohen, R.M, Weingartner, H., Smallberg, S.A., Pickar, D., & Murphy, D.L. (1982). Effort and cognition in depression. *Archives of General Psychiatry, 39*, 593-597.

Costanzo, P.R., & Hasher, L. (1989). Mood and memory: A reconsideration. In D. Kuiken (Ed.), Mood and memory: Theory, research, and applications [Special Issue]. *Journal of Social Behavior and Personality, 4*, 71-78.

Coyne, J.C., & Gotlib, I.H. (1983). The role of cognition in depression: A critical appraisal. *Psychological Bulletin, 94*, 472-505.

Easterbrook, J.A. (1959). The effect of emotion on cue utilization and the organization of behavior. *Psychological Review, 66*, 183-201.

Edmunson, E.D., & Nelson, D.L. (1976). Anxiety, imagery, and sensory interference. *Bulletin of the Psychonomic Society, 8*, 319-322.

Ellis, H.C., & Ashbrook, P.W. (1988). Resource-allocation model of the effects of depressed mood states on memory. In K. Fiedler & J. Forgus (Eds.), *Affect, cognition, and social behavior: New evidence and integrative attempts* (pp. 25-43). Toronto: Hogrefe.

Ellis, H.C., Thomas, R.L., McFarland, A.D., & Lane, W. (1985). Emotional mood states and retrieval in episodic memory. *Journal of Experimental Psychology: Learning, Memory, and Cognition, 11*, 363-370.

Ellis, H.C., Thomas, R.L., & Rodriguez, I.A. (1984). Emotional mood states and memory: Elaborative encoding, semantic processing, and cognitive effort. *Journal of Experimental Psychology: Learning, Memory, and Cognition, 10*, 470-482.

Eysenck, M.W. (1982). *Attention and arousal: Cognition and performance*. New York: Springer-Verlag.

Eysenck, M.W., MacLeod, C., & Mathews, A. (1987). Cognitive functioning in anxiety. *Psychological Research, 49*, 189-195.

Foa, E.B., & Kozak, M.J. (1986). Emotional processing of fear: Exposure to corrective information. *Psychological Bulletin, 99*, 20-35.

Geen, R.G. (1980). Test anxiety and cue utilization. In I.G. Sarason (Ed.), *Test anxiety: Theory, research, and applications* (pp. 43-62). Hillsdale, NJ: Erlbaum.

Greenberg, M.S., & Beck, A.T. (1989). Depression versus anxiety: A test of the content-specificity hypothesis. *Journal of Abnormal Psychology, 98*, 9-13.

Hasher, L., Rose, K.C., Zacks, R.T., Sanft, H., & Doren, B. (1985). Mood, recall, and selectivity effects in normal college students. *Journal of Experimental Psychology: General, 114*, 104-118.

Hasher, L., & Zacks, R.T. (1979). Automatic and effortful processes in memory. *Journal of Experimental Psychology: General*, 108, 356-388.

Herrmann, D.J., & Searleman, A. (1990). The new multi-modal approach to memory improvement. In G. Bower (Ed.), *Advances in learning and motivation* (Vol. 26, pp. 175-205). New York: Academic Press.

Hertel, P.T., & Hardin, T.S. (1990). Remembering with and without awareness in a depressed mood: Evidence for deficits in initiative. *Journal of Experimental Psychology: General, 119*, 45-59.

Hertel, P.T., & Rude, S.S. (1991a). Depressive deficits in memory: Focusing attention improves subsequent recall. *Journal of Experimental Psychology: General, 120*, 301-312.

Hertel, P.T., & Rude, S.S. (1991b). Recalling in a state of natural or experimental depression. *Cognitive Therapy and Research, 15*, 103-127.

Ingram, R.E. (1984). Toward an information-processing analysis of depression. *Cognitive Therapy and Research, 8*, 443-478.

Ingram, R.E. (1989). External validity issues in mood and memory research. In D. Kuiken (Ed.), Mood and memory: Theory, research, and applications [Special Issue]. *Journal of Social Behavior and Personality, 4*, 57-62.

Ingram, R.E. (1990). Attentional nonspecificity in depressive and generalized anxious affective states. *Cognitive Therapy and Research, 14*, 25-35.

Ingram, R.E., & Kendall, P.C. (1987). The cognitive side of anxiety. *Cognitive Therapy and Research, 11*, 523-536.

Ingram, R.E., Kendall, P.C., Smith, T.W., Donnell, C., & Ronan, K. (1987). Cognitive specificity in emotional distress. *Journal of Personality and Social Psychology, 53*, 734-742.

Isen, A.M. (1984). Toward understanding the role of affect in cognition. In R. Wyer & T. Srull (Eds.), *Handbook of social cognition* (Vol. 3, pp. 179-236). Hillsdale, NJ: Erlbaum.

Jacoby, L.L., & Kelley, C.M. (1987). Unconscious influences of memory for a prior event. *Personality and Social Psychology Bulletin, 13*, 314-336.

Johnson, M.H., & Magaro, P.A. (1987). Effects of mood and severity on memory processes in depression and mania. *Psychological Bulletin, 101*, 28-40.

Kahneman, D. (1973). *Attention and effort*. Englewood Cliffs, NJ: Prentice-Hall.

Klatzky, R.L. (1984). *Memory and awareness: An information-processing perspective* (p. 137). New York: Freeman.

Kolers, P.A., & Roediger, H.L., III (1984). Procedures of mind. *Journal of Verbal Learning and Verbal Behavior, 23*, 425-449.

Krames, L., & MacDonald, M.R. (1985). Distraction and depressive cognitions. *Cognitive Therapy and Research, 9*, 561-573.

Kuhl, J., & Helle, P. (1986). Motivational and volitional determinants of depression: The degenerated-intention hypothesis. *Journal of Abnormal Psychology, 95*, 247-251.

Leight, K.A., & Ellis, H.C. (1981). Emotional mood states, strategies, and state dependency in memory. *Journal of Verbal Learning and Verbal Behavior, 20*, 251-266.

Mathews, A., Mogg, K., May, J., & Eysenck, M. (1989). Implicit and explicit memory bias in anxiety. *Journal of Abnormal Psychology, 98*, 236-240.

Mueller, J.H. (1976). Anxiety and cue utilization in human learning and memory. In M. Zuckerman & C.D. Spielberger (Eds.), *Emotions and anxiety: New concepts, methods and applications* (pp. 197-229). Hillsdale, NJ: Erlbaum.

Poon, L.W. (1980). A systems approach for the assessment and treatment of memory problems. In J.M. Ferguson & C.B. Taylor (Eds.), *The comprehensive handbook of behavioral medicine* (Vol. 1, pp. 193-212). New York: Spectrum.

Postman, L., & Brown, D.R. (1952). Perceptual consequences of success and failure. *Journal of Abnormal and Social Psychology*, *47*, 213-221.

Rehm, L.P. (1982). Self-management in depression. In P. Karoly & F.H. Kanfer (Eds.), *Self-management and behavior change: From theory to practice* (pp. 522-567). New York: Pergamon.

Richards, P.M., & Ruff, R.M. (1989). Motivational effects on neuropsychological functioning: Comparison of depressed versus nondepressed individuals. *Journal of Consulting and Clinical Psychology*, *57*, 396-402.

Riskind, J.H. (1989). Will the field ultimately need a more detailed analysis of mood-memory? In D. Kuiken (Ed.), Mood and memory: Theory, research, and applications [Special Issue]. *Journal of Social Behavior and Personality*, *4*, 39-44.

Rodrigue, J.R., Olson, K.R., & Markley, R.P. (1987). Induced mood and curiosity. *Cognitive Therapy and Research*, *11*, 101-106.

Roy-Byrne, P.P., Weingartner, H., Bierer, L.M., Thompson, K., & Post, R.M. (1986). Effortful and automatic cognitive processes in depression. *Archives of General Psychiatry*, *43*, 265-267.

Russell, P.W., & Beekhuis, M.E. (1976). Organization in memory. *Journal of Abnormal Psychology*, *85*, 527-534.

Silberman, E.K., Weingartner, H., & Post, R.M. (1983). Thinking disorder in depression. *Archives of General Psychiatry*, *40*, 775-780.

Small, S.A., & Robins, C.J. (1988). The influence of induced depressed mood on visual recognition thresholds: Predictive ambiguity of associative network models of mood and cognition. *Cognitive Therapy and Research*, *12*, 295-306.

Teasdale, J.D. (1983). Negative thinking in depression: Cause, effect, or reciprocal relationship? *Advances in Behaviour Research and Therapy*, *5*, 27-49.

Teasdale, J.D., Fennell, M.J.V., Hibbert, G.A., & Amies, P.L. (1984). Cognitive therapy for major depressive disorders in primary care. *British Journal of Psychiatry*, *144*, 400-406.

Watkins, M.J. (1990). Mediationism and the obfuscation of memory. *American Psychologist*, *45*, 328-335.

Watts, F.N., & Cooper, Z. (1989). The effects of depression on structural aspects of the recall of prose. *Journal of Abnormal Psychology*, *98*, 150-153.

Watts, F.N., MacLeod, A.K., & Morris, L. (1988a). A remedial strategy for memory and concentration problems in depressed patients. *Cognitive Therapy and Research*, *12*, 185-193.

Watts, F.N., MacLeod, A.K., & Morris, L. (1988b). Associations between phenomenal and objective aspects of concentration problems in depressed patients. *British Journal of Psychology*, *79*, 241-250.

Weingartner, H., Cohen, R.M., Murphy, D.L., Martello, J., & Gerdt, C. (1981). Cognitive processes in depression. *Archives of General Psychiatry*, *38*, 42-47.

Williams, J.M.G., Watts, F.N., MacLeod, C., & Mathews, A. (1988). *Cognitive psychology and emotional disorders*. New York: Wiley.

Wine, J.D. (1980). Cognitive-attentional theory of text anxiety. In I.G. Sarason (Ed.), *Test anxiety: Theory, research, and applications* (pp. 349-385). Hillsdale, NJ: Erlbaum.

Improving Memory: The Possible Roles of Metamemory

Christopher Hertzog

Psychologists interested in memory have become increasingly aware of the potential role of metamemory in the acquisition and retention of to-be-remembered information (Cavanaugh & Green, 1990; Cavanaugh, Morton, & Tilse, 1989; Hertzog, Dixon, & Hultsch, 1990a; Schneider & Pressley, 1989). The term metamemory can be defined broadly as cognitions about memory (e.g., Wellman, 1983). As such, it is one aspect of a broader concept of metacognition--or cognitions about all aspects of cognition. Metamemory is actually a label for multiple specific concepts, including knowledge, beliefs, and behaviors related to memory (Cavanaugh, Kramer, Sinnott, Camp, & Markley, 1985; Dixon, 1989; Gilewski & Zelinski, 1986; Hultsch, Hertzog, Dixon, & Davidson, 1988). Hultsch et al. (1988) identified four broad aspects of metamemory: (a) factual knowledge about memory tasks and memory processes--defined as knowledge about both how memory functions and the viability of strategic behaviors for tasks requiring memory processes; (b) memory monitoring--defined as awareness of how one typically uses memory as well as the current state of one's memory system; (c) memory self-efficacy--defined as one's sense of mastery or capability to use memory effectively in memory-demanding situations; and (d) memory-related affect--defined as a variety of emotional states that may be related to or generated by memory demanding situations, including anxiety, depression, and fatigue.

Recognition of the multidimensional nature of metamemory is crucial for understanding the role metamemory plays in remembering, both in the laboratory and in everyday life. As discussed briefly by Pressley and El-Dinary (this volume), declarative knowledge about the potential utility of memory strategies--one aspect of the metamemory system--is necessary but not sufficient for effective strategy formation and utilization in memory-demanding situations. Other aspects of metamemory, including beliefs about one's ability to use a particular strategy effectively, also come into play. Moreover, metamemory can help to explain affect in memory-demanding situations and as such, has the potential for explaining some of the relationships observed between affect and memory task performance.

This chapter selectively reviews the literature on metamemory/memory performance relationships, focusing primarily on results from studies of adults of varying ages. This focus reflects the area of interest and expertise of the author, but it seems appropriate for another reason. Age-related changes in memory functioning may be, to some degree, influenced by age-related variability in metamemory. Intervention programs seeking to enhance effective cognitive functioning of adults have recently begun to attend to two issues regarding metacognition: (a) the possible role of metacognition in influencing the magnitude of cognitive training effects and (b) the possible benefits of concomitant training in both cognition and metacognition.

Metamemory in Adult Populations

Metamemory: Knowledge, Self-Awareness, and Strategic Behavior

The original usage of metamemory in the developmental literature emphasized the connotations of awareness of or knowledge about memory, focusing on metamemory as a possible explanation for developmental changes in episodic memory task performance during the transition from early to late childhood (e.g., Flavell & Wellman, 1977; Schneider, 1985; Schneider & Pressley, 1989; Wellman, 1983). Developmental changes in intentional remembering were attributed in part to increased knowledge of the causal linkage between different behaviors during encoding and retrieval and the subsequent probability of successful recall. Moreover, as children grow older, they are better able to monitor the extent to which they have successfully attained a representation of a to-be-remembered informational unit in memory. Some of the improvements in performance were therefore attributed to the volitional application of effective strategies, due in large part to (a) the emerging knowledge that such strategies exist and can be effective and (b) the awareness that behaviors designed to enhance encoding and/or retrieval are required, given the current state of the memory system. This perspective led to a metacognitive version of the production deficiency hypothesis: Deficient memory performance in individual children, or specialized subgroups such as the learning disabled, might be attributed to deficient metamemory, and in particular, suboptimal use of memory strategies, rather than to any inherent deficiencies in basic memory processes themselves (e.g., Belmont, 1978; Borkowski, Carr, & Pressley, 1987; Brown, 1978).

As in the child development literature, some gerontologists have argued that deficient metamemory knowledge and awareness might determine inefficient memory task strategies in older persons and in turn, produce observed age differences in memory task performance (Lachman & Lachman, 1980; Perlmutter, 1978). Some studies have suggested less spontaneous and effective use of appropriate mnemonic strategies by older persons, including organizational strategies at encoding and maintenance strategies prior to recall (e.g., Hulicka & Grossman, 1967; Hultsch, 1969, 1975; Treat, Poon, Fozard, & Popkin, 1978), and there is some evidence that such effects may be related to metamemory. For example, Sanders, Murphy, Schmitt, and Walsh (1980) compared adults on a free recall task using categorizable nouns, both with and without explicit instructions to rehearse. Young persons shifted from serial to category rehearsal in the latter part of list presentation, but old subjects showed no increase in categorically clustered rehearsals across items. Similarly, Murphy, Sanders, Gabriesheski, and Schmitt (1981) found age differences in study time in a serial recall task, which they attributed to an age-related memory monitoring deficiency: Older adults were less aware of readiness to recall and hence did not select an optimal study time. In both paradigms, older adults improved their utilization of study time and rehearsal under explicit strategy instructions, with benefits for memory performance (Murphy, Schmitt, Caruso, & Sanders, 1987; Schmitt, Murphy, & Sanders, 1981). Training that makes explicit the link between strategy and performance may be necessary for modifying strategic behavior by older adults. Providing additional opportunities and encouragement to utilize strategies is, by itself, insufficient to guarantee optimal strategy utilization (Rabinowitz, 1989).

Brigham and Pressley (1988) presented persuasive evidence for a link between metacognitive deficiencies and deficient strategy utilization in older persons. They required subjects to learn new, esoteric vocabulary after exposure to two alternative mnemonic strategies: keyword generation and semantic context generation. Subjects predicted performance levels before study, evaluated performance by postdicting performance after recall, and indicated which strategy they would choose if asked to learn a new vocabulary list. Young subjects were more likely to adjust their postdictions to reflect differences in strategy effectiveness and were more likely to nominate the superior keyword method for subsequent use. Older persons were apparently less aware of the relative superiority of the keyword strategy, even after employing it. As in the rest of the literature, however, the study did not suggest that age differences in recall could be attributed solely to metacognitive deficits in strategy selection and utilization. Age differences in recall were actually larger when subjects were forced to encode the items using the superior keyword method.

In general, then, the literature suggests that memory tasks can be constructed which maximize the probability of performance being influenced by strategies during acquisition and that such tasks will adversely affect performance of older adults, relative to younger adults (Craik & Rabinowitz, 1984). Although age differences on memory tasks are at least partly due to age-related, structural deficiencies in memory mechanisms, such differences can be amplified by age differences in strategy selection and utilization during acquisition and maintenance of information in memory prior to retrieval. Metamemory, in turn, may be a contributing factor to deficient strategy utilization by older persons in two ways: (a) failure to construct and/or identify the strategic behaviors necessary to optimize task performance, perhaps secondary to deficient knowledge of task strategies and their effectiveness and (b) inadequate ability to monitor the contents of memory. Deficient memory monitoring would reduce the likelihood of (a) selective application of encoding, maintenance, and retrieval enhancing processes to the information at greatest risk for subsequent forgetting and (b) adaptive selection of alternative, appropriate strategies given the state of the memory system.

As in the Brigham and Pressley (1988) study, memory predictions have often been conceptualized as an index of knowledge about one's own memory (Cavanaugh & Perlmutter, 1982; Schneider, 1985). The implicit logic is as follows: the more accurate the prediction, the better one's knowledge about one's own memory and how it functions. There is a complex literature on age differences in prediction accuracy. Several studies have suggested that old subjects are less accurate in their performance predictions than younger adults (Brigham & Pressley, 1988; Bruce, Coyne, & Botwinick, 1982; Coyne, 1985; Lachman and Jelalian, 1984; Lovelace & Marsh, 1985; Murphy et al., 1981). In contrast, other studies have found relatively accurate memory task predictions by older adults (Camp, Markley, & Kramer, 1983; Lachman, Steinberg, & Trotter, 1987; Perlmutter, 1978). Moreover, there seems to be relatively little age difference in either (a) accuracy of predictions of future performance based on item-by-item ratings of memorability (Lovelace & Marsh, 1985; Rabinowitz, Ackerman, Craik, & Hinchley, 1982) or (b) feeling of knowing judgments collected during or after the study phase of a memory task but prior to recall (e.g., Lachman, Lachman, & Thronesbery, 1979; Butterfield, Nelson, & Peck, 1988). The different pattern of age differences across prediction paradigms suggests that general performance ratings after instructions or practice but prior to the study of memory task materials may measure a different aspect of metamemory than other prediction paradigms (Lovelace & Marsh, 1985). Be that as it may, these types of prediction paradigms offer little evidence of meaningful age differences in ability to assess the status of one's own memory. It appears, therefore, that deficiencies in utilization of strategies in laboratory tasks by older adults are not necessarily a simple function of deficits in monitoring the current status of the memory system.

An implicit assumption of most prediction studies is that prediction accuracy is determined by both (a) accuracy of declarative knowledge about one's own memory system and (b) the degree of awareness of current status of information held in memory. Accurate knowledge about one's own memory system implies accurate knowledge about how memory functions in general.

How accurate is the knowledge adults of different ages have about memory systems? Shaw and Craik (1989) and Rabinowitz et al. (1982) demonstrated that neither young nor old subjects vary predicted item recall to accurately reflect the influence of experimentally manipulated variables on subsequent recall. Brigham and Pressley (1988) found that both young and old subjects failed to show a preference for the keyword strategy after being introduced to it but prior to actually using it to study vocabulary items. Such findings suggest that experimental psychologists may make unwarranted assumptions about the extent of knowledge subjects have about memory functioning, as well as the degree to which individuals can evaluate the memory-processing demands of tasks with which they have little or no prior experience (e.g., Glenberg, Sanocki, Epstein, & Morris, 1987; Herrmann, Grubs, Sigmundi, & Grueneich, 1986).

Metamemory as a Belief System

Sehulster (1981) was one of the earliest cognitive psychologists interested in self-reported memory to advocate a conceptualization of metamemory as a set of beliefs (see also Herrmann, 1982, 1990). He characterized perceptions of memory ability as components of a self-theory of memory and argued that beliefs about one's memory ought to be viewed as a subset of one's beliefs about self. Sehulster emphasized that use of the concept of memory self-theory had multiple advantages. First, it grounded metamemory within the larger framework of self-theory, rendering the burgeoning findings regarding self-conceptions and theories relevant to the understanding of how beliefs about memory are formed and maintained. Second, the concept of belief calls into question the veridicality of beliefs about memory (Langer, 1981). Third, the concept of memory beliefs suggests that certain behaviors (e.g., the amount of risk one takes in situations perceived as demanding memory) may be more highly related to memory beliefs than actual memory ability (Sehulster).

Many gerontologists now accept the importance of differentiating knowledge about memory mechanisms and processes from beliefs about one's own memory abilities, strengths, and weaknesses, which can be subsumed under the term *memory self-efficacy* (e.g., Berry, West, & Dennehy, 1989; Cavanaugh et al., 1985; Dixon & Hertzog, 1988; Hultsch et al., 1988; Perlmutter et al., 1987). Memory self-efficacy is the set of beliefs regarding one's own capability to use memory effectively in different situations (Bandura, 1989). Memory self-efficacy can in turn be viewed as one aspect of a larger, multidimensional self-concept as currently discussed in theories of social cognition (Markus & Wurf, 1987). The differentiation of knowledge about memory functions from memory self-efficacy allows for the possibility that an older individual may have extensive and accurate knowledge about how memory functions but may also believe that his or her ability to remember in a given context is poor.

The modal approach for measuring memory beliefs has been the use of self-report questionnaires. There are a large number of questionnaires available for work with adults (for reviews, see Dixon, 1989; Gilewski & Zelinski, 1986; and Herrmann, 1982). The construct of memory self-efficacy helps to explain much of the observed age differences in multidimensional metamemory questionnaire responses. The most robust finding in the literature is that the greatest age differences are observed on measures of perceived change in memory ability during adulthood (Hultsch, Hertzog, & Dixon, 1987; Perlmutter, 1978). It also appears that measures of current memory complaints and perceived memory ability show age differences, with lower perceived memory capacity and a greater degree of memory complaints by older persons (Dixon & Hultsch, 1983; Hultsch et al., 1987; Zelinski, Gilewski, & Anthony-Bergstone, 1990), although some studies have failed to find age differences in current memory complaints (e.g., Chaffin & Herrmann, 1983). It appears that questionnaire measures of perceived frequency of forgetting may be less likely to show age differences than scales measuring perceived memory ability (Hultsch et al., 1987), but different results with identical instruments across different samples suggest that mean age differences in perceived memory functioning vary across persons and may be influenced by moderator variables that have not yet been identified and understood.

The Memory in Adulthood (MIA; see Dixon, Hultsch, & Hertzog, 1988) questionnaire contains three subscales that seem closely related to the concept of memory self-efficacy: Capacity--measuring perceived ability, Change--measuring perceived change in memory ability, and Locus--measuring perceived control over one's memory. Hertzog, Hultsch, and Dixon (1989) showed that these scales from the MIA and the memory complaint scales from the Memory Functioning Questionnaire (MFQ: Zelinski et al., 1990), principally the Frequency of Forgetting scale, converged to measure a factor they identified as Memory Self-Efficacy (MSE). Cavanaugh and Poon (1989) also found convergence between these MIA scales and measures of frequency of forgetting from another metamemory questionnaire. Several studies have found that there are reliable age differences on the MIA scales related to MSE (Cavanaugh & Poon; Carroll & Drevenstedt, 1987; Dixon & Hultsch, 1983, Hultsch et al., 1987; Loewen, Shaw, & Craik, 1990). MSE may account, then, for the bulk of age differences in scales measuring aspects of metamemory. Age differences on other scales from the MIA, especially the Task scale, which measures general knowledge about memory functions, have been found, but not as consistently. Age differences in self-reported strategy use are usually not found, although Loewen et al. suggest that older persons may report greater use of external aids and lower use of mnemonic strategies.

The literature on memory complaints in adult populations supports the notion that memory self-efficacy beliefs are often inaccurate. One common method for evaluating this hypothesis is to examine correlations of memory self-efficacy measures and memory task performance, although there are some valid reasons to be concerned about this operational definition of accuracy (e.g., Rabbitt & Abson, 1990). These correlations are generally weak in both normal and memory-impaired adult populations (e.g., Cavanaugh & Poon, 1989; Hertzog et al., 1990a; O'Hara, Hinrichs, Kohout, Wallace, & Lemke, 1986; Rabbitt & Abson; Sunderland, Harris, & Baddeley, 1983; Sunderland, Watts, Baddeley, & Harris, 1986; Zelinski et al., 1990). These correlations generally range between 0 and .3 in normal adult populations. The magnitude of the MSE/memory performance correlations may be influenced by a number of factors, including type of memory task and correspondence between domain of self-reported memory and memory tasks. Larrabee, West, and Crook (1991) correlated tasks simulating everyday memory demands (e.g., dialing a newly learned phone number) with self-reported frequency of forgetting in the same contexts, and also found relatively small associations between self-reports and performance. Some studies have suggested that memory complaints are more likely to be related to depressive affect than actual memory functioning (Popkin, Gallagher, Thompson, & Moore, 1982; West, Boatwright, & Schleser, 1984; Zarit, Cole, & Guider, 1981).

As noted by Herrmann (1982), the lack of strong relationships between questionnaire measures and memory performance might be attributed to low reliability and construct validity of metamemory questionnaires (see also Dixon, 1989; Gilewski & Zelinski, 1986). This does not appear to be the case. Most recent work suggests adequate internal consistency for metamemory questionnaire scales (Gilewski & Zelinski). In addition to the evidence for strong convergent validity across different questionnaires, the available evidence suggests that metamemory questionnaires also have adequate discriminant validity. Metamemory scales do show some significant correlations with measures of personality, depression, affective states, and general measures of self-efficacy and locus of control (Broadbent, Cooper, Fitzgerald, & Parkes, 1982; Cavanaugh & Murphy, 1986; Hertzog et al., 1990a; Niederehe & Yoder, 1989; Rabbitt & Abson, 1990; Zelinski et al., 1990), which is to be expected on theoretical grounds. However, these correlations are sufficiently small to support the argument that MSE and other metamemory factors are related to but distinct from constructs such as extraversion, neuroticism, depressive affect, and general self-efficacy beliefs. Regarding speculations that memory complaints are actually a manifestation of depressive affect, recent studies by Hertzog et al. (1990a) and Zelinski et al. suggest that, although negative affect such as depression and anxiety do correlate with memory complaints, they can explain neither age differences in perceived memory ability nor the modest correlations of memory beliefs and memory performance. It appears that questionnaires may give relatively valid reflections of memory beliefs but that individual differences in MSE beliefs are not necessarily valid reflections of relative memory ability, at least as measured by experimental tasks (see also Herrmann, 1990).

In contrast to treatments of performance predictions as reflections of knowledge about memory functioning, predictions may be conceptualized as self-efficacy judgments that are specific to the immediate memory-demanding context (Berry et al., 1989; Lachman & Jelalian, 1984). Knowledge about effective strategies and their relevance for the memory task at hand may influence such efficacy judgments, in that an individual *may* consciously appraise the task and its requirements in the process of forming a task-specific efficacy judgment. On the other hand, task-specific efficacy judgments may be predominantly influenced by generic memory self-efficacy unless and until one has specific experience performing on the particular memory task in question.

Hertzog, Dixon, & Hultsch (1990b) reported evidence that initial performance predictions in a multitrial recall paradigm correlated significantly with the MIA Capacity, MIA Change, and MFQ Frequency of Forgetting scales but showed lower correlations with measures of declarative knowledge about memory and use of memory strategies. The correlations between predictions and MSE measures were largest for the first prediction but then appeared to decline slightly across trials. Prediction/recall correlations for word recall and text recall increased over trials, and structural equation models suggested that this phenomenon was best understood as a post-hoc upgrading of task-specific self-efficacy as a function of task experience.

A crucial issue for understanding memory self-efficacy beliefs is the extent to which they are derived from inferences about actual memory-related experiences or internalization of stereotypes about persons as rememberers. There is little question that such generalized beliefs about memory and the memory skills of different person-types, exist, and develop early in life (e.g., Crawford, Herrmann, Holdsworth, Randall, & Robbins, 1989; Wellman, 1983). A key to understanding the memory-related aspects of the self-theories of adults may be the implicit theories people have about cognition and memory as either enduring traits or entities that are relative fixed indications of ability or, alternatively, skills that can be improved through learning (Dweck & Leggett, 1988). Furthermore, implicit theories about memory will differ in terms of the expected effects of aging on memory (Langer, 1981; Perlmutter et al., 1987; Person & Wellman, 1988; Ryan, 1990). To the extent that individuals believe that memory is a biologically fixed entity, or ability, and that biologically determined decline in functioning is impending, they may internalize the stereotype of decline (Elliott & Lachman, 1989; Langer, 1981). This could lead individuals to believe their memory has declined, irrespective of any age-related changes in actual frequency of memory successes or failures. On the other hand, beliefs of inevitable memory decline may make incidents of forgetting more salient and bias older adults to attribute memory failures to age-related loss of effective functioning. It is therefore reasonable to ask about the extent to which memory self-efficacy beliefs identified by metamemory questionnaires are influenced by biased interpretations of everyday events determined by schematic beliefs about memory and its age-related changes.

Beliefs about the potential efficacy of strategies for remembering may also have a major effect on whether and how strategies are utilized. Fabricius and Hagen (1984) showed that children's beliefs and attributions about strategies they are exposed to affect subsequent likelihood of strategy utilization and, indirectly, actual memory performance. Fabricius and Cavalier (1989) further demonstrated that the nature of children's causal conceptions of how strategies work were related to their strategic behavior.

Metamemory, Affect, and Memory Performance

As ably reviewed by Hertel (this volume), there are a number of different relationships between affective state and memory. One important area is the relationship between anxiety and memory task performance. Several studies suggest that older persons' performance on memory tasks are negatively influenced by test anxiety (e.g., Eisdorfer, 1968; Whitbourne, 1976), although it appears unlikely that age differences in memory performance are in any meaningful sense an artifact of age differences in text anxiety (Kausler, 1990).

Under what conditions are individuals likely to experience anxiety in performance situations? Bandura (1986, 1988) has argued that anxiety is a direct outcome of individuals' low self-efficacy beliefs. If one believes that failure is likely in a performance situation, then one experiences anxious affect, phobic desires to avoid the failure experience, and self-protective cognitions and postperformance attributions. The literature on text anxiety and classroom performance clearly implicates low self-efficacy beliefs as a determinant of test anxiety and indirectly, poor classroom performance (Covington & Omelich, 1988; Pintrich & DeGroot, 1990; Zimmerman & Martinez-Pons, 1990). Other theorists in the area acknowledge the importance of efficacy beliefs in determining anxiety but emphasize the primacy of anticipated outcomes, as defined within expectancy-value theory, as determinants of situational anxiety (e.g., Paris & Oka, 1986; Wigfield & Eccles, 1989).

Cognitive performance, whether in an assessment setting or in the real world, can be viewed as a complex, self-regulated, behavior (Borkowski et al., 1987; Kanfer, 1987; Zimmerman & Schunk, 1989). Self-regulation theory argues that optimal performance requires individuals to define performance goals, formulate plans or strategies for achieving these goals, and monitor degree of success to enable adaptive changes in behavior, if needed, to maximize the degree of success. Beliefs about the nature of the task and its processing requirements--whether or not they are based upon a conscious appraisal of the task and its demands--will influence the formation of performance goals and plans, as will beliefs about one's own ability to achieve performance goals through action.

Self-efficacy beliefs can influence cognitive performance in several ways. First, self-efficacy beliefs influence the construction of effective plans of action for attaining performance goals. Second, high self-efficacy beliefs lead to higher levels of effort and persistence in the face of initial failure (Bandura, 1986). Third, high self-efficacy beliefs limit the experience of concurrent negative affect (depression and anxiety), whereas low self-efficacy beliefs lead to increased levels of performance anxiety in the testing situation. Anxiety in the performance situation may then influence the extent to which individuals effectively monitor their performance. To the extent that individuals are preoccupied with their affective state or are dealing with the consequences of negative ideation associated with anxiety regarding failure, they may be less likely to attend to the implications of goal/performance discrepancies for potential modifications of task strategies (Bandura, 1989; Berry et al., 1989; Zimmerman & Schunk, 1989). Although it is clear that cognitive self-efficacy beliefs may influence cognitive task performance without being mediated by negative mood states in the performance situation, induced performance anxiety is envisaged as one of the principal paths by which low self-efficacy can inhibit older persons' performance. Moreover, given that individuals actually experience anxiety due to low self-efficacy beliefs, their beliefs about whether performance can be improved by managing themselves and their affective reactions to performance stress may moderate the effects of anxiety on performance.

Self-reported anxiety about memory performance is substantially correlated with memory self-efficacy beliefs (e.g., Hertzog et al., 1989) and does predict recall in elderly samples (Dixon & Hultsch, 1983). Davidson, Dixon, and Hultsch (in press) recently reported evidence that domain-specific anxiety about memory (a) is more highly related to recall performance than measures of state anxiety and (b) may be a better predictor of actual memory task performance in older adults than in middle-aged and younger adults. The differential relationship with memory task performance occurred in a sample in which there were no overall mean age differences in memory-related anxiety and higher levels of self-reported state anxiety in younger adults.

Memory self-efficacy and memory-related anxiety may therefore help to explain why studies have often failed to observe strong relationships between measures of trait anxiety and memory performance in older adults. The degree of anxiety experienced in cognitive performance settings may vary in different samples of older, middle-aged, and younger persons, depending upon the cognitively related belief system of the individuals actually sampled. Moreover, the domain-specific construct of anxiety about cognitive performance, *not trait anxiety*, may be the proximal determinant of performance anxiety. Finally, the effects of anxiety on performance may be moderated by the efforts of individuals to regulate their affective responses, and this self-regulation process will likewise be strongly influenced by the belief system of the individuals. From this perspective, then, adequate explication of anxiety/performance relationships in older adults must account for individual differences in belief systems that both mediate and moderate the relationships between age, anxiety, and performance. As such, cognitive representations of self and memory task become crucial to understanding how emotion affects performance.

Possible Relations of Metamemory to Memory Improvement

The potential relationship of metamemory to memory improvement depends in part upon the domain of metamemory being discussed. Certainly, memory improvement can be achieved by increasing individuals' knowledge of memory-enhancing strategies, including both mnemonics and external aids. As pointed out by Pressley and El-Dinary (this volume), strategy training requires shaping changes in both knowledge and behavior, as well as concomitant intervention to influence the attributions and beliefs individuals have about strategy effectiveness. The major problem with strategy training, though, is that strategy training may be most effective in circumscribed domains (e.g., study skills for classroom examinations) and may show relatively short-term maintenance and limited generalization across classes of memory-demanding situations.

In theory, memory could be improved by training individuals to effectively use their memory-monitoring skills to regulate their learning and subsequent efforts to recall. Effective memory monitoring should affect adaptive strategic behavior to acquire and retain new information. There seems to be little difference in memory-monitoring ability across different age groups, but there may be differences in the effective use of memory-monitoring capability to evaluate the costs and benefits of particular memory strategies in the memory-demanding situation. Interventions targeted at developing alternative mental models for memory-demanding situations as problem-solving tasks, in which individuals must consciously attempt to access the status of the memory system and evaluate the effectiveness of different strategies, may be crucial to developing more effective memory-related behaviors. The problem can be cast as one of developing a style of consistent self-monitoring of the memory system and using this monitoring process to guide efforts at acquisition and retrieval. As such, it resembles the concept of mindfulness articulated by Langer (1989), in which an emphasis is placed on training individuals to become more aware of self and environment. Langer (1989) emphasizes the importance of consciously appraising self and situation rather than routinely or automatically behaving on the basis of schema-driven processing. Although strategy-training interventions often indirectly target memory-monitoring behavior, greater emphasis on changing the appraisal processes of individuals may be crucial to increasing the likelihood that individuals will correctly perceive the need for efforts to enhance memory when it exists.

Certainly, addressing the issue of belief systems about memory, including memory self-efficacy, may be a fruitful avenue for improving effective memory functioning. Causal theories about memory and memory self-efficacy beliefs are probably stable and enduring schemata held in long-term memory and hence--like negative beliefs and ideational patterns in general--may be difficult to change. Nevertheless, several gerontologists have suggested that intervention studies designed to identify and ameliorate negative self-efficacy beliefs and dysfunctional attributional patterns may both improve affect related to self-concept and enhance the effective memory functioning of the individual (Rebok & Balcerak, 1989; Elliott & Lachman, 1989; Zarit, 1982). Elliott and Lachman have drawn parallels between these kinds of interventions and cognitive therapy for depression, arguing that a fundamental cognitive restructuring is needed to identify and modify dysfunctional beliefs about memory that impair effective functioning. Initial studies attempting to modify attributional processes and memory self-efficacy beliefs have achieved some changes in beliefs and attributional patterns but have not been found to be differentially effective in improving memory (e.g., Rebok & Balcerak; Weaver & Lachman, 1989). Of course, the limited impact of these initial studies on memory performance may be a function of multiple factors, including especially (a) the limited scope of the intervention relative to the difficulty in changing beliefs and thought patterns that have become firmly rooted in the individual's self-concept and (b) the choice of laboratory memory tasks, as opposed to everyday memory behaviors, for criterion tasks.

Interventions designed to address negative self-efficacy beliefs may also be crucial for reducing negative affect in testing situations. There is evidence that training older persons to use memory strategies is enhanced by the concomitant training of relaxation techniques to reduce anxiety in memory performance situations (Yesavage, 1985). This approach may be further enhanced by attempts to identify and ameliorate negative self-efficacy beliefs, particularly when those beliefs appear to be inconsistent with levels of memory skills. An integrated intervention approach that simultaneously targets beliefs, affect, and the strategic repertoire of the individual may hold the most promise for improving memory in everyday life.

Endnote 1

The author was supported by a Research Career Development Award from the National Institute on Aging (K04-AG00335).

I want to give thanks to my friends and colleagues, Roger Dixon and Dave Hultsch, who have collaborated with me in a program of research on this general topic. Most of the ideas expressed in this paper have evolved over the course of years of discussions regarding metamemory between the three of us.

Correspondence regarding the chapter may be sent to the School of Psychology, Georgia Institute of Technology, Atlanta, GA 30332-0170; BITNET address: PSCKHCH@GITVM1.

References

Bandura, A. (1986). *Social foundation of thought and action: A social cognitive theory*. Englewood Cliffs, NJ: Prentice Hall.

Bandura, A. (1988). Self-efficacy conception of anxiety. *Anxiety Research*, *1*, 77-98.

Bandura, A. (1989). Regulation of cognitive processes through perceived self-efficacy. *Developmental Psychology*, *25*, 729-735.

Belmont, J.M. (1978). Individual differences in memory: The cases of normal and retarded development. In M.M. Gruneberg & P. Morris (Eds.), *Aspects of memory* (pp. 153-185). London: Methuen.

Berry, J.M., West, R.L., & Dennehy, D.M. (1989). Reliability and validity of the Memory Self-Efficacy Questionnaire (MSEQ). *Developmental Psychology*, *25*, 701-713.

Borkowski, J.G., Carr, M., & Pressley, M. (1987). "Spontaneous" strategy use: Perspectives from metacognitive theory. *Intelligence*, *11*, 61-75.

Brigham, M.C., & Pressley, M. (1988). Cognitive monitoring and strategy choice in younger and older adults. *Psychology and Aging*, *3*, 249-257.

Broadbent, D.E., Cooper, P.F., Fitzgerald, P., & Parkes, K.R. (1982). The Cognitive Failures Questionnaire (CFQ) and its correlates. *British Journal of Clinical Psychology*, *21*, 1-16.

Brown, A.L. (1978). Knowing when, where, and how to remember: A problem in metacognition. In R. Glaser (Ed.), *Advances in instructional psychology* (pp.77-165). Hillsdale, NJ: Erlbaum.

Bruce, P.R., Coyne, A.C., & Botwinick, J. (1982). Adult age differences in metamemory. *Journal of Gerontology*, *37*, 354-357.

Butterfield, E.C., Nelson, T.O., & Peck, V. (1988). Developmental aspects of the feeling of knowing. *Developmental Psychology*, *24*, 654-663.

Camp, C.J., Markley, R.P. & Kramer, J.J. (1983). Spontaneous use of mnemonics by elderly individuals. *Educational Gerontology*, *9*, 57-71.

Carroll, J.D., & Drevenstedt, J. (1987). *Metamemory in adulthood: Age differences and predictive validity*. Unpublished manuscript.

Cavanaugh, J.C., & Green, E.E. (1990). I believe, therefore I can: Self-efficacy beliefs in memory aging. In E.A. Lovelace (Ed.), *Aging and cognition: Mental processes, self-awareness, and interventions*. Amsterdam: Elsevier.

Cavanaugh, J.C., Kramer, D.A., Sinnott, J.D., Camp, C.J., & Markley, R.P. (1985). On missing links and such: Interfaces between cognitive research and everyday problem solving. *Human Development*, *27*, 146-168.

Cavanaugh, J.C., Morton, K.R., & Tilse, C.S. (1989). A self-evaluation framework for understanding everyday memory aging. In J.D. Sinnott (Ed.), *Everyday problem solving: Theory and application* (pp. 266-283). New York: Praeger.

Cavanaugh, J.C., & Murphy, N.Z. (1986). Personality and metamemory correlates of memory performance in younger and older adults. *Educational Gerontology, 12*, 385-394.

Cavanaugh, J.C., & Perlmutter, M. (1982). Metamemory: A critical examination. *Child Development, 53*, 11-28.

Cavanaugh, J.C. & Poon, L.W. (1989). Metamemorial predictors of memory performance in young and old adults. *Psychology and Aging, 4*, 365-368.

Chaffin R., & Herrmann, D.J. (1983). Self-reports of memory ability by old and young adults. *Human Learning, 2*, 17-28.

Covington, M.V., & Omelich, C.L. (1988). Achievement dynamics: The interaction of motives, cognitions, and emotions over time. *Anxiety Research, 1*, 165-183.

Coyne, A.C. (1985). Adult age, presentation time, and memory performance. *Experimental Aging Research, 11*, 147-149.

Craik, F.I.M., & Rabinowitz, J.C. (1984). Age differences in the acquisition and use of verbal information: A tutorial review. In H. Bouma & D. G. Bouwhuis (Eds.), *Attention and Performance X* (pp. 471-499). Hillsdale, NJ: Erlbaum.

Crawford, M., Herrmann, D.J., Holdsworth, M.J., Randall, E.P., & Robbins, D. (1989). Gender and beliefs about memory. *British Journal of Psychology, 80*, 391-401.

Davidson, H.A., Dixon, R.A., & Hultsch, D.F. (in press). Memory anxiety and memory performance in adulthood. *Applied Cognitive Psychology*.

Dixon, R.A. (1989). Questionnaire research on metamemory and aging: Issues of structure & function. In L.W. Poon, D.C. Rubin, & B.A. Wilson (Eds.), *Everyday cognition in adulthood and late life* (pp. 394-415). New York: Cambridge University Press.

Dixon, R.A. & Hertzog, C. (1988). A functional approach to memory and metamemory development in adulthood. In F.E. Weinert & M. Perlmutter (Eds.), *Memory development: Universal changes and individual differences* (pp. 293-330). Hillsdale, NJ: Erlbaum.

Dixon, R.A., & Hultsch, D.F. (1983). Metamemory and memory for text relationships in adulthood: A cross-validation study. *Journal of Gerontology, 38*, 689-694.

Dixon, R.A., Hultsch, D.F., & Hertzog, C. (1988). The Metamemory in Adulthood (MIA) Questionnaire. *Psychopharmacology Bulletin, 24*, 671-688.

Dweck, C.S., & Leggett, E.L. (1988). A social-cognitive approach to motivation and personality. *Psychological Review, 95*, 256-273.

Eisdorfer, C. (1968). Arousal and performance: Experiments in verbal learning and a tentative theory. In G.A. Talland (Ed.), *Human aging and behavior: Recent advances in research and theory* (pp. 189-216). New York:

Academic Press.
Elliott, E., & Lachman, M.E. (1989). Enhancing memory by modifying control beliefs, attributions, and performance goals in the elderly. In P.S. Fry (Ed.), *Psychological perspectives on helplessness and control in the elderly* (pp. 339-367). Amsterdam: Elsevier.
Fabricius, W.V., & Cavalier, L. (1989). The role of causal theories about memory in young children's memory strategy choice. *Child Development, 60*, 298-308.
Fabricius, W.V., & Hagen, J.W. (1984). Use of causal attributions about recall performance to assess metamemory and predict strategic memory behavior in young children. *Developmental Psychology, 20*, 975-987.
Flavell, J.H., & Wellman, H.M. (1977). Metamemory. In R.V. Kail & J.W. Hagen (Eds.), *Perspectives on the development of memory and cognition*. Hillsdale, NJ: Erlbaum.
Gilewski, M.J., & Zelinski, E.M. (1986). Questionnaire assessment of memory complaints. In L.W. Poon (Ed.), *Handbook for clinical memory assessment of older adults* (pp. 93-107). Washington, DC: American Psychological Association.
Glenberg, A.M., Sanocki, T., Epstein, W., & Morris, C. (1987). Enhancing calibration of comprehension. *Journal of Experimental Psychology: General, 116*, 119-136.
Herrmann, D.J. (1982). Know thy memory: The use of questionnaires to assess and study memory. *Psychological Bulletin, 92*, 434-452.
Herrmann, D.J. (1990). Self perceptions of memory performance. In K.W. Schaie (Ed.), *Self directedness and efficacy: Causes and effects throughout the life course*. Hillsdale, NJ: Erlbaum.
Herrmann, D.J., Grubs, L., Sigmundi, R., & Grueneich, R. (1986). Awareness of memory ability before and after relevant memory experience. *Human Learning, 5*, 91-107.
Hertzog, C., Dixon, R.A., & Hultsch, D.F. (1990a). Metamemory in adulthood: Differentiating knowledge, belief, and behavior. In T. M. Hess (Ed.), *Aging and cognition: Knowledge organization and utilization*. Amsterdam: Elsevier.
Hertzog, C., Dixon, R.A., & Hultsch, D.F. (1990b). Relationships between metamemory, memory predictions, and memory task performance in adults. *Psychology and Aging, 5*, 215-227.
Hertzog, C., Hultsch, D.F., & Dixon, R.A. (1989). Evidence for the convergent validity of two self-report metamemory questionnaires. *Developmental Psychology, 25*, 687-700.
Hulicka, I.M., & Grossman, J.L. (1967). Age group comparisons for the use of mediators in paired associate learning. *Journal of Gerontology, 22*, 46-51.
Hultsch, D.F. (1969). Adult age differences in the organization of free recall. *Developmental Psychology, 1*, 673-678.
Hultsch, D.F. (1975). Adult age differences in retrieval: Trace-dependent and

cue-dependent forgetting. *Developmental Psychology*, *11*, 197-201.

Hultsch, D.F., Hertzog, C., & Dixon, R. (1987). Age differences in metamemory: Resolving the inconsistencies. *Canadian Journal of Psychology*, *41*, 193-208.

Hultsch, D.F., Hertzog, C., Dixon, R.A., & Davidson, H. (1988). Memory self-knowledge and self-efficacy in the aged. In M.L. Howe & C.J. Brainerd (Eds.), *Cognitive development in adulthood: Progress in cognitive development research* (pp. 65-92). New York: Springer-Verlag.

Kanfer, R. (1987). Task-specific motivation: An integrative approach to issues of measurement, mechanisms, processes, and determinants. *Journal of Social and Clinical Psychology*, *5*, 237-264.

Kausler, D.H. (1990). Motivation, human aging, and cognitive performance. In J.E. Birren & K.W. Schaie (Eds.), *Handbook of the psychology of aging* (3rd ed., pp. 171-182). San Diego: Academic Press.

Lachman, J.L., & Lachman, R. (1980). Age and actualization of world knowledge. In L.W. Poon, J.L. Fozard, L.S. Cermak, D. Arenberg, & L.W. Thompson (Eds.), *New directions in memory and aging* (pp. 285-311). Hillsdale, NJ: Erlbaum.

Lachman, J.L., Lachman, R., & Thronesbery, C. (1979). Metamemory through the adult life span. *Developmental Psychology*, *15*, 543-551.

Lachman, M.E. & Jelalian, E. (1984). Self-efficacy and attributions for intellectual performance in young and elderly adults. *Journal of Gerontology*, *39*, 557-582.

Lachman, M.E., Steinberg, E.S., & Trotter, S.D. (1987). Effects of control beliefs and attributions on memory self-assessments and performance. *Psychology and Aging*, *2*, 266-271.

Langer, E. (1981). Old age: An artifact? In J. McGaugh & S. Kiesler (Eds.), *Aging: Biology and behavior* (pp. 255-282). New York: Academic Press.

Langer, E. (1989). *Mindfulness*. Reading, MA: Addison-Wesley.

Larrabee, G.J., West, R.L., & Crook, T.H. (1991). The association of memory complaint with computer-simulated everyday memory performance. *Journal of Clinical and Experimental Neuropsychology*, *13*, 466-478.

Loewen, E.R., Shaw, R.J., & Craik, F.I.M. (1990). Age differences in components of metamemory. *Experimental Aging Research*, *16*, 43-48.

Lovelace, E.A., & Marsh, G.R. (1985). Prediction and evaluation of memory performance by young and old adults. *Journal of Gerontology*, *40*, 192-197.

Markus, H., & Wurf, E. (1987). The dynamic self-concept: A social psychological perspective. *Annual Review of Psychology*, *38*, 299-338.

Murphy, M.D., Sanders, R.E., Gabriesheski, A.S., & Schmitt, F.A. (1981). Metamemory in the aged. *Journal of Gerontology*, *36*, 185-193.

Murphy, M.D., Schmitt, F.A., Caruso, M.J., & Sanders, R.E. (1987). Metamemory in older adults: The role of monitoring in serial recall. *Psychology and Aging*, *2*, 331-339.

Niederehe, G., & Yoder, C. (1989). Metamemory perceptions in depressions of young and older adults. *The Journal of Nervous and Mental Disease*, *177*,

4-14.
O'Hara, M.W., Hinrichs, J.V., Kohout, F.J., Wallace, R.B., & Lemke, J.H. (1986). Memory complaint and memory performance in the depressed elderly. *Psychology and Aging, 1*, 208-214.
Paris, S.G., & Oka, E. (1986). Children's reading strategies, metacognition, and motivation. *Developmental Review, 6*, 25-86.
Perlmutter, M. (1978). What is memory aging the aging of? *Developmental Psychology, 14*, 330-345.
Perlmutter, M., Adams, C., Berry, J., Kaplan, M., Person, D., & Verdonik, F. (1987). Aging and memory. In K.W. Schaie (Ed.), *Annual review of gerontology and geriatrics* (Vol. 7, pp. 57-92). New York: Springer-Verlag.
Person, D.C., & Wellman, H.M. (1988). *Older adults' theories of memory difficulties*. Unpublished manuscript.
Pintrich, P.R., & DeGroot, E.V. (1990). Motivational and self-regulated learning components of classroom academic performance. *Journal of Educational Psychology, 82*, 33-40.
Popkin, S.J., Gallagher, D., Thompson, L.W., & Moore, M. (1982). Memory complaint and performance in normal and depressed older adults. *Experimental Aging Research, 8*, 141-145.
Rabbitt, P., & Abson, V. (1990). "Lost and found": Some logical and methodological limitations of self-report questionnaires as tools to study cognitive ageing. *British Journal of Psychology, 81*, 1-16.
Rabinowitz, J.C. (1989). Age deficits in recall under optimal study conditions. *Psychology and Aging, 4*, 378-380.
Rabinowitz, J.C., Ackerman, B.P., Craik, F.I.M., & Hinchley, J.L. (1982). Aging and metamemory: The roles of relatedness and imagery. *Journal of Gerontology, 37*, 688-695.
Rebok, G.W., & Balcerak, L.J. (1989). Memory self-efficacy and performance differences in young and old adults: Effects of mnemonic training. *Developmental Psychology, 25*, 714-721.
Ryan, E.B. (1990). *Beliefs about memory changes across the lifespan*. Unpublished manuscript.
Sanders, R.E., Murphy, M.D., Schmitt, F.A., & Walsh, K.K. (1980). Age differences in free recall rehearsal strategies. *Journal of Gerontology, 35*, 550-558.
Schmitt, F.A., Murphy, M.D., & Sanders, R.E. (1981). Training older adult free recall rehearsal strategies. *Journal of Gerontology, 36*, 329-337.
Schneider, W. (1985). Developmental trends in the metamemory-memory behavior relationship: An integrative review. In D.L. Forrest-Pressley, G.E. MacKinnon, & T.G. Waller (Eds.), *Cognition, metacognition, and human performance* (Vol. 1, pp. 57-109). New York: Academic Press.
Schneider, W., & Pressley, M. (1989). *Memory development between 2 and 20*. New York: Springer-Verlag.
Sehulster, J.R. (1981). Structure and pragmatics of a self-theory of memory.

Memory & Cognition, *9*, 263-276.
Shaw, R.J., & Craik, F.I.M. (1989). Age differences in predictions and performance on a cued recall task. *Psychology and Aging*, *4*, 131-135.
Sunderland, A., Harris, J.E., & Baddeley, A.D. (1983). Do laboratory tests predict everyday memory? A neuropsychological study. *Journal of Verbal Learning and Verbal Behavior*, *22*, 341-357.
Sunderland, A., Watts, K., Baddeley, A.D., & Harris, J.E. (1986). Subjective memory assessment and test performance in elderly adults. *Journal of Gerontology*, *41*, 376-384.
Treat, N.J., Poon, L.W., Fozard, J.L., & Popkin, S.J. (1978). Toward applying cognitive skill training to memory problems. *Experimental Aging Research*, *4*, 305-319.
Weaver, S.L., & Lachman, M.E. (1989, August). *Enhancing memory self-conceptions and strategies in young and old adults*. Paper presented at the 97th Annual Meeting of the American Psychological Association, New Orleans, LA.
Wellman, H.M. (1983). Metamemory revisited. In M.T.H. Chi (Ed.), *Trends in memory development research* (pp. 31-51). Basel: Karger.
West, R.L., Boatwright, L.K., & Schleser, R. (1984). The link between memory performance, self-assessment, and affective status. *Experimental Aging Research*, *10*, 197-200.
Whitbourne, S.K. (1976). Test anxiety in elderly and young adults. *International Journal of Aging and Human Development*, *7*, 201-210.
Wigfield, A., & Eccles, J. (1989). Test anxiety in elementary and secondary school students. *Educational Psychologist*, *24*, 159-183.
Yesavage, J.A. (1985). Nonpharmacologic treatments for memory losses with normal aging. *American Journal of Psychiatry*, *142*, 600-605.
Zarit, S.H. (1982). Affective correlates of self-report about memory in older adults. *International Journal of Behavioral Geriatrics*, *1*, 25-34.
Zarit, S.H., Cole, K.D., & Guider, R.L. (1981). Memory training strategies and subjective complaints of memory in the aged. *The Gerontologist*, *21*, 158-164.
Zelinski, E.M., Gilewski, M.J., & Anthony-Bergstone, C.R. (1990). Memory functioning questionnaire: Concurrent validity with memory performance and self-reported memory failures. *Psychology and Aging*, *5*, 388-399.
Zimmerman, B.J., & Martinez-Pons, M. (1990). Student differences in self-regulated learning: Relating grade, sex, and giftedness to self-efficacy and strategy use. *Journal of Educational Psychology*, *82*, 51-59.
Zimmerman, B.J., & Schunk, S.H. (1989). *Self-regulated learning and academic achievement*. New York: Springer-Verlag.

Memory Strategy Instruction that Promotes Good Information Processing

Michael Pressley and Pamela Beard El-Dinary

Like many other cognitive psychologists, we have been interested in the role of cognitive strategies in facilitating cognitive performances. Strategies used by proficient thinkers to accomplish diverse intellectual goals have been identified, including effective reading comprehension, essay composition, and mathematical problem-solving procedures (see McCormick, Miller, & Pressley, 1989; Pressley & Associates, 1990; Pressley & Levin, 1983a, 1983b). Strategies used by good memorizers have been determined as well. Thus, there are large literatures about how proficient learners use rehearsal when studying lists of single items, reorganization while processing categorizable lists, and elaborative mnemonic procedures during associative learning (for a review, see Pressley, Heisel, McCormick, & Nakamura, 1982; also, Schneider & Pressley, 1989).

Nature of Strategies

Despite much empirical progress in detailing the strategies used by good learners, recent years have witnessed a substantial amount of debate about the fundamental nature of strategic competence, centering on a debate about what constitutes a strategy. Our view is that strategies are "...composed of cognitive operations over and above the processes that are a natural consequence of carrying out [a] task, ranging from one such operation to a sequence of interdependent operations. Strategies achieve cognitive purposes (e.g., memorizing) and are potentially conscious and controllable activities" (Pressley, Forrest-Pressley, Elliott-Faust, & Miller, 1985, p. 4). This perspective on strategies differs from that of others who argue that strategies are always conscious and controlled (e.g., Bjorklund & Harnishfeger, 1990;

Paris, Lipson, & Wixson, 1983); according to these authors, when the processes that constitute a conscious strategy become automatized and automatically activated in appropriate situations, the processing is a skill more than a strategy.

We are unconvinced. What Paris et al. (1983) refer to as skills look like the same processes and serve the same functions as what Paris et al. refer to as strategies, except that skills are executed more efficiently (e.g., more quickly) and more certainly. Moreover, it is easy to identify processes that appear automatic and not consciously controlled (although they are potentially controllable) that are considered strategies by those using (as well as those researching) them--for instance, see Lundeberg's (1987) analysis of the strategies used by lawyers as they read cases. If the form of "skills" is just a fast version of the form of "strategies," if function is identical for skills and strategies, and if laymen and researchers close to "skilled" processing (i.e., they either do it or study it) consider it to be strategic, is there any good reason to maintain separate categories for skills and strategies? It seems to us that if it looks like a duck, waddles, and quacks, it's a duck--both when it is swimming slowly and quietly in the reeds, deliberately and effectively hiding from hunters, and when it is flying swiftly and mindlessly, scouting efficiently for minnows just below the surface of the water.

Others who have worked with both nonautomatic and automatic cognitive processes agree:

> Nowadays...the term strategy has a considerably broader connotation, loosely "how some task is performed mentally." Though some current research preserves the notion that a strategy is a deliberate and conscious mental procedure, an equally valid case can be made that strategies need not be deliberate or conscious in order for the term to be applied meaningfully. Indeed, this change in connotation is almost literally forced upon us by the evidence that formerly conscious or controlled processes could achieve a substantial degree of automaticity with practice (Posner & Snyder, 1975; Shiffrin & Schneider, 1977). Thus, in order to accommodate the far broader range of behavior and mental processing now being investigated in the area of cognitive development, and to accommodate empirical effects such as the growth of automaticity, the term strategy must be redefined. It must also be liberalized to include not only the deliberate and conscious but also the nondeliberate and automatic processes and procedures by which various mental events take place (Ashcraft, 1990, p. 186).

Howe and O'Sullivan (1990) went even further in acknowledging both automatic and controlled strategies, arguing that maintaining a distinction between them may actually be counterproductive, undermining progress in the understanding of human information processing:

> ...the extent to which processing is effortful is more a matter of degree, with different processes or processing components lying on a continuum ranging from *predominantly automatic* to *predominantly controlled*. When aspects of memory development are dissected in an all-or-none manner, rather than viewed as variations on a continuum, we effectively isolate (both empirically and theoretically) what are integral components of the behavior under study. In order to understand how an individual "solves" a memory problem, we must take into account those processes that are executed effortfully, and the way in which processes that vary in degree of effortfulness conjoin to produce organized (strategic) behavior. By simply focussing on one set of processes at a time, we may tend to ignore the emergent properties inherent in strategy use (p. 132).

In summary, those who reject arbitrary distinctions between deliberate and more automatic strategies have presented powerful arguments in favor of their position. To date, no effective counters to these arguments have been presented by those who argue for preserving the distinction between strategies and skills.

Introduction to the Nature of Memory Strategy Instruction

The main purpose of this chapter is to discuss the nature of memory strategy instruction, instruction that is aimed at the ultimate development of automatic, appropriate use of a number of memory strategies--the development of good information processing. The most extensive instructional research, especially with student populations (our principal concern), has been conducted with the same small set of strategies used to study the development of strategic competence (i.e., rehearsal, reorganization, elaboration, etc.), strategies intended to facilitate learning in a small set of laboratory memory tasks. For the most part, those doing this work pursued entirely theoretical issues (see Belmont & Butterfield, 1977), rather than development and instruction of strategies that might be valuable as mediators of realistic learning tasks. Our current view of instructional research contrasts with this traditional perspective.

Our Approach to Memory Strategy Instruction

We believe that one of the most important activities for researchers interested in enhancing memory is to design and validate new strategies, especially ones that might mediate memory tasks commonly experienced in the world. As researchers interested in areas other than memory developed strategies to facilitate performance on complicated academic tasks, such as composing entire essays (McGoldrick, Cariglia-Bull, Symons, & Pressley, 1990) or increasing understanding of textbook-length presentations (e.g., Education Development Center, 1988), the failure of the vast majority of memory researchers (albeit, not all; see Gruneberg, Morris, & Sykes, 1988) to devise methods for dealing with ecologically valid memory problems became ever more apparent. To emphasize our commitment to and methods for investigating ecologically valid memory strategies, the next section summarizes our recent work on improving memory for materials representative of factual content presented as part of learning in school.

Memory Strategy Instruction that Mediates an Ecologically-Valid Memory Demand: Facilitation of Fact Learning Using Elaborative Interrogation

Although there are many educators who decry that memorization should not be at the heart of schooling, it is (e.g., Goodlad, 1984). Students are expected to master many sets of facts. Rarely are these facts completely divorced from the learner's prior knowledge, although sometimes associations to prior knowledge may be sufficiently remote that they do not occur automatically to the learner when new facts are presented for study. Our recent work and that of some colleagues has been concerned with the development of strategies to deal with such situations.

Elaborative interrogation is one strategy that seems especially promising as a mediator of fact learning. It involves asking students to think beyond facts as stated and to construct reasons why the factual relationships make sense. The assumption is that learners often fail to make use of prior knowledge they possess that could be used to understand new facts and thus, facilitate learning of facts.

The pragmatic value of elaborative interrogation has been easy to prove, as will be obvious in the review that follows. This program of research has also provided support for the theoretical assumptions that stimulated the research and has permitted some additional theoretical insights about memory, memory development, and strategy use.

Empirical Advances: Experiments on Elaborative Interrogation

In Pressley, Symons, McDaniel, Snyder, and Turnure (1988, Experiment 3), Canadian university students studied pieces of information about each of the Canadian provinces (e.g., "British Columbia is the province with the highest proportion of its population in unions," "The first schools for deaf children were established in Quebec"). The most important finding in these experiments was that memory of such facts was greatly improved when students answered why-questions about each piece of information (e.g., "Why would it make sense that the first educational radio station was in Alberta?").

More recent studies have involved learning facts embellished in paragraph-length prose. In Woloshyn, Willoughby, Wood, and Pressley (1990), Canadian university students were presented one-paragraph descriptions of five Canadian universities. Each paragraph contained six facts about a particular campus. For example, the University of Calgary was described as follows:

> The park-like atmosphere at the University of Calgary is partially maintained by the school's policy that no cars be allowed on campus. Some of Canada's best research institutes, like the Arctic Institute of North America, are located on or near the campus. The university also has a wilderness information and communication center on campus. The school has a theatre that is modeled on Stratford. The school's art museum has a very fine collection of ancient coins. Unfortunately, the school offers very few intramural sports.

Students in an elaborative interrogation condition were taught to treat each of the six facts as why-questions (e.g., "Why are some of the country's best research institutes located on or near this campus?"). They answered each of these why-questions aloud, experiencing little difficulty doing so. Students in a reading control condition read and studied the paragraphs for the same amount of time that elaborative interrogation participants processed the passages. The elaborative interrogation instructions greatly facilitated memory of the facts presented in prose. Collapsing over two experiments, the recall advantage in the elaborative interrogation condition was 1.07 *SD*s (relative to the means and variabilities in control conditions; see Cohen's, 1988, discussion of effect sizes).

Wood, Pressley, and Winne (1990) demonstrated that elaborative interrogation can benefit younger students (i.e., in Grades 4 through 8). Their participants were presented paragraphs containing information about animals. Each contained six pieces of information about an animal, as in the following example:

> The Western Spotted Skunk lives in a hole in the ground. The skunk's hole is usually found on a sandy piece of farmland near crops. Often the skunk lives alone, but families of skunks sometimes stay together. The skunk mostly eats corn. It sleeps just about any time except between three o'clock in the morning and sunrise. The biggest danger to this skunk is the great horned owl.

Students in the elaborative interrogation condition responded to each factual statement in the passages as a why-question (e.g., "Why does it make sense that the skunk lives alone?" "Why do families of skunks sometimes stay together?"). Reading control participants read the text for the entire time that corresponded to reading and question answering in the elaborative interrogation condition. The criterion task was to provide the name of the animal associated with each fact when the fact was provided on a test (e.g., "Which animal lives in a hole in the ground?" Answer: Western Spotted Skunk or skunk). Elaborative interrogation subjects answered 59% of these questions correctly, compared to 49% in the reading control condition, a 0.85 *SD* difference.

Theoretical Advances: What Research on Elaborative Interrogation Reveals About Strategy Instruction and Naturalistic Fact Learning

A great deal about the nature and probable development course of fact learning has been acquired during this program of research.

Elaboration without why-question prompting is far from complete.
When children and adults are presented factual material to learn, their elaboration of it is less complete than it could be. If learners automatically activated their prior knowledge about information related to facts as stated, then the why-question effects would be minimal. That is, learners would already be processing in a fashion consistent with the elaborative processing that why-questioning stimulates. Our conclusion that even bright adults, such as university students, do not elaborate factual information as completely as they could is consistent with data and conclusions produced in other paradigms involving acquisition of expository content (e.g., Britton, Van Dusen, Glynn, & Hemphill, 1990; Britton, Van Dusen, Gulgoz, & Glynn, 1989; Christopoulos, Rohwer, & Thomas, 1987; Graesser, 1981; Spires, Donley, & Penrose, 1990).

Our preferred explanation for elaborative interrogation effects as due to why-questions stimulating activation of prior knowledge, activation that does not occur in the absence of the why-questions, could be challenged, however, something we have known since the beginning of this program of research (see Pressley, McDaniel, Turnure, Wood, & Ahmad, 1987). Elaborative interrogation gains might reflect the "generation effect," that materials are acquired better when learners must generate information in response to them (e.g., Slamecka & Graf, 1978). Elaborative interrogation might also be effective by inducing conscious processing of materials, producing arousal, requiring cognitive effort, or promoting deep encodings (Jacoby, 1978; Slamecka & Graf; Tyler, Hertel, McCallum, & Ellis, 1979).

We are beginning to produce research, however, that challenges most, if not all, of the alternatives to prior knowledge activation as the active ingredient. For instance, in Martin and Pressley (in press), Canadian adults were asked to answer why-questions about facts pertaining to Canadian provinces. The directions for answering the why-questions varied between the four questioning conditions in the study. The subjects were to answer either by referring only to information about (a) the province in question or (b) other provinces. In addition, subjects were asked either to specify why each fact was (a) "expected" or (b) "unexpected." Thus, the questioning conditions could be conceived as 2 (same province, other provinces) x 2 (expected, unexpected) design.

The four why-question conditions varied systematically with respect to how much subjects were directed to search for information supporting versus interfering with to-be-learned facts. Consider the two most extreme questioning conditions. Subjects directed to indicate why a fact was expected by referring only to the province in question were assumed to be engaging in an elaborative search highly supportive of memory for the new fact; they were directed to activate information in long-term memory consistent with the fact as stated. So, for example, for the fact, "The first Canadian-based farm protest organization was formed in Manitoba," one acceptable answer would have been, "Farmers in Manitoba are concentrated in the lower half of the province and have easy access to each other in terms of organizing a protest group. Manitoba is also a province known for social reform and socialized government." (Notably, the processing in the expected/refer-to-the-province-in-question condition was most similar to processing in the elaborative interrogation conditions of studies reviewed earlier.) In contrast, subjects trying to explain why facts were unexpected in terms of information about other provinces presumably searched information much less related to facts as stated. An acceptable answer in that condition would have been, "Provinces such as Ontario and Quebec should have had the first protest organization since agriculture is a large part of their economies, and they had the first established farms in the country."

Generally, the results were as expected. There was clear facilitation in the expected/refer-to-the-province-in-question condition relative to a fifth condition, a control condition outside the 2 x 2 layout. There was no facilitation in the unexpected/other province condition relative to this control condition. Performances in the other two questioning conditions were intermediate, as was expected, because they were intermediate in the extent they prompted attention to relevant prior knowledge. In short, answering why-questions facilitated learning to the extent that the questions stimulated activation of prior knowledge consistent with the to-be-learned fact. Arousal, effort, and other general factors should have occurred in all questioning conditions and thus, would be unlikely to account for differences in performance between the why-questions conditions.

Developmental differences in elaborative interrogation benefits.

All of the participants in studies of elaborative interrogation discussed until this point have been 7 years old or older. When younger children have been asked to answer questions requiring elaborative answers, learning gains have been less apparent. For instance, in Miller and Pressley (1989), learning was impaired in some instances when 4- to 6-year-old children answered why-questions about to-be-learned facts. In particular, in some cases in that study, why-questions led children to pay attention to information that was largely irrelevant to the important factual content that was to be acquired, even though the questions were designed to point children to supportive prior knowledge. Yedlicka, Wood, and Miller (1990) have continued this line of research but have yet to produce striking elaborate interrogation benefits with children 4 to 6 years of age. When these results are combined with Wood et al. (1990), discussed earlier, and then compared to the amount of facilitation observed in adults, there is good reason to hypothesize that elaborative interrogation instructions may increase in potency from early childhood to adulthood. Determining mechanisms that might mediate such a developmental progression could be an important direction for future research. One possibility is that it is due to more extensive or accessible prior knowledge in adults compared to children. (See Pressley and Forrest-Pressley, 1985, for a review of evidence that questioning interventions with primary-grade children generally produce small effects.)

How Can Memory Strategies Be Taught So that They Are Used Generally

Perhaps the most frequent criticism of strategy instruction is that it does not generalize, that students do not continue to use strategies following instruction unless they are cued explicitly to do so (e.g., Borkowski, Carr, & Pressley, 1987; Brown, Bransford, Ferrara, & Campione, 1983) or at least they do not use them as extensively as they could (e.g., Pressley & Dennis-Rounds, 1980). This conclusion follows from many studies in which a strategy was taught in one situation with students then failing to use it when presented another task, one in which students would benefit from using the trained strategy. What is apparent from these experiments is that the training typically employed in such research is not sufficient to promote general use of most strategies.

Such transfer failures stimulated a number of researchers to search for a "missing ingredient" that might produce transfer. Some progress was made in understanding strategy generalization using this approach (see Pressley, Forrest-Pressley, & Elliott-Faust, 1988), especially in identifying a number of components that had at least some impact on transfer in some situations: (a) Practice of strategies facilitates continued use of strategies, presumably by making strategy use more automatic or easier and thus, more appealing (e.g., Guttentag, 1984); (b) adding information to instruction about where and when to apply strategies increases appropriate generalization (e.g., O'Sullivan & Pressley, 1984); (c) disadvantaged learners benefit from explicit instruction that they can do better by using strategies they are taught, that their disadvantage is more a function of poor strategies they have been using than some deficiency in ability (e.g., Clifford, 1984; Reid & Borkowski, 1987); and (d) teaching self-testing in conjunction with a main strategy of interest can increase durable use of the main strategy. When students are taught to compare their performances before and after using a strategy like elaborative interrogation, the self-test makes obvious the potency of the new strategy and increases understanding of why the strategy should continue to be used (see Ghatala, 1986; Pressley & Ghatala, 1990); see Neuringer (1981) for an impressive commentary on the real-world utility of self-testing and teaching students to do it.

Despite these successes, no one could review these experiments evaluating single components and conclude that really good information processing (Pressley, Borkowski, & Schneider, 1989) had been shaped up by adding any one component to traditional strategy instruction. Fortunately, at the same time that the single-component evaluations were being conducted, other researchers took a different approach--one less analytical but one that was definitely more fruitful. Their tactic was to add everything to instruction that they thought might facilitate transfer, including many of the single components that eventually would prove their worth in studies of single ingredients.

For instance, a group at Kansas, headed by Deshler and Schumaker (1988), designed these types of complex instructional packages. The transfer components in the current version of their teaching model include the following: (a) Contracts are made with students--students promise to apply to their regular coursework what they are learning as part of strategy instruction in the resource room; (b) students have a role in determining which strategies and academic goals they intend to improve; (c) practice is provided in flexibly adapting instructed procedures to tasks that are different from the original training tasks; (d) students are taught to instruct themselves to use strategies consistently and reward themselves when they do so; (e) information about when and where to use instructed procedures is provided from early in the instructional process; (f) reinforcement is provided for transfer activities; (g) the assistance of classroom teachers in promoting transfer to the classroom is solicited by the resource room personnel who do the original strategy training; and (h) there is long-term follow-up, including "booster shots" of instruction.

The Kansas approach has been tested both formally and informally and has proven successful in producing strategy transfer, including transfer of powerful mnemonic procedures (Deshler & Lenz, in press; Deshler & Schumaker, 1988; Schmidt, Deshler, Schumaker, & Alley, 1989). It is one of several successful multiple-component models (Deshler & Schumaker; Duffy et al., 1987; Pressley et al., in press).

Interestingly, a consistent portrayal of how to do strategy instruction so that effects are general emerges from these varying approaches: Introducing strategies one at a time is essential if they are to be explained well to students, although instruction must eventually lead students to coordinate use of a number of strategies. The strategy instructor should model use of a new strategy, doing so repeatedly and with a number of tasks that could be accomplished using it. For example, the strategy of summarizing to aid comprehension and memory of text could be modeled in the context of reading social studies content, class assignments, and science texts. Much of the modeling involves the teacher thinking aloud, providing extensive explanations about how the strategy could be applied to different situations. Modeling and explaining are not sufficient, however. Frequent and extensive reexplanations are absolutely essential, for students usually will misunderstand at least some part of strategy instruction. Good instruction depends largely on good instructor diagnosis of what students do not understand followed by tailored reinstruction. Such teaching continues as a student practices a strategy until he or she can execute the procedure with a high level of confidence. Students should be made explicitly aware of improvements in their performance as a function of strategy use, perhaps by teaching them to monitor their improvements via instruction in self-testing. Instruction should include explicit tuition about when and where a strategy can be used, with practice of the strategy across a wide range of appropriate application situations.

In summary, strategy instruction that produces general effects is extensive and intensive instruction. It must be so if it is to develop the coordination of components that is required for memory strategy use that is good information processing.

The Ultimate Goal of Strategy Instruction: Good Information Processing

Some of the more important components of good information processing are reviewed in this section, culminating with illustrative discussion of how the various components can act in concert to produce good information processing.

Intact Neurology

Cognitive strategies and other cognitive processes depend on intact neurology. For instance, language is neurologically determined to a great degree (e.g., Caplan, 1987; Caplan & Hildebrandt, 1987). Short-term memory, a capacity that is crucial for execution of more complex memory strategies (e.g., Cariglia-Bull & Pressley, 1990; Pressley, Cariglia-Bull, Deane, & Schneider, 1987), is determined in part by neurology (e.g., Baddeley, 1986).

Strategies

Strategies are one class of symbol-manipulation rules; that is, they are algorithms that specify how other knowledge can be manipulated, something like computer programs (e.g., Pylyshyn, 1984, Ch. 4). For example, the mnemonic keyword method for learning the meaning of a foreign vocabulary word can be specified as a rule composed of five parts: (a) Identify a portion of the foreign word that physically resembles an English word (i.e., in the case of native English speakers)--thus, for the Spanish word *carta* meaning letter, the *cart-* portion could be identified, and *cart* would be the keyword for *carta*; (b) retrieve an image of the keyword referent, in this case, an image of a cart; (c) retrieve an image of the referent of the foreign word translation, in this case an image of a letter; (d) identify a semantically meaningful context that includes both the keyword and translation referents, perhaps a letter in a mailman's cart; and (e) use the images of the keyword and translation referents to construct an image consistent with the semantically meaningful context (e.g., imagine a letter in a mailman's cart).

In summary, the mnemonic-keyword rules specify how verbal and imaginal symbols can be manipulated: The foreign word can be recoded to another item, the keyword; the keyword and translation can be recoded as images; and the separate images can be transformed to an integrated meaningful image consistent with the semantically meaningful context linking the keyword to the translation. See Pressley and Levin (1978) for validation of this multiple-step characterization of keyword mnemonics.

Good information processors know many different memory strategies, as well as other types of strategies. Each strategy is only appropriate to particular goals and circumstances, however. Understanding when to apply the strategies that are known is metacognitive knowledge possessed by good information processors.

Metacognitive Knowledge About Strategies

Good information processors possess extensive knowledge about when and where to use the strategic procedures they know; they also know how to adapt the strategies they possess to new circumstances and tasks. Most contemporary views of self-regulated strategy use posit such metacognitive information (or a form of representation functionally similar to it) as crucial for appropriate, generalized use of strategies to occur (e.g., Ashman & Conway, 1989; Singley & Anderson, 1989).

Nonstrategic Prior Knowledge: Knowledge of the World

Strategies interact with and often depend on the nonstrategic knowledge base--the many concepts that can be known about the world and interrelations between these concepts. Consider, for example, two ways that prior knowledge can affect use of the elaborative interrogation strategy introduced earlier.

(1.) What would happen if a student with no knowledge of the University of Calgary, of Calgary, or of Canada were given the description of the University of Calgary presented earlier? An instruction to use the elaborative interrogation strategy to learn the passage would probably produce a great deal of frustration, since it would be difficult, if not impossible, to generate explanations going beyond the content of the passage without some knowledge of Calgary.

Research is beginning to appear substantiating that elaborative interrogation effects depend on relevant prior knowledge. For instance, Woloshyn, Pressley, and Schneider (1990) presented both Canadian and German students with facts to learn about both Canadian provinces and German states. If elaborative interrogation is effective because it results in activation of relevant background knowledge, then an elaborate interrogation advantage should be greater when the learner possesses prior knowledge relevant to the to-be-learned materials. That is, elaborative interrogation should promote learning more when German students study information about German states and when Canadian students study facts about Canadian provinces than when German students study facts about Canadian provinces or Canadian students study about German states. That was the pattern observed by Woloshyn, Pressley, and Schneider.

(2.) Suppose a student at the University of Calgary were given the same passage. With substantial knowledge about the University readily accessible, there might be no need to ask oneself explicitly why each statement made sense. In fact, associations might spring from mere mention of each characteristic. Thus, suggestions of a "park-like atmosphere" might immediately call to mind spring days throwing the frisbee. The comment on the "no cars" policy might automatically remind the learner of all the hassles associated with commuting to the campus. An image of one or more of the research institute facilities might come to mind when they were mentioned. Automatic elaboration might occur for the student with extensive prior knowledge (e.g., Kee & Davies, 1988). Thus, new learning does not occur simply via the symbol manipulations specified by strategies but also occurs via associative mechanisms. That is, although mind sometimes operates in a classical computer-like fashion (e.g., Fodor & Pylyshyn, 1988), with program-like strategies manipulating information in the knowledge base, mind also sometimes works in a more connectionistic, associativistic fashion (e.g., Rumelhart, 1989). The more related prior knowledge possessed by a learner, the more likely presentation of a new piece of information will trigger associations at all and the more associations triggered once the process begins. As far as fact learning is concerned, automatic activation of substantial prior knowledge often is more than enough to mediate acquisition of facts related to that prior knowledge.

Motivational beliefs and attitudes

Even otherwise capable learners--those possessing extensive strategies, substantial metacognitive knowledge about the strategies they possess, and vast networks of prior knowledge--can have motivational beliefs that undermine maximally efficient use of their cognitive resources. Capable students sometimes believe they are academic frauds, that they have succeeded thus far because tasks are easy or they exerted inordinate effort (e.g., Kolligian, 1990). Some have a tendency to attribute any task failure, no matter how difficult the task, as an indicator of low ability (e.g., Covington, 1985). Such beliefs can definitely undermine cognitive efforts (e.g., see Borkowski, Carr, Rellinger, & Pressley's, 1990, analysis).

A more positive outlook is that effort expended *using task-appropriate strategies and prior knowledge related to to-be-learned content* is often a much surer determinant of capable performance than ability alone (e.g., Clifford, 1984). Such a belief can fuel continued use of appropriate strategies and prior knowledge. The most impressive demonstrations of the potency of such beliefs have been provided by Borkowski and his colleagues. They have succeeded in showing more durable effects of strategy training when it includes highlighting to students that performance gains are due to use of effort expended on trained strategies rather than to intellectual effort only (Borkowski, Weyhing, & Carr, 1988; Reid & Borkowski, 1987).

Motivation to use memory strategies sometimes involves more than just knowledge about their effects on performance, however. In fact, even people who know very well the potency of memory strategies often fail to use them. For example, Park, Smith, and Cavanaugh (1990) provided a telling piece of data on this point. They asked a group of cognitive psychologists how much they used memory strategies, such as mnemonic imagery. Surprising though it may seem, this group of individuals, most of whom were presumably aware of the benefits of classical memory strategies, reported that they almost never used such procedures.

Consider another example. Brigham and Pressley (1988) permitted younger (i.e., 20s & 30s) and older (i.e., 50s and up) adults an opportunity to try two memory strategies and observe the effects of the strategies on memory. One was a powerful imagery mnemonic and the other an inefficient rote procedure. As in previous investigations (e.g., Pressley, Levin, & Ghatala, 1984), the younger adults realized that they learned much more with the powerful mnemonic procedure than with the rote method; this realization guided subsequent decisions to use the mnemonic rather than the rote approach (i.e., when given memory tasks similar to the one encountered during the initial comparison of the two strategies, they elected the mnemonic strategy). More surprising were the outcomes with the older adults. Although many of the older participants recognized they had done better objectively with the imagery mnemonic, many rejected it as a preferred strategy on subsequent tasks when it could have been helpful. They cited reasons such as lack of familiarity and that the imagery strategy required too much effort.

In short, for some people, knowing a strategy works is not enough to guarantee that the strategy will be used. One of the real challenges for those interested in training memory strategies is to devise methods that motivate people to use strategies they know.

Other Components

Good information processors have a number of other characteristics. Because strategy planning and execution require time (as do other aspects of good information processing, such as retrieval of information from long-term memory), good information processors are *reflective* rather than impulsive. Because anxiety impairs functioning of short-term memory (e.g., Eysenck, 1979), efficient thinkers have *low anxiety*. Good information processors are *appropriately attentive* to tasks, selectively attending to the most informative aspects of information presented to them and resisting distractions. Good information processors are *highly aware* how they are doing on important tasks (i.e., they monitor). Moreover, good information processors *elect themselves into situations likely to increase what they want to know*. Thus, the academically-oriented good information processor may read books and articles, go to the library and theatre, and hang out with academically-oriented peers and older, more knowledgeable adults. More mechanically-oriented good information processors might digest all of *Popular Mechanics* each month, seek out after-school employment in a garage or auto parts store, and interact extensively with local Mr. Fix-Its.

An Illustration of Components in Interaction: Good Use of Memory Strategies

Intact neurology permits storage of strategies, metacognitive knowledge about strategies, conceptual knowledge, and motivational beliefs in long-term memory. The conscious use of this knowledge takes place in short-term memory, which is also determined in part by biological structures.

A good information processor who is confronted with a demanding memory task is often well armed to do so. One such task would be giving a speech without notes. A variety of mnemonic strategies (e.g., first-letter mnemonics) can be used to remember the general categories of information that are to be covered and the order of mention. Thus, the chairperson's talk to his faculty about the upcoming year's tasks might include commentary on undergraduate teaching, graduate teaching, a departmental evaluation, university research money, a job search, and departmental social functions. A first-letter mnemonic encoding the order of mention could be TUG at 'EM So Softly (i.e., *T*eaching, *U*ndergraduate and *G*raduate, *E*valuation, *M*oney, *S*earch,

Social). Because the person giving such a speech would have the pieces of information for each category integrated as part of prior knowledge, recalling the category labels would be enough to elicit retrieval of the contents to be conveyed at the meeting. The first-letter mnemonic would be used because the good information processor would know its utility for memory tasks requiring recall of order.

A good information processor would deploy other memory strategies for other memory tasks; for instance, summarization and story grammar strategies might be deployed in order to encode and remember some of the contents of long narratives (see Pressley, Johnson, Symons, McGoldrick, & Kurita, 1989). Memory of such narratives also would be facilitated by associations with prior knowledge--associations that would affect memory by first improving comprehension. Thus, understanding and memory of a good information processor's first encounter with Shakespeare's *Timon of Athens* is affected by knowledge of other Shakespearean tragedies, including *King Lear*, which shares some plot elements (e.g., both protagonists give away their possessions to loved ones, with reasons to regret their decisions later). Details of the play more specific than the overall plot structure may require more deliberate memorization efforts, however--perhaps some type of mnemonic strategy to remember the lists of friends who shun Timon once he is without fortune. The main point is that a good information processor who needed to remember the play would use a mix of prior knowledge and strategies to acquire different aspects of the information presented in the text.

The use of these memory strategies would proceed calmly, both when the good information processor is encoding the content and when retrieving it. Responding would not be rushed but would be carried out at a pace permitting the strategies to be used effectively. Motivation to use appropriate strategies and prior knowledge would be high. The result would be more thorough understanding and memory of the material than would have occurred without strategies and use of prior knowledge. This in turn would increase the amount and quality of prior knowledge available to mediate future encounters with text and motivate the continued use of the strategies and styles that just permitted the successful encoding of text.

Closing Comments

Teaching that improves memory and memorizing abilities must be multifaceted. At a minimum, strategies should be taught along with information about when and where to use them; every effort should be made to motivate continued use of strategies. The effects of strategies on performances should be made obvious to the strategy learner, although much more may be required to obtain long-term commitment from learners.

Because a number of different memory strategies are required for the many memory tasks that learners face, effective memory strategy instruction must be long-term. In addition, because strategy functioning depends on extensive conceptual knowledge, strategy instruction cannot be so demanding of instructional resources that it takes substantial time away from acquisition of nonstrategic content. It is best if instruction is arranged so that new strategies can be practiced with content that is essential for the learner to know. That way content does not have to be sacrificed to teach process; in fact, using efficient strategies to learn such material should improve mastery of it, if anything. Sometimes treatment for impulsivity, anxiety, or attention deficit should accompany (or precede) strategy instruction, since overly rapid responding, high anxiety, and low attention are all incompatible with strategy use.

In short, what is proposed here is a different type of strategy instruction than put forward in the past. Rather than the quick fix, the strategy instruction advocated here is more like a curriculum, one intermingled with other curricula. Thus, our view is that memory strategies may be taught best in the context of ongoing tasks--traditional academic tasks for children and on-the-job or in-the-home demands for adults. If done so, the relevance of strategies to important tasks should be more obvious than when strategy training is done as a stand-alone course, reducing some of the problems associated with recognizing when to use strategies and being motivated to use them.

Our belief is that this different approach to instruction is also going to require a different approach to research and evaluation. For the most part, strategy instructional research has focused on performances occurring shortly after initial instruction of a strategy. There is much less data on strategy use after people have had opportunity to work with and practice strategies. A real need exists for longitudinal research documenting shifts in strategy competence from first learning a strategy to use of it after some practice to proficient and perhaps, automatic use of the trained procedure in interaction with other procedures.

One of the best reasons for doing such research is that even the most effective instruction of novices will produce some individual differences in understanding of strategies. Learners will vary in how well they can execute various aspects of the procedures, how well they understand where and when to use the strategies, and how motivated and committed they are to continue using strategies. This situation alone would be expected to lead to increasing individual differences in use of an instructed strategy. Following the logic of *Chaos* (Gleick, 1987), initial differences, no matter how small, tend to magnify with additional time and experience. Thus, two people who begin in extremely similar behavioral states almost invariably differ more if measured several days, months, or years later. This effect is accentuated to the extent that different environments are encountered. Even for two students in the same classroom, the functional environments are going to differ somewhat so that use of trained strategies should differ quite a bit with the passage of time. Studying such long-term changes should provide insights into the many ways that ultimately proficient strategy use develops. Moreover, it should provide important information about how and why only certain learners become fully proficient and committed to particular strategies. In addition, it might also provide insights as to how to measure proficient learners' use of strategies in order to map out variabilities in strategy functioning even among those who are very proficient. In short, rather than focusing attention on how strategies can create a type of efficient, common functioning (which has been a typical focus in studies of expertise; see Chi, Glaser, & Farr, 1988), the time seems ripe to begin to take more seriously the diversity in functioning that follows particular forms of strategy instruction.

Finally, in arguing for study for long-term strategy instruction, instruction of multiple components, and study of individual differences that emerge during extended use of strategies, we are not arguing against continuing short-term evaluations of the potency of particular strategies. Quite the contrary, our point of departure for this chapter was that far too little attention has been paid to strategies that can be applied to ecologically valid tasks. Thus, there is a great deal of work to do in order to identify procedures that facilitate memory situations, with short-term instructional studies likely to continue as a principal method of evaluating new strategies (e.g., Pressley, Woloshyn, Lysynchuk, Martin, Wood, & Willoughby, 1990). Study of realistic tasks, when coupled with study of long-term development of strategic competence following instruction, should result in more interesting contemporary views of memory development than what is currently available (see Bjorklund, 1990; also Schneider & Pressley, 1989)--views informed mostly by short-term studies of tasks that rarely occur in the real world.

References

Ashcraft, M.H. (1990). Strategic processing in children's mental arithmetic: A review and proposal. In D.F. Bjorklund (Ed.), *Children's strategies: Contemporary views of cognitive development* (pp. 185-211). Hillsdale, NJ: Erlbaum.

Ashman, A.F., & Conway, R.N.F. (1989). *Cognitive strategies for special education*. London: Routledge.

Baddeley, A. (1986). *Working memory*. New York: Oxford University Press.

Belmont, J.M., & Butterfield, E.C. (1977). The instructional approach to developmental cognitive research. In R.V. Kail & J.W. Hagen (Eds.), *Perspectives on the development of memory and cognition* (pp. 437-481). Hillsdale, NJ: Erlbaum.

Bjorklund, D.F. (Ed.). (1990). *Children's strategies: Contemporary views of cognitive development*. Hillsdale, NJ: Erlbaum.

Bjorklund, D.F., & Harnishfeger, K.K. (1990). Children's strategies: Their definitions and origins. In D.F. Bjorklund (Ed.), *Children's strategies: Contemporary views of cognitive development* (pp. 309-323). Hillsdale, NJ: Erlbaum.

Borkowski, J.G., Carr, M., & Pressley, M. (1987). "Spontaneous" strategy use: Perspectives from metacognitive theory. *Intelligence, 11*, 61-75.

Borkowski, J.G., Carr, M., Rellinger, E., & Pressley, M. (1990). Self-regulated cognition: Interdependence of metacognition, attributions, and self-esteem. In B.F. Jones & L. Idol (Eds.), *Dimensions of thinking and cognitive instruction* (pp. 53-92). Hillsdale, NJ: Erlbaum.

Borkowski, J.G., Weyhing, R.S., & Carr, M. (1988). Effects of attributional retraining on strategy-based reading comprehension in learning-disabled children. *Journal of Educational Psychology, 80*, 46-53.

Brigham, M.C., & Pressley, M. (1988). Cognitive monitoring and strategy choice in younger and older adults. *Psychology and Aging, 3*, 249-257.

Britton, B.K., Van Dusen, L., Glynn, S.M., & Hemphill, D. (1990). The impact of inferences on instruction text. In A.C. Graesser & G.H. Bower (Eds.), *Inferences and text comprehension* (pp. 53-87). San Diego: Academic Press.

Britton, B.K., Van Dusen, L., Gulgoz, S., & Glynn, S.M. (1989). Instructional texts rewritten by five expert teams: Revision and retention improvements. *Journal of Educational Psychology, 81*, 226-239.

Brown, A.L., Bransford, J.D., Ferrara, R.A., & Campione, J.C. (1983). Learning, remembering and understanding. In J.H. Flavell & E.M. Markman (Eds.), *Handbook of child psychology: Vol. 3. Cognitive development* (pp. 77-166). New York: Wiley.

Caplan, D. (1987). *Neurolinguistic and linguistic aphasiology: An introduction*. New York: Cambridge University Press.

Caplan, D.N., & Hildebrandt, N. (1987). *Disorders of syntactic comprehension*. Cambridge, MA: MIT Press.

Cariglia-Bull, T., & Pressley, M. (1990). Short-term memory differences between children predict imagery effects when sentences are read. *Journal of Experimental Child Psychology, 49*, 384-398.

Chi, M.T.H., Glaser, R., & Farr, M.J. (1988). *The nature of expertise*. Hillsdale, NJ: Erlbaum.

Christopoulos, J.P., Rohwer, W.D., Jr., & Thomas, J.W. (1987). Grade level differences in students' study activities as a function of course characteristics. *Contemporary Educational Psychology, 12*, 303-323.

Clifford, M.M. (1984). Thoughts on a theory of constructive failure. *Educational Psychologist, 19*, 108-120.

Cohen, J. (1988). *Statistical power analysis for the behavioral sciences*. Hillsdale, NJ: Erlbaum.

Covington, M.V. (1985). Anatomy of failure-induced anxiety: The role of cognitive mediators. In R. Schwarzer (Ed.), *Self-related cognitions in anxiety and motivation* (pp. 247-263). Hillsdale, NJ: Erlbaum.

Deshler, D.D., & Lenz, B.K. (in press). The strategies instructional approach. *International Journal of Disability, Development, and Education*.

Deshler, D.D., & Schumaker, J.B. (1988). An instructional model for teaching students how to learn. In J.L. Graden, J.E. Zins, & M.J. Curtis (Eds.), *Alternative educational delivery systems: Enhancing instructional options for all students* (pp. 391-411). Washington DC: National Association of School Psychologists.

Duffy, G.G., Roehler, L.R., Sivan, E., Rackliffe, G., Book, C., Meloth, M., Vavrus, L., Wesselman, R., Putman, J., & Bissiri, D. (1987). The effects of explaining the reasoning associated with using reading strategies. *Reading Research Quarterly, 22*, 347-368.

Education Development Center (1988, February). *Improving textbook usability*. Conference Report. Newton MA: Education Development Center.

Eysenck, M.W. (1979). Anxiety, learning, and memory: A reconceptualization. *Journal of Research in Personality, 13*, 363-385.

Fodor, J.A., & Pylyshyn, Z.W. (1988). Connectionism & cognitive architecture: A critical analysis. *Cognition: International Journal of Cognitive Science, 28*, 1-72.

Ghatala, E.S. (1986). Strategy-monitoring training enables young learners to select effective strategies. *Educational Psychologist, 21*, 43-54.

Gleick, J. (1987). *Chaos: Making a new science*. New York: Penguin Books.

Goodlad, J.I. (1984). *A place called school*. New York: McGraw-Hill.

Graesser, A.C. (1981). *Prose comprehension beyond the word*. New York: Springer-Verlag.

Gruneberg, M., Morris, P., & Sykes, R.N. (Eds.). (1988). *Practical aspects of memory*. Chichester: Wiley.

Guttentag, R.E. (1984). The mental effort requirement of cumulative rehearsal: A developmental study. *Journal of Experimental Child Psychology, 37*, 92-106.

Howe, M.L., & O'Sullivan, J.T. (1990). The development of strategic memory: Coordinating knowledge, metamemory, and resources. In D.F. Bjorklund (Ed.), *Children's strategies: Contemporary views of cognitive development* (pp. 129-155). Hillsdale, NJ: Erlbaum.

Jacoby, L.L. (1978). On interpreting the effects of repetition: Solving a problem versus remembering a solution. *Journal of Verbal Learning and Verbal Behavior, 17*, 649-667.

Kee, D.W., & Davies, L. (1988). Mental effort and elaboration: A developmental analysis. *Contemporary Educational Psychology, 13*, 221-228.

Kolligian, J., Jr. (1990). Perceived fraudulence as a dimension of perceived incompetence. In R.J. Sternberg & J. Kolligian, Jr. (Eds.), *Competence considered* (pp. 261-285). New Haven, CT: Yale University Press.

Lundeberg, M.A. (1987). Metacognitive aspects of reading comprehension: Studying understanding in legal case analysis. *Reading Research Quarterly, 22*, 407-432.

Martin, V.L., & Pressley, M. (in press). Elaborative interrogation effects depend on the nature of the question. *Journal of Educational Psychology*.

McCormick, C.B., Miller, G.E., & Pressley, M. (Eds.). (1989). *Cognitive strategy research: From basic research to educational applications*. New York:

Springer-Verlag.

McGoldrick, J.A., Cariglia-Bull, T., Symons, S., & Pressley, M. (1990). Writing. In M. Pressley & Associates (Eds.), *Cognitive strategy instruction that really improves children's academic performance* (pp. 117-152). Cambridge, MA: Brookline Books.

Miller, G.E., & Pressley, M. (1989). Picture versus question elaboration on young children's learning of sentences containing high- and low-probability content. *Journal of Experimental Child Psychology, 48,* 431-450.

Neuringer, A. (1981). Self-experimentation: A call for change. *Behaviorism, 9,* 79-94.

O'Sullivan, J.T., & Pressley, M. (1984). Completeness of instruction and strategy transfer. *Journal of Experimental Child Psychology, 38,* 275-288.

Paris, S.G., Lipson, M.Y., & Wixson, K.K. (1983). Becoming a strategic reader. *Contemporary Educational Psychology, 8,* 293-316.

Park, D.C., Smith, A.D., & Cavanaugh, J.C. (1990). Metamemories of memory researchers. *Memory & Cognition, 18,* 321-327.

Posner, M.I., & Snyder, C.R.R. (1975). Facilitation and inhibition in the processing of signals. In P.M.A. Rabbit & S. Dornic (Eds.), *Attention and Performance V* (pp. 669-682). New York: Academic Press.

Pressley, M., & Associates. (1990). *Cognitive strategy instruction that really improves children's academic performance.* Cambridge, MA: Brookline Books.

Pressley, M., Borkowski, J.G., & Schneider, W. (1989). Good information processing: What it is and how education can promote it. *International Journal of Educational Research, 13,* 868-878.

Pressley, M., Cariglia-Bull, T., Deane, S., & Schneider, W. (1987). Short-term memory, verbal competence, and age as predictors of imagery instructional effectiveness. *Journal of Experimental Child Psychology, 43,* 194-211.

Pressley, M., & Dennis-Rounds, J.(1980). Transfer of a mnemonic keyword strategy at two age levels. *Journal of Educational Psychology, 72,* 575-582.

Pressley, M., & Forrest-Pressley, D.L. (1985). Questions and children's cognitive processing. In A. Graesser & J. Black (Eds.), *Psychology of questions* (pp. 277-296). Hillsdale, NJ: Erlbaum.

Pressley, M., Forrest-Pressley, D.L., & Elliott-Faust, D. (1988). How to study strategy instructional enrichment: Illustrations from research on children's prose memory and comprehension. In F. Weinert & M. Perlmutter (Eds.), *Memory development: Universal changes and individual differences* (pp. 101-130). Hillsdale, NJ: Erlbaum.

Pressley, M., Forrest-Pressley, D.L., Elliott-Faust, D., & Miller, G.E. (1985). Children's use of cognitive strategies, how to teach strategies, and what to do if they can't be taught. In M. Pressley & C.J. Brainerd (Eds.), *Cognitive learning and memory in children* (pp. 1-47). New York: Springer-Verlag.

Pressley, M., Gaskins, I.W., Cunicelli, E.A., Burdick, N.A., Schaub-Matt, M., Lee, D.S., & Powell, N. (in press). Strategy instruction at Benchmark

School: A faculty interview study. *Learning Disabilities Quarterly*.
Pressley, M., & Ghatala, E.S. (1990). Self-regulated learning: Monitoring learning from text. *Educational Psychologist, 25*, 19-33.
Pressley, M., Heisel, B.E., McCormick, C.G., & Nakamura, G.V. (1982). Memory strategy instruction with children. In C.J. Brainerd & M. Pressley (Eds.), *Progress in cognitive development research: Vol. 2. Verbal processes in children* (pp. 125-159). New York: Springer-Verlag.
Pressley, M., Johnson, C.J., Symons, S., McGoldrick, J.A., & Kurita, J.A. (1989). Strategies that improve children's memory and comprehension of text. *Elementary School Journal, 90*, 3-32.
Pressley, M., & Levin, J.R. (1978). Developmental constraints associated with children's use of the keyword method for foreign language vocabulary learning. *Journal of Experimental Child Psychology, 26*, 359-372.
Pressley, M., & Levin, J.R. (1983a). *Cognitive strategy research: Educational applications*. New York: Springer-Verlag.
Pressley, M., & Levin, J.R. (1983b). *Cognitive strategy research: Psychological foundations*. New York: Springer-Verlag.
Pressley, M., Levin, J.R., & Ghatala, E.S. (1984). Memory strategy monitoring in adults and children. *Journal of Verbal Learning and Verbal Behavior, 23*, 270-288.
Pressley, M., McDaniel, M.A., Turnure, J.E., Wood, E., & Ahmad, M. (1987). Generation and precision of elaboration: Effects on intentional and incidental learning. *Journal of Experimental Psychology: Learning, Memory, and Cognition, 13*, 291-300.
Pressley, M., Symons, S., McDaniel, M.A., Snyder, B.L., & Turnure, J.E. (1988). Elaborate interrogation facilities acquisition of confusing facts. *Journal of Educational Psychology, 80*, 268-278.
Pressley, M., Woloshyn, V., Lysynchuk, L.M., Martin, V., Wood, E., & Willoughby, T. (1990). *Educational Psychology Review, 2*, 1-58.
Pylyshyn, Z.W. (1984). *Computation and cognition: Toward a foundation for cognitive science*. Cambridge, MA: MIT Press.
Reid, M.K., & Borkowski, J.G. (1987). Causal attributions of hyperactive children: Implications for training strategies and self-control. *Journal of Educational Psychology, 79*, 296-307.
Rumelhart, D.E. (1989). The architecture of mind: A connectionist approach. In M.I. Posner (Ed.), *Foundations of cognitive science* (pp. 133-159). Cambridge, MA: MIT Press.
Schmidt, J.L., Deshler, D.D., Schumaker, J.B., & Alley, G.R. (1989). Effects of generalization instruction on the written language performance of adolescents with learning disabilities in the mainstream classroom. *Journal of Reading, Writing, and Learning Disabilities, 4*, 291-309.
Schneider, W., & Pressley, M. (1989). *Memory development between 2 and 20*. New York: Springer-Verlag.
Shiffrin, R.M., & Schneider, W. (1977). Controlled and automatic human information processing: II. Perceptual learning, automatic attending, and

a general theory. *Psychological Review, 84*, 127-190.

Singley, M.K., & Anderson, J.R. (1989). *The transfer of cognitive skill.* Cambridge, MA: Harvard University Press.

Slamecka, N.J., & Graf, P. (1978). The generation effect: Delineation of a phenomenon. *Journal of Experimental Psychology: Human Learning and Memory, 5*, 592-604.

Spires, H.A., Donley, J., & Penrose, A.M. (1990, April). *Prior knowledge activation: Inducing text engagement in reading to learn.* Paper presented at the annual meeting of the American Educational Research Association, Boston, MA.

Tyler, S.W., Hertel, P.T., McCallum, M.C., & Ellis, H.C. (1979). Cognitive effort and memory. *Journal of Experimental Psychology: Human Learning and Memory, 5*, 607-617.

Woloshyn, V.E., Pressley, M., & Schneider, W. (1990). Manuscript in preparation. University of Western Ontario: London, Ontario.

Woloshyn, V.E., Willoughby, T., Wood, E., & Pressley, M. (1990). Elaborative interrogation facilitates adult learning of factual paragraphs. *Journal of Educational Psychology, 82*, 513-524.

Wood, E., Pressley, M., & Winne, P.H. (1990). Elaborative interrogation effects on children's learning of factual content. *Journal of Educational Psychology, 82*, 741-748.

Yedlicka, J., Wood, E., & Miller, G.E. (1990, August). *Elaborative interrogation effects on children's memory.* Paper presented at the annual meeting of the American Psychological Association, Boston.

External Memory Aids: Effects and Effectiveness

Margaret Jean Intons-Peterson and George L. Newsome, III

Do external memory aids improve memory? Our tentative answer is yes, some of the time. Research on external memory aids still is in its infancy and, as such, offers partial information. The use of devices external to people, such as shopping lists, calendar entries, and alarm clocks, to aid memory has only recently been of interest to psychologists, perhaps because the devices have been considered incidental, peripheral, or even unrelated to traditional memory. Indeed, one can ask whether memory is involved when we consult our grocery list or a dental appointment noted in our (electronic) calendars. We conclude that the use of external memory aids is widespread and that their use both influences and is influenced by memory.

We define an *external memory aid* as any device or mechanism, external to the person, whose purpose is to facilitate memory in some way. The rest of the chapter develops the implications of this definition. The first part considers various attributes of external memory aids and some prototypical methodologies for investigating their use and effectiveness. The second part evaluates the effectiveness of various external memory aids. The third part probes the effects of memory aids on memory, per se, and the theoretical implications of the effectiveness of external memory aids.

Why should we study external memory aids? The first and most obvious reason is that many people claim to use them (Cavanaugh, Grady, & Perlmutter, 1983; Cavanaugh & Morton, 1988; Ellis, 1988; Grueneich, Herrmann, & Allen, 1985; Harris, 1980; Intons-Peterson & Fournier, 1986; Jackson, Bogers, & Kerstholt, 1988; Petro, Herrmann, Burrows, & Moore, 1990; Poon, 1980; West, 1988). A second reason is that the apparent reciprocity between the use of external memory aids and memory has theoretical implications. Another reason is that if these aids are effective, they could be applied to memory-training procedures. Such procedures might be particularly beneficial for law enforcement agencies (Yuille, 1984), for the elderly, or for others with memory problems (Cavanaugh & Morton; Cohen,

1988; Herrmann, Rea, & Andrzejewski, 1988; Light, 1988; Petro et al.; Poon). The general assumption appears to be that these aids can be used profitably.

Attributes and Methodology

Attributes

Noncommercial and commercial aids.
External memory aids come in many forms, both noncommercial (Harris, 1980; Grueneich, et al., 1985; Intons-Peterson & Fournier, 1986) and commercial (Herrmann & Petro, in press). Noncommercial aids include various kinds of notes (e.g., taking notes in a lecture, preparing shopping lists, entering appointments in a calendar, writing on one's hand), different types of timers (e.g., all clocks, oven timers, computer timers), photographs, drawings, maps, and the like. Putting objects in a conspicuous place and asking someone else are used as external memory aids. Commercial external memory aids now are available to do everything from beeping to signal an unlatched seat belt to "telling" the user to do something (Herrmann & Petro).

Cues for past (retrospective) memories and for future (prospective) remembering.
External memory aids are used to retrieve memories from the past (retrospective memory). Photographs may be used to "jog" memories for former classmates or of holiday trips. Perhaps even more common is the use of external memory aids to facilitate remembering in the future (prospective memory). We prepare shopping lists, write notes in the calendar, and set timers to help us remember some intention or act.

Cues for verbal and spatial memories.
Some external memory aids are distinctly verbal in nature (e.g., reminder notes, calendar entries); others are more spatial (e.g., pictures, maps).

Situational specificity.
External memory aids typically are specific to certain kinds of situations (e.g., the timers), but some are more general (e.g., tying a string around one's finger, putting a ring on a different finger, tying a knot in a handkerchief, writing reminder notes). To illustrate, let us consider first noncommercial memory aids, then commercial ones. Following Harris's (1980) work, Intons-Peterson and Fournier (1986) asked college students to indicate how often they used various kinds of memory aids in 32 different situations. The situations, modified from Herrmann and Neisser's (1978) Inventory of Memory Experiences, covered both past and future remembering in situations that contained primarily verbal or spatial components. We found that although

all respondents claimed to use external memory aids in some situations, even the most commonly employed external memory aid, asking someone else, was used in only 14 to 16.7% of the situations. The external memory aid employed least often, a timer, was used in 0.7 to 3% of the situations (p.271).

Commercial aids show a similar specificity (Herrmann & Petro, in press). Herrmann and Petro report that the manufacturers of the 254 aids they identified had designed the aids for specific functions (e.g., shopping, using the telephone, keeping track of possessions). Some functions (e.g., key finder) are limited; others (memo stickers) are more versatile. The commercial memory aids, like noncommercial ones, tend to be situationally specific.

Other attributes.
Noncommercial external memory aids also vary in flexibility, reliability, and versatility. In the Intons-Peterson and Fournier (1986) research, the claimed use of aids ranged from two or fewer times to three to five times in the last two weeks. Further, the aids varied in their dependability, ease of use, accuracy (of cuing particular memories), and preference. Similar variations appeared in Herrmann and Petro's (in press) analysis of commercial aids.

The very diversity of external memory aids defies a simple classification of them, save their defining characteristic as devices external to the person that are intended to facilitate memory. We must keep in mind the situational dependencies of external memory aids and their variations in frequency of use and reliability as we consider their effectiveness.

Methodology

Three general types of methods have been used to obtain information about the identification and use of external memory aids: self-report, naturalistic diary, and experimentation.

Self-report.
Self-report assumes various forms from simple questions such as, "What would you do to be sure that you remember to bring skates to school tomorrow?" (Kreutzer, Leonard & Flavell, 1975), to substantial questionnaires about memory aids people use to remember (Harris, 1980), to listings of memory failures (Reason & Mycielska, 1982). Self-report has been used with single situations (e.g., Kreutzer et al.; Perlmutter, 1978) and multiple situations (Intons-Peterson & Fournier, 1986; Jackson et al., 1988). The standard finding is a preference for making notes or lists of various kinds.

Diaries.
The obvious problem with all of the self-report research is the absence of a validity check. Self-report affords no information about how often people

actually use memory aids in their daily lives. To get around this problem, Cavanaugh et al. (1983) had people keep diaries. Corroborating typical findings with self-report, they noted that writing lists was the most commonly used aid. Further supporting self-report results, external memory aids were used more often than internal memory aids, such as mnemonic devices, repetition, and other forms of rehearsal. This technique has been used to study memory lapses (Reason & Lucas, 1984; Reason & Mycielska, 1982), strategies to try to recall intentions (Ellis, 1988), and autobiographical memories (Brewer, 1988).

Experimentation.
The third method is experimentation. Clearly, the most persuasive way to assess the effectiveness of external memory aids is to compare memory performance accompanied or not accompanied by external memory aids. Experimental studies of the effectiveness of external memory aids are unfortunately rare, and a number do not have the appropriate aid-absent control.

Meacham and Leiman (1982) had subjects put tags on their key chains to help them remember to mail postcards over as many as 32 days. Other investigators have asked people to mail back postcards after certain intervals (e.g., Levy & Loftus, 1984), to come for an appointment (Levy & Clark, 1980), or to monitor time when a clock was strategically placed to highlight clock checking (Ceci, Baker, & Bronfenbrenner, 1988; Ceci & Bronfenbrenner, 1985; Harris & Wilkins, 1982; Meacham & Colombo, 1980). Brewer (1988) combined the diary and experimental methods. He cued subjects at random intervals using a beeper system. They were to immediately stop their activities and to record their memories. None of these studies included the important aid-absent controls, which are included in some other research, primarily that on notetaking.

Comparisons of methods.
The three methods have their advantages and disadvantages. The use of diaries seems more ecologically valid than self-report and experimentation. The use of diaries also offers the possibility of divulging aspects of everyday memory not tapped by more circumscribed and artificial methods. It suffers from the disadvantage of being highly selective and intrusive. The times selected for memory examination may be atypical. These selections may be biased by general societal events recognized by the experimenter as well as the participants. The selection also may be biased by private events in the rememberers' lives that are unknown to the experimenter. Another problem is that the participant's decision process about whether or not to record episodes is relatively unconstrained. This problem also afflicts self-report. Finally, the requirement to halt other activity to record the use of a memory aid or a memory failure intrudes on regular activities and may distort the results. The experimenter has no way of knowing how often the participants

chose to continue their activities rather than record their use of memory aids or their memory failures.

Self-report is relatively easy to administer, does not require a substantial investment of participants' time, and affords fairly easy manipulation of the situations. It is artificial, however, and in itself, does not guarantee that respondents actually use memory aids in the manner they claim. Further, some questionnaires are more reliable or valid than others (Herrmann, 1982, 1984; Martin, 1988; Martin & Jones, 1984; Morris, 1984) and assess different factors (Martin). Finally, questions on the questionnaires call for responses that often depend on accurate remembering (Martin; Poon, 1980; Wilson, Baddeley, & Cockburn, 1988). For example, the only way to accurately answer a question about how often one forgets one's keys is to *remember* how often one forgot the keys! This requirement is particularly troublesome when dealing with the memory impaired. It is a difficulty shared with the other methods, as well, of course. For us to have much confidence in the results of self-report, the results need validation.

With the more artificial methods, self-report and experimentation, the experimenter has control over the breadth of the described situations but loses the spontaneity of the diary method. Participants may respond quite differently in the more stilted and unfamiliar artificial environment. Fortunately, these problems are not invalidating, for all three methods appear to produce quite similar results.

This brief, nonexhaustive survey of methods is intended to identify the methods most commonly used and to point to several advantages and disadvantages of each. Since there is no single ideal method, it clearly is desirable to use a variety of approaches.

The Effectiveness of External Memory Aids

The effective use of external memory aids depends on a complex set of processes to select, apply, and implement memory aids that are compatible with the situation at hand. These high-level processes require at least some of the following memory-related processes:

1. Recognition of the need for a memory aid of some kind, presumably identified via the monitoring of memory.
2. The selection of a memory aid, given recognition of a need.
3. Application of the memory aid, an encoding and possibly recoding process (as when items in a list are reclassified by categories).
4. Retrieval of the cues provided by the external memory aid, a decoding process (e.g., a calendar must be consulted if its entries are to jog memory).
5. Interpretation of the memory aid's cues, an easy task for a highly circumscribed set of cues (e.g., a listing of errands to run) but a more difficult one for vague cues (e.g., those represented by a knotted handkerchief).

6. Expression of the interpretation as a memory for a particular intention, action, fact, and so forth.

Each of these stages could be further subdivided.

Not all memory aids depend on all stages (e.g., asking someone else presumably rarely depends on the encoding stages), but breakdowns at requisite stages are likely to jeopardize memory aid effectiveness and, therefore, retention. Since multiple stages are essential to the success of external memory aids, it is not surprising that external memory aids, like other memorial strategies, are fallible.

It should be obvious that research is unlikely to disclose simple and reliable guides about how and when to use particular memory aids. Such an enterprise is thwarted by the varied nature of external memory aids, their situational specificity, and their dependence on various processes for effective use.

We begin with memory monitoring. Are people able to detect the need for memory aids? Not very well, as it turns out. Aptitude appears to increase with age, at least up to adulthood.

Memory Monitoring

After reviewing research on prospective memory with preschoolers, Beal (1988) concluded that children have confidence in their ability to remember. They do not seem to recognize the need to prepare for future retrieval, nor do they easily identify effective aids, even though their memory is demonstrably faulty.

Another, more sophisticated group, college students, should be experts at monitoring their needs for memory assistance and at selecting effective, efficient external memory aids. To test this hypothesis, the first author read aloud a list of 36 verb-noun pairs to 25 individual college students. The verb-noun pairs described actions common among a college population, such as "buy gas" and "write home." She told the students that (a) after they had heard all of the pairs, she would ask them to write down all of the pairs and (b) if, while she was reading the pairs, a time came when they were afraid that they would not be able to remember all of the pairs they should stop her. If they stopped her, she then asked what they wanted her to do to help them remember, citing as possibilities their making notes, her repeating the pairs, and so forth. This open-ended technique seemed to be an effective device for showcasing their memory-monitoring talents.

Eighteen (72%) of the 25 students stopped her before she had finished reading all 36 pairs. Stopping occurred after a range of from 4 to 28 pairs and after a mean of 12.61 and a median of 10 pairs. In brief, about one-third of the way through the pairs, more than half of the students recognized that they needed help. All of these students wanted to take notes to help themselves remember. This strategy appeared to be effective, in the sense that they remembered more than twice as many pairs after they began taking notes (mean = 6.28) as before (mean = 2.72), $F(1, 17) = 15.11$, $p < .001$. Students who took notes were not allowed to look at those notes during the immediate free recall test.

The remaining seven apparently thought that they did not need help, and they affirmed in postexperimental discussion that they "just trusted to memory." This strategy did not serve them well, however, for their mean performance on items in serial positions 13 through 36 (the latter two-thirds of the items) was 4.31, markedly below that of the notemakers. Analyses of retention of early pairs indicated that the difference could not be attributed to the possibility that nonnotemakers had poorer memories than the notemakers.

These results suggest that some college students effectively monitor their memories and recognize the need to use memory aids. Others have such confidence in their memories that they do not perceive a need for memory aids even though their memories are imperfect. This confidence seems to wane as adulthood advances, however. The literature is replete with reports of how the elderly complain about their memories (Martin, 1988; Moscovitch, 1982; Poon, 1980; Poon & Schaffer, 1982; but see West, 1988).[1]

We come now to the heart of this chapter, the assessment of the effectiveness of various types of external memory aids. In this assessment, we focus on the situational dependencies of external memory aids. Obviously, we would not expect timers to be effective cues for meeting an appointment in 3 months' time or for the name of a former acquaintance.

Our review of the relevant literature yielded a fair amount of information about various kinds of notetaking. Information about other kinds of external memory aids was sparse.

Notes

We take notes in many different situations. The purpose may be the same--that of aiding retention of the information--but the conditions of preparation and use of the aids vary substantially. In the lecture situation, for example, we attempt to transform another person's predominantly verbal input to a written record. In most cases, this transformation occurs under time pressure. Further, most investigations study high school or college students in a classroom setting. In contrast, when we prepare a shopping list or similar kind of note, we often commit our own thoughts, plans, or intended actions to paper, although others may offer additions to the list. Typically, this type of note is prepared somewhat more leisurely than those produced under the standard fast pace of a lecture. The latter type of notes, made by people of many ages and occupations, usually occurs in various everyday settings. The differences between these extremes are so marked that it is possible that the same principles may not hold. To avoid confusion, we will refer to the standard lecture- or prose-type of notetaking as "notetaking" and to the shopping list-type of notetaking as "listmaking." These terms are not particularly apt, to be sure, but they suffice to convey important distinctions. We consider notetaking first.

Notetaking.

Notetaking might facilitate remembering through one or two general types of effects: the recording and related memorial functions that are elicited during or by the recording process and the review of notes after they have been recorded. The evidence is somewhat contradictory, although on balance, both processes appear to aid performance. In a recent review, Kiewra (1985) found that the process of simply taking notes was beneficial in 33 of 56 studies, ineffective in 21, and dysfunctional in 2. Review of the notes helped in 17 of 22 studies and had no effect in 5. Similar results have emerged from other reviews (e.g., Carrier & Titus, 1979; Hartley, 1983).

The above research did not always take account of the rate of speech during a lecture or of the density of information being delivered. It appears that rapid speech (Peters, 1972), high density information (Aiken, Thomas, & Shennum, 1975), and poor organization of the presented material (prose: Annis, 1979; Schultz & DiVesta, 1972; Shimmerlick & Nolan, 1976; and lecture: Howe, 1977) reduce the effectiveness of notetaking, even when participants are allowed to review notes of prose material (Hayes-Roth & Walker, 1979; Waern, 1981). Organization facilitated notetaking in all of the studies cited. In brief, notetaking is more likely to be beneficial when the rate of speech is slower than faster, the density of information is not particularly high, and the material is well organized.

In addition, characteristics of the notetakers are important. High performers tend to take more notes than lower achieving students (Kiewra & Fletcher, 1984). Compared to lower achievers, high achievers tend to use more words (e.g., Fisher & Harris, 1973) and to capture the most important ideas (Einstein, Morris, & Smith, 1985).

Listmaking.

Listmaking is one of the preferred external memory aids (e.g., Cavanaugh et al., 1983; Harris, 1980; Intons-Peterson & Fournier, 1986). Lists are used as reminder notes, often to prepare for future remembering. This pattern appears to be quite extensive, since it has been found with college students (Intons-Peterson & Fournier), some slightly older adults (Harris, 1980), and elderly subjects (Cavanaugh et al.). Commercial forms of lists, such as checkable grocery lists also are available (Herrmann & Petro, in press; Petro et al., 1990).

Despite its apparent popularity, experimental evidence about the effectiveness of listmaking is rare. Intons-Peterson and Fournier (1986, Experiment 3) found that college students who had taken notes during presentation of lists of grocery store (or department store) items recalled more than subjects who had not made lists, even though the listmakers were not allowed to review their lists. McEvoy and Moon (1988) reported that memory training that included listmaking reduced the number of complaints made by elderly subjects about memory failures on routine tasks.

These studies do not assess the effectiveness of lists in actual everyday performance, of course. Koriat and Ben-Zur (1988) used interviews to probe output monitoring (the monitoring of whether an action has been completed). They found that their respondents frequently reported the use of external aids such as checking off items on a list or throwing a list away. Obviously, the original preparation of the lists was intended to cue memory for the intended action.

Despite the frequency of its use, listmaking is not always optimal. Bennett (1983) found that waitresses who went from table to table to obtain drink orders in bars remembered most effectively when they imagined the drinks in particular locations and least effectively then they made lists of the orders. Listmaking may not be effective for the young or the memory impaired, who may forget to prepare and use lists or who cannot do so (Naugle, Naugle, Prevey, & Delaney, 1988). Thus, even listmaking, which seems to be among the most widespread and effective external memory aids, is not always beneficial.

Calendar Entries

Calendar entries in both written and electronic form seem to be ideal to prompt execution of an act or intention after a time lapse. Learning to use calendar entries to facilitate keeping appointments reduced subsequent complaints about appointment-keeping memory failures (McEvoy & Moon, 1988), but once again, the effective use of a calendar entry requires both notation of the event and subsequent checking of the calendar (Naugle et al., 1988), memorial activities that may be difficult for the young or memory impaired.

Timing Devices

Also important as external memory aids are clocks and other types of electronic and mechanical timers. These memory aids are appropriate for monitoring shorter lengths of time than are usually involved in calendar entries, although some watches (e.g., Casio's Module 563) can record a substantial number of appointments. In some cases, timers are quiet and passive, not intruding on or alerting the potential rememberer.

For example, when adults focus on a timing interval, they may use clocks even though they were not told to do so. Harris and Wilkins (1982) asked adults to raise placards to indicate the time remaining in a waiting period. A clock was placed in the back of the room so that a confederate could record turning to look at the clock. The subjects learned to monitor their "psychological time" so that they did not have to turn to look at the clock until close to the end of the period. The subjects usually responded on time, but more than half failed on at least one occasion. Ceci and Bronfenbrenner (1985) found similar results with children who were to take cupcakes from an oven in exactly 30 minutes.

Another example is the medicine-dispensing device. These devices do not necessarily attract attention and are heavily memory dependent. In these cases, the user or caretaker has to remember to fill the device, as Harris (1984) points out. Clocks and other passive timers require attention if they are to be effective.

Presumably more effective are the alerting timers. These mechanisms are designed to attract the attention of the rememberer to the need to remember or to do something. One example is the telephone call. Gates and Colborn (1976) and Shepard and Moseley (1976) found that subjects who were reminded by telephone or mail were more likely to keep appointments than subjects who were not reminded. Even the reminded subjects did not always keep their appointments, however. The success rates were slightly higher for mail-prompted subjects (83.7%) than for phone-prompted ones (80%; Gates & Colborn, 1976). Some 55% of the nonreminded controls arrived for their appointments.

These results suggest that the effectiveness of timers increases with their ability to attract attention. When subjects do not attend to the timing device, they may not remember. The effectiveness of timers also requires remembering to set them, to interpret the meaning of the signal, and to reset them. Sometimes these devices, such as the Casio Module 563 (or "Data Bank") can be used effectively with the memory impaired given sufficient training (Naugle et al., 1988). These caveats underscore the dependence of memory aid effectiveness on memory.

Organizational Techniques

External memory aids also manifest themselves as conspicuous locational placements, files, and even hierarchical organizational systems exemplified by computers. Putting to-be-remembered items in an obvious place is a tactic grade school children say they would use to remember to bring skates to school (Kreutzer et al., 1975). Adults agree that this aid is useful for future remembering (Harris, 1980; Intons-Peterson & Fournier, 1986). Further, McEvoy and Moon (1988) noted that training with this technique reduced the frequency of their elderly subjects' complaints about misplacements of possessions. Preschoolers, however, have difficulty developing and implementing such a strategy (Beal, 1988).

Organizational memory aids also may be filing cabinets, books, and the like. Hertel (1988) found that her colleagues' confidence in their knowledge was correlated with the estimated depth (in inches) of their office files, the number of books in their offices, the number of books read, the years they had been collecting, and the overall organizational structure of their offices. We reserve judgment about the effectiveness of these organizational aids, because confidence in knowledge is not necessarily the same as actual possession of the knowledge.

Today's electronic capabilities deliver many kinds of external memory aids, but the effective use of these aids typically requires memory. With computers, for example, abbreviated file names are used as external memory aids to access information about the contents of the file. It seems reasonable to assume that the closer the semantic relation between the file name and the contents of the file, the more effective the aid (file name) will be. Schönpflug (1988) tested this possibility by allowing subjects to choose their own file names or by using experimenter-chosen file names with high or lower semantic fit to file contents. The subjects did well with the first two, high fit, conditions compared to the last, lower fit ones. These results suggest that the effectiveness of an external memory aid may depend on its semantic kinship to the to-be-remembered material.

Similar situational constraints may occur with the care of patients. Consider home care, for example. Different caregivers may need to learn the techniques to be used with a particular patient. The use of videotapes may be an effective, accurate instructional tool (Smith, Dutton, Diver, & Gray, 1989). Videotapes offer the advantages of being tailored to the patient, providing both visual and auditory cues, and being available (for some people). They also have disadvantages. The film may become outdated as the patient's status changes. The filmmakers may have limited filming proficiency, caretakers may not attend to the films, and so forth.

Nonspecific Memory Aids

Does tying a string on one's finger really help? We might expect such nonspecific external memory aids to be effective to the extent that they remind the person that something is to be remembered. Subjects do not claim to use these aids as often as more specific ones when tested by self-report and diary. Nevertheless, the aids may be effective in as least some circumstances. Meacham and Leiman's (1982) subjects were able to use tags on their key chains to help them to remember to mail back postcards. Similar results have been reported by others for calling telephone numbers (Moscovitch, 1982; Poon & Schaffer, 1982), although not all subjects in these studies were successful. The nonspecific peal of memory bank wrist watches is sometimes elaborated by a short prompt to identify the item to be remembered (Naugle et al., 1988). This option undoubtedly helps the memorially proficient but may be too abbreviated to satisfactorily cue the memorially less proficient. These studies typically did not test aid-absent controls, however, so the effectiveness of these devices is not clear.

Other Types of External Memory Aids

External aids take many forms, including those of the sizes and shapes of drinking glasses. Beach (1988) found that glass sizes help experienced bartenders keep drink orders in mind. Inexperienced bartenders tend to rehearse the ordered drinks. As the bartenders become more experienced, this rehearsal strategy gives way to one of placing a distinctive glass on the bar rail when the drink is ordered.

Summary of Studies of Effectiveness of Memory Aids

Although self-report and diaries provide testimonials for the widespread use of external memory aids, actual tests of the effectiveness of these aids are relatively rare. The most extensive information comes from notetaking. In this case, the evidence is mixed, although it mirrors a feature of the analyses of the other memory aids, the need for specificity. Under some, but not necessarily all circumstances, notetaking may be helpful. This conclusion applies to all of the external memory aids surveyed. In brief, external memory aids claim to be used extensively, but they are not infallible.

It seems likely that the noncommercial memory aids often are beneficial, as signalled by their common endorsement. If people found these aids to fail, they probably would not use them. Although the effectiveness of commercial external memory aids have not been explored to any great extent, their situational specificity should make their effectiveness easy to evaluate. Some of these aids are quite complex, with memory and comprehension demands that may limit their utility. For example, the need to remember the sequence of steps needed to program some of the reminder watches or timers may tax the abilities of some users. In general, the effective use of most or all external memory aids depends on memory.

Most important is the highly specific nature of external memory aids. No external memory aid seems to have universal applicability and many are markedly limited. This seems to be particularly and deliberately true of commercial memory aids (Herrmann & Petro, in press; Petro et al., 1990).

Taken as a whole, the results of the survey reflect a strong belief in the effectiveness of external memory aids, given a propitious combination of aid, circumstance, and user. Our inclination, in turn, is to believe in the beliefs described by the informants--at least until compelling contradictions convince us to the contrary.

Memory Aids and Memory: Theoretical Implications

External memory aids clearly function as external storage units that have cuing properties, but do external memory aids have other functions? Do they affect memory in some way? If external memory aids serve solely as cues, they probably have no greater role in memory theory than other contextual cues. These cues often figure prominently in retrieval, to be sure, but the theoretical implications of external memory aids would be enhanced if external-aid cues also affected memory itself.

Functions of External Memory Aids

Storage and cuing properties.
The storage and cuing functions of external memory aids are obviously important. The entry on a calendar substitutes for memory in the head. It relieves us of the need to try to keep track of the appointment. External memory aids cue our intention or our behavior. These consequential functions are worthy of exploration in their own right even if memory aids have no additional memorial functions. We need to know which kinds of external storage devices are the most effective and efficient. Memory aids have additional functions, however.

Interdependence between external memory aids and memory.
The effective use of external memory aids relies on memory in various ways. First, we must recognize when we need an external memory aid. This implies knowledge of what can be effectively allocated to an aid. It implies knowledge of how an external memory aid can be used, as well as the likelihood and ease of retrieving the information. Most important, it implies the ability to use the external memory aid. In short, external memory aids depend upon memory and may reflect the organization of memory.

Conversely, memory may be affected by the encoding and recoding of material that occurs when external memory aids are prepared. For example, when college students were allowed to make lists during the presentation of a list of items that could be bought at a grocery store, they remembered more items than nonlistmakers even though they were not allowed to review their lists prior to test (Intons-Peterson & Fournier, 1986, Experiment 3). These results suggest that it helps to write out a grocery list even if we leave the list at home. Presumably this result reflects the impact of the generation of the list on memory. Further, the listmakers tended to categorize their lists into meat, vegetables, and so forth, even though the items were read in a randomized order. This reorganization imposed during the generation of lists (notes) also may aid retrieval by providing additional access or priming cues for the original input and other, associated memories (Bahrick & Phelps, 1988; Intons-Peterson & Fournier, 1986).

External memory aids may affect memory in still other ways. It is likely that review of external memory aids elicits rehearsal of the material in memory. Moreover, external memory aids may assist the monitoring of what has been done (Koriat & Ben-Zur's, 1988, "output monitoring"). Items on reminder lists may be checked off, the reminder lists may be discarded, and so forth, to indicate that an intended action has been executed. Without such a system, we might repeatedly check the latches on doors, call to check appointment dates, and generally engage in inefficient and unnecessary memory checks.

Situational Specificity

Situational specificity increases the cue validity of external memory aids. The meaning of a knot in a handkerchief is ambiguous but the meaning of an oven timer's peal usually is not. The differences in the situational specificity of external memory aids both enhance the value of aids taken in toto as cues and complicate their theoretical role. To the extent that external memory aids generally function as cues for recoding, for retrieval, and so forth, they could be classified as context cues and incorporated into contextual theories (e.g., Raaijmakers & Shiffrin, 1981). However, this approach is somewhat misleading because certain kinds of relatively nonspecific external memory aids (string-tied fingers) trigger a general memory search, whereas the more specific aids (list entries) point toward a particular memory address and often, associated action. Furthermore, external aids differ in cue value from the role customarily assigned to contextual cues in that they are chosen, prepared, and used deliberately, a combination of functions that triggers various perceptual, motivational, and memorial processes.

The Role of Age

As already noted, preschoolers appear to have difficulty identifying effective external memory aids (Beal, 1988). Adolescents and adults obviously endorse them. Do the elderly use them even more than younger adults so that we are dealing with a monotonic relation between age and the use of external memory aids? This possibility has received some support (Jackson et al., 1988; Martin, 1988; Perlmutter, 1978; Poon, 1980; Zelinski, Gilewski, & Thompson, 1980) but has been challenged (Chaffin & Herrmann, 1983; West, 1988). West reported that when the type of situation is taken into account, older adults show patterns of use that are similar to those of younger adults. It should be noted that the dependence of many external memory aids on memory may limit their utility to the memory impaired, a group that stands to benefit from extensive use of the aids. These considerations argue for the use of relatively simple external memory aids (e.g., listmaking, postable notes) when feasible.

Harris's Test-Wait-Test-Exit (TWTE) Model

We found only one model addressed explicitly to remembering to do something, Harris's (1984; Harris & Wilkins, 1982) Test-Wait-Test-Exit model, and it is identified by Harris as a descriptive--not explanatory--model. Harris divides remembering to do things into two principal categories, remembering to keep appointments and remembering sequential acts. As Harris says, "The essence of remembering to do something is that it cannot be done straightaway; there is a relative cost associated with doing it too early (or, of course, too late)" (1984, p. 83). He proposes that a monitoring process occurs in which tests are made to see if the time is right for execution of an action. If the test is negative, the person waits a little longer and then tests again. This loop will be repeated until a positive test induces action and an exit from the monitoring process.

Note that this kind of model readily accommodates the situational specificity of external memory aids. It does not, however, specify in advance how the costs and benefits of the use of any particular external memory aid will be assessed or will function in a given situation or what governs the decisions made at each stage. At present, then, the model seems incomplete. This criticism was further articulated by Ellis (1988) and Morris (1984).

The critique of Harris's (1984) model pinpoints some major problems that confront research on external memory aids. We need persuasive evidence of the conditions under which external memory aids do and do not facilitate memory. We need information about the relation of these conditions to age and other subject characteristics. We need to know the decision rules that contribute to memory aid selection. Perhaps most important, we need information about the interdependence between general memory functioning and the use of external memory aids.

Our assessment of the current evidence is that the role of external memory aids is important and should be accommodated by a comprehensive model of memory. External memory aids play a significant role in our everyday lives. Like other memory strategies, they do not invariably produce accurate retention, but they add to the devices that can be used to facilitate memory. External memory aids function as cues for encoding, recoding, reorganizing, rehearsing, and retrieving. In brief, they appear to contribute to most recognized memory functions.

Endnote 1

Alternatively, deficient memory monitoring might reflect unsatisfactory psychometric properties of the scales (Gilewski & Zelinski, 1986; Herrmann, 1982; Herrmann & Neisser, 1978; Johnson & Anderson, 1988; Martin, 1988; Reige, 1982). Herrmann, Grubs, Sigmundi, and Grueneich (1986) assessed the possibility that the low correlations between memory monitoring or metamemorial assessments and performance were due to low validity of the measurements by obtaining metamemorial judgments before and after performing the tasks. The judgments improved noticeably, suggesting that the customary low correlations were not due to invalid measures of metamemory. The low correlations appear to be due, instead, to the low opinions adults have about their memories. The results index the *lack* of confidence adults seem to have in their memorial abilities unless they are confronted with success in a specific task or set of tasks. These results imply that confidence in one's memorial abilities declines with age. This decline in confidence appears to be accompanied by increased reliance on memory aids.

References

Aiken, E.G., Thomas, G.S., & Shennum, W.A. (1975). Memory for lecture: Effects of notes, lecture rate, and information density. *Journal of Educational Psychology*, *67*, 439-444.

Annis, L.F. (1979). Effect of cognitive style and learning passage organization on study technique effectiveness. *Journal of Educational Psychology*, *71*, 620-626.

Bahrick, H.P., & Phelps, E. (1988). The maintenance of marginal knowledge. In U. Neisser & E. Winograd (Eds.), *Remembering reconsidered: Ecological and traditional approaches to the study of memory* (pp. 178-192). Cambridge: Cambridge University Press.

Beach, K. (1988). The role of external memory symbols in acquiring an occupation. In M. M. Gruneberg, P. E. Morris, & R. N. Sykes (Eds.), *Practical aspects of memory: Current research and issues* (Vol. 1, pp. 342-346). Chichester: Wiley.

Beal, C.R. (1988). The development of prospective memory skills. In M.M. Gruneberg, P.E. Morris, & R.N. Sykes (Eds.), *Practical aspects of memory: Current research and issues* (Vol. 1, pp. 366-370). Chichester: Wiley.

Bennett, H.L. (1983). Remembering drink orders: The memory skills of cocktail waitresses. *Human Learning*, *2*, 157-169.

Brewer, W.F. (1988). Memory for randomly sampled autobiographical events. In U. Neisser & E. Winograd (Eds.), *Remembering reconsidered: Ecological and traditional approaches to the study of memory* (pp. 21-90). Cambridge: Cambridge University Press.

Carrier, C.A., & Titus, A. (1979). The effects of notetaking: A review of studies. *Contemporary Educational Psychology, 4*, 299-314.

Cavanaugh, J.C., Grady, J.G., & Perlmutter, M. (1983). Forgetting and use of memory aids in 20 to 70 year olds' everyday life. *International Journal of Aging and Human Development, 17*, 113-122.

Cavanaugh, J.C., & Morton, K.R. (1988). Older adults' attributions about everyday memory. In M.M. Gruneberg, P.E. Morris, & R.N. Sykes (Eds.), *Practical aspects of memory: Current research and issues* (Vol. 1, pp. 209-214). Chichester: Wiley.

Ceci, S.J., Baker, J.G., & Bronfenbrenner, U. (1988). Prospective remembering, temporal calibration, and context. In M.M. Gruneberg, P.E. Morris, & R.N. Sykes (Eds.), *Practical aspects of memory: Current research and issues* (Vol. 1, pp. 360-365). Chichester: Wiley.

Ceci, S.J., & Bronfenbrenner, U. (1985). Don't forget to take the cupcakes out of the oven: Prospective memory, strategic time-monitoring, and context. *Child Development, 56*, 152-164.

Chaffin, R., & Herrmann, D.J. (1983). Self-reports of memory abilities by old and young adults. *Human Learning, 2*, 17-28.

Cohen, G. (1988). Memory and aging: Toward an explanation. In M.M. Gruneberg, P.E. Morris, & R.N. Sykes (Eds.), *Practical aspects of memory: Current research and issues* (Vol. 2, pp. 78-83). Chichester: Wiley.

Einstein, G.O., Morris, J., & Smith, S. (1985). Notetaking, individual differences, and memory for lecture information. *Journal of Educational Psychology, 77*, 522-532.

Ellis, J.A. (1988). Memory for future intentions: Investigating pulses and steps. In M.M. Gruneberg, P.E. Morris, & R.N. Sykes (Eds.), *Practical aspects of memory: Current research and issues* (Vol. 1, pp. 371-376). Chichester: Wiley.

Fisher, J.L., & Harris, M.B. (1973). Effect of note taking and review on recall. *Journal of Educational Psychology, 65*, 321-325.

Gates, S.J., & Colborn, D.K. (1976). Lowering appointment failures in a neighborhood health center. *Medical Care, 14*, 263-267.

Gilewski, M.J., & Zelinski, E.M. (1986). Questionnaire assessment of memory complaints. In L.W. Poon (Ed.), *Clinical memory assessment of older adults* (pp. 93-107). Washington, DC: American Psychological Association.

Grueneich, R., Herrmann, D.J., & Allen, L.A. (1985). The development of self-reports about everyday memory in children and adolescents. *Human Learning, 4*, 179-185.

Harris, J.E. (1980). Memory aids people use: Two interview studies. *Memory & Cognition, 8*, 31-38.

Harris, J.E. (1984). Remembering to do things: A forgotten topic. In J.E. Harris & P.E. Morris (Eds.), *Everyday memory, actions, and absent-mindedness* (pp. 71-92). London: Academic Press.

Harris, J.E., & Wilkins, A.J. (1982). Remembering to do things: A theoretical framework and an illustrative experiment. *Human Learning, 1*, 123-136.

Hartley, J. (1983). Notetaking research: Resetting the scoreboard. *Bulletin of the British Psychological Society, 36*, 13-14.

Hayes-Roth, B., & Walker, C. (1979). Configural effects in human memory: The superiority of memory over external information sources as a basis for inference verification. *Cognitive Science, 3*, 119-140.

Herrmann, D.J. (1982). Know thy memory: The use of questionnaires to assess and study memory. *Psychological Bulletin, 92*, 434-452.

Herrmann, D.J. (1984). Questionnaires about memory. In J.E. Harris & P.E. Morris (Eds.), *Everyday memory, actions, and absent-mindedness* (pp. 133-151). London: Academic Press.

Herrmann, D.J., Grubs, L., Sigmundi, R.A., & Grueneich, R. (1986). Awareness of memory ability before and after relevant memory experience. *Human Learning, 5*, 91-107.

Herrmann, D.J., & Neisser, U. (1978). An inventory of everyday memory experiences. In M.M. Gruneberg, P.E. Morris, & R.N. Sykes (Eds.), *Practical aspects of memory* (pp. 35-51). London: Academic Press.

Herrmann, D.J., & Petro, S.J. (in press). Commercial memory aids. *Applied Cognitive Psychology.*

Herrmann, D., Rea, A., & Andrzejewski, S. (1988). The need for a new approach to memory training. In M.M. Gruneberg, P.E. Morris, & R.N. Sykes (Eds.), *Practical aspects of memory: Current research and issues* (Vol. 2, pp. 415-420). Chichester: Wiley.

Hertel, P.T. (1988). Monitoring external memory. In M.M. Gruneberg, P.E. Morris, & R.N. Sykes (Eds.), *Practical aspects of memory: Current research and issues* (Vol. 1, pp. 221-226). Chichester: Wiley.

Howe, M.J. (1977). Learning and the acquisition of knowledge by students: Some experimental investigations. In M.J. Howe (Ed.), *Adult learning: Psychological research and applications* (pp. 145-160). London: Wiley.

Intons-Peterson, M.J., & Fournier, J. (1986). External and internal memory aids: When and how often do we use them? *Journal of Experimental Psychology: General, 115*, 267-280.

Jackson, J.L., Bogers, H., & Kerstholt, J. (1988). Do memory aids aid the elderly in their day to day remembering? In M.M. Gruneberg, P.E. Morris, & R.N. Sykes (Eds.), *Practical aspects of memory: Current research and issues* (Vol. 2, pp. 137-142). Chichester: Wiley.

Johnson, J.W., & Anderson, N.S. (1988). A comparison of four metamemory scales. In M.M. Gruneberg, P.E. Morris, & R.N. Sykes (Eds.), *Practical aspects of memory: Current research and issues* (Vol. 1, pp. 543-548). Chichester: Wiley.

Kiewra, K.A. (1985). Investigation notetaking and review: A depth of processing alternative. *Educational Psychologist, 20*, 23-32.

Kiewra, K.A., & Fletcher, H.J. (1984). The relationship between levels of notetaking and achievement. *Human Learning, 3*, 273-280.

Koriat, A., & Ben-Zur, H. (1988). Remembering that I did it: Processes and deficits in output monitoring. In M.M. Gruneberg, P.E. Morris, & R.N. Sykes, (Eds.) *Practical aspects of memory: Current research and issues* (Vol. 1, pp. 203-208). Chichester: Wiley.

Kreutzer, M.A., Leonard, C., & Flavell, J.H. (1975). An interview study of children's knowledge about memory. *Monographs of the Society for Research in Child Development, 40* (1, Serial No. 159).

Levy, R.L., & Clark, H. (1980). The use of an overt commitment to enhance compliance: A cautionary note. *Journal of Behavior Therapy and Experimental Psychiatry, 11*, 105-107.

Levy, R.L., & Loftus, G.R. (1984). Compliance and memory. In J.E. Harris & P.E. Morris (Eds.), *Everyday memory, actions, and absent-mindedness* (pp. 93-112). London: Academic Press.

Light, L.L. (1988). Preserved implicit memory in old age. In M.M. Gruneberg, P.E. Morris, & R.N. Sykes (Eds.), *Practical aspects of memory: Current research and issues* (Vol. 2, pp. 90-95). Chichester: Wiley.

Martin, M. (1988). Individual differences in everyday memory. In M.M. Gruneberg, P.E. Morris, & R.N. Sykes (Eds.), *Practical aspects of memory: Current research and issues* (Vol. 1, pp. 466-471). Chichester: Wiley.

Martin, M. & Jones, G.V. (1984). Cognitive failures in everyday life. In J.E. Harris & P.E. Morris (Eds.), *Everyday memory, actions, and absent-mindedness* (pp. 173-190). London: Academic Press.

McEvoy, C.L., & Moon, J.R. (1988). Assessment and treatment of everyday memory problems in the elderly. In M.M. Gruneberg, P.E. Morris, & R.N. Sykes (Eds.), *Practical aspects of memory: Current research and issues* (Vol. 2, pp. 155-160). Chichester: Wiley.

Meacham, J., & Colombo, J.A. (1980). External retrieval cues facilitate prospective remembering in children. *Journal of Educational Research, 73*, 299-301.

Meacham, J.A., & Leiman, B. (1982). Remembering to perform future actions. In U. Neisser (Ed.), *Memory observed: Remembering in natural contexts* (pp. 327-336). San Francisco: Freeman.

Morris, P.E. (1984). The validity of subjective reports on memory. In J.E. Harris & P.E. Morris (Eds.), *Everyday memory, actions, and absent-mindedness* (pp. 153-172). London: Academic Press.

Moscovitch, M. (1982). A neuropsychological approach to memory and perception in normal and pathological aging. In F.I.M. Craik & S. Trehub (Eds.), *Aging and cognitive processes* (pp. 55-78). New York: Plenum.

Naugle, R., Naugle, C., Prevey, M., & Delaney, R. (1988, July/August). New digital watch as a compensatory device for memory dysfunction. *Cognitive Rehabilitation*, pp. 22-23.

Perlmutter, M. (1978). What is memory aging the aging of? *Developmental Psychology, 14*, 330-345.

Peters, D.L. (1972). Effects of notetaking and rate of presentation on short term objective test performance. *Journal of Educational Psychology, 63*, 276-280.

Petro, S.J., Herrmann, D.J., Burrows, D., & Moore, C.M. (1990). Usefulness of commercial memory aids as a function of age. Manuscript under review.

Poon, L.W. (1980). A systems approach for the assessment and treatment of memory problems. In J.M. Ferguson & C.B. Taylor (Eds.), *The comprehensive handbook of behavioral medicine* (Vol. 1, pp. 191-212). New York: Spectrum.

Poon, L.W., & Schaffer, G. (1982, August). Prospective memory in young and elderly adults. Paper presented at the meeting of the American Psychological Association, Washington, DC.

Raaijmakers, J.G.W., & Shiffrin, R.M. (1981). Search of associative memory. *Psychological Review*, *88*, 93-134.

Reason, J.T., & Lucas, D. (1984). Using cognitive diaries to investigate naturally occurring memory blocks. In J.E. Harris & P.E. Morris (Eds.), *Everyday memory, actions, and absentmindedness* (pp. 53-70). London: Academic Press.

Reason, J.T., & Mycielska, K. (1982). *Absent minded? The psychology of mental lapses and everyday errors*. Englewood Cliffs, NJ: Prentice-Hall.

Reige, W.H. (1982). Self-report and tests of memory aging. *Clinical Gerontologist*, *1*, 23-36.

Schönpflug, W. (1988). Retrieving texts from an external store: The effects of an explanatory context and of semantic fit between text and address. *Psychological Research*, *50*, 19-27.

Schultz, C.B., & DiVesta, F.J. (1972). Effects of passage organization on the selection of clustering strategies and recall of textual materials. *Journal of Educational Psychology*, *63*, 244-252.

Shepard, D.S., & Moseley, T.A. (1976). Mailed vs telephoned appointment reminders to reduce broken appointments in a hospital outpatient department. *Medical Care*, *14*, 268-273.

Shimmerlick, S.M., & Nolan, J.D. (1976). Organization and recall of prose. *Journal of Educational Psychology*, *68*, 779-786.

Smith, M.J., Dutton, M., Diver, D., & Gray, J. (1989, March/April). Augmenting discharge teaching with the use of audiovisual aids. *Cognitive Rehabilitation*, pp. 28-30.

Waern, Y. (1981). On the relation between comprehension and memory of a complex text. *Scandinavian Journal of Educational Research*, *25*, 21-37.

West, R.L. (1988). Prospective memory and aging. In M.M. Gruneberg, P.E. Morris, & R.N. Sykes (Eds.), *Practical aspects of memory: Current research and issues* (Vol. 2, pp. 119-125). Chichester: Wiley.

Wilson, B.A., Baddeley, A.D., & Cockburn, J. (1988). Trials, tribulations, and triumphs in the development of a test of everyday memory. In M.M. Gruneberg, P.E. Morris, & R.N. Sykes (Eds.), *Practical aspects of memory: Current research and issues* (Vol. 2, pp. 249-254). Chichester: Wiley.

Yuille, J.C. (1984). Research and teaching with police: A Canadian example. *International Review of Applied Psychology*, *33*, 5-23.

Zelinski, E.M., Gilewski, M.J., & Thompson, L.W. (1980). Do laboratory tests relate to self assessment of memory ability in the young and old? In L.W. Poon, J.L. Fozard, L.S. Cermak, D. Arenberg, & L.W. Thompson (Eds.), *New directions in memory and aging* (pp. 519-544). Hillsdale, NJ: Erlbaum.

The Role of Social Interaction in Memory Improvement

Deborah L. Best

During the past several years, my 3 1/2-year-old son and I have made a number of trips to visit my sister, who lives several hours away, and my husband has not been able to go with us on many of these occasions. My sister's house is different from ours, since she has a swimming pool in the backyard and two teenage daughters. As most parents know or remember, there is an enormous amount of child-care paraphernalia that must be taken on such trips, especially when the home you are visiting is not equipped for young children. Invariably, I forget something essential that my sister no longer has, such as a booster seat or tippy cups. Recently while packing for one of our visits, I overheard my son tell his father, who was going to accompany us on this trip, how we make sure that we "don't forget my floaties. You have to pretend that you are walking through Aunt Dee's house, and first you come to the room where I sleep. That's where my clothes are... and my cot and my pillow. Next you come to the bathroom, and we put my toothbrush there. And, what goes in the kitchen? My toys go in the den. Then we go outside and my floaties and, uh uh, and pool toys go there." I was amazed to hear that my son had learned the strategy that I had developed in order to remember the things that we must take on our visits. I had made no attempt to teach it to him. I had usually involved him in my little game to keep him entertained while I made my last minute mental check of what we had packed before we pulled out of the driveway.

Even though parents seldom attempt to teach memory strategies directly to children, children may benefit from observing and imitating what their parents do in situations that have memory demands. This form of learning may be even more provocative for a child than intentional instructional situations because of the established emotional relationship between parent and child based upon numerous social interactions that have taken place in the past.

Also, an intentional instructional situation may be more stressful, less motivating, and less interesting for a child than simply imitating parental behavior as they choose.

In this chapter, I will address the role of social interaction in memory improvement, a role that has only recently been recognized by cognitive researchers, perhaps receiving new attention as a result of the rebirth of interest in Vygotsky's (1978; 1981) theory of psychological development and social psychologists' recent attention to social cognition. Social interactions are viewed differently by researchers investigating memory development in children and those concerned with improving memory difficulties experienced by older adults. Researchers studying children have treated social interaction as one aspect of the normal course of acquiring improved mnemonic skills. In contrast, those concerned about intervention with older adults have considered social interaction to be a relatively unimportant contributor to adult cognitive functioning, especially in the context of training cognitive strategies. As a consequence of these differing views of the role of social interaction in memory, I will review these two areas of research, memory development and memory improvement, separately and will then address common themes that emerge from the two.

Memory Development and Social Interaction

Early Social Interactions and Memory

From birth, humans are social animals. By 2 weeks of age, babies prefer to look at faces rather than other patterned figures (Fagan, 1979), and they prefer their own mother's face to that of a female stranger (Carpenter, Tecce, Stechler, & Friedman, 1968). Recognition of mother's face is one of the most impressive memory feats of the neonate, demonstrating memory for a complex stimulus that has been seen through blurry eyes only a relatively small number of times. Babies quickly learn many other things about the people in their world, such as mother's voice (DeCasper & Fifer, 1980) and breast smell (Macfarlane, 1978), suggesting the importance of social contact from birth.

Development of Scripts and Event Representations

By 7 months of age, babies show evidence of recall of caretaking routines or scripts, such as teeth brushing and baths, and social interactions, such as peek-a-boo games (Ashmead & Perlmutter, 1980). Even young children are able to construct a script of an event after participating in it only a few times (Fivush, 1984; Fivush, Hudson, & Nelson, 1984; Nelson, 1978). Scripts constitute an important form of social learning, representing widely shared cultural knowledge for both private (teeth brushing) and public events (eating in a restaurant). Assuming that others share scripted knowledge has important consequences for how individuals communicate and interact.

Understanding of causal relations may develop in the domain of social behavior before developing in the physical domain, since social figures may ease the memory demands required to understand causality (Ashmead & Perlmutter, 1980). Parents adjust their styles of interaction to the level of the child, thereby guiding the development of the child's scripts or generalized event representations (Nelson & Gruendel, 1981). For example, while looking at picture books with their 17- to 22-month-old children, mothers have shown that they are sensitive to their children's level of knowledge, asking questions when the child indicated understanding of a word ("What's that?") and providing labels when the child did not know the word ("Where is the doll?"; Ninio, 1983). By 2 to 3 years of age, both old and new routines are readily recalled. As children get older, parents require them to generate more and more stored information verbally, which promotes children's ability to regulate their own memory (Price, 1984).

Parental Memory Demands and Children's Memory Development

While belief-behavior links are often complicated and unclear, parent's beliefs concerning their children's mnemonic abilities most likely influence the way they guide their children's mnemonic activities (Miller, 1988). In spite of abundant memory development research, only one study (Bird & Berman, 1985) has examined parental beliefs about children's mnemonic abilities, and no research has examined how such beliefs may directly influence the way that parents guide or interact with their children in mnemonic contexts (Miller, 1988). Clearly, this area needs further research to illuminate the way in which children's mnemonic performance is influenced by parental beliefs about children's competence.

The development of intentional memory also shows improvement that is attributable to social interactions, most often with parents. When parents ask 2- to 4-year-old children to remind them to do something in the future, even 2-year-olds remember to remind their parents of promised treats 80% of the time without prompts (Somerville, Wellman, & Cultice, 1983). This strong performance, sometimes with delayed recall of 1/2 day or more, contrasts with the often poor performance of 2- to 3-year-olds on formal laboratory-type memory tasks. While there are a number of explanations for the differential performance in the two settings, such as lack of familiarity with the setting and lack of awareness of how to apply memory strategies to new stimuli, the social aspect of the task has too often been ignored. In most cases laboratory tasks require children to interact with an unfamiliar person in a context where the rewards for performance are unclear and the reinforcement history with that person has not been established. Understanding the context of the task and interacting with someone with whom the relationship is predictable may strengthen children's mnemonic performance. For example, there is some evidence, though not consistent (Weissberg & Paris, 1986), to suggest that children may remember more in the context of a game than in a laboratory task context (Ceci, Bronfenbrenner, & Baker, 1988; Istomina, 1975).

Ratner (1980) observed 2- and 3-year-olds and their mothers to see what kinds of everyday memory demands mothers place upon their children and the role that these demands play in children's memory development. She found that mothers expect their children to remember a vast array of information, such as the location of objects, social routines, and past events. Children's memory performance was limited and largely nonstrategic even in the familiar setting of their own homes. Mothers occasionally instructed their children how to use their memory abilities, but children demonstrated little sensitivity to memory processes. For 2-year-olds, there was no relationship between the mother's memory questions and the child's memory on laboratory tasks. However, by 3 years of age, children of mothers who asked event and knowledge questions performed better on the memory tasks. Children whose mothers asked questions about past events, requiring long-term memory information retrieval, outperformed those children whose mothers asked for long-term memory information pertaining only to present events. While mothers' memory demands appear to influence the performance of 3-year-olds, it is not clear how such demands foster memory development and how responsibility for memory performance shifts from joint to independent functioning.

Zone of Proximal Development

According to Vygotsky's (1978; 1981) theory, the learning that takes place in social interactions serves as the foundation for cognitive development. As the child learns a task and its requirements, the distance between current and potential understanding of the task becomes apparent. Vygotsky labeled this interval the zone of proximal development, the distance between a child's "actual development level as determined by independent problem solving [and the higher level of] potential development as determined through problem solving under adult guidance or in collaboration with more capable peers" (Vygotsky, 1978, p. 86). Task requirements that fall within this zone, such as knowledge about strategies and their attributes, are gradually mastered, and with the assistance and supervision of an adult, these cognitive skills are eventually internalized. Finally, the child successfully completes a task within the zone using elementary strategies that have been assimilated into the repertoire. According to Vygotsky:

> The very mechanism underlying higher mental functions is a copy from social interaction; all higher mental functions are internalized social

> relationships....Their composition, genetic structure, and means of action [forms of mediation]--in a word, their whole nature--is social. Even when we turn to mental [internal] processes, their nature remains quasi-social. In their own private sphere, human beings retain the functions of social interaction. (1981, p. 164)

Belmont (1989) has recently suggested that the reason that many memory strategy training studies with children have shown little maintenance or generalization of strategy use may be due to the level of instruction relative to the child's zone of proximal development. For example, children who respond to memory strategy instruction but later fail to use the instructed strategy without prompting have been introduced to a strategy in the upper end of their zone. Those who maintain the strategy but do not generalize its use have been instructed in their midzone, and those who both maintain and generalize are in the lower end of their zone, close to the point where spontaneous strategy use would have soon occurred without instruction. Although this explanation is plausible, no memory-training studies have been conducted as yet to validate this framework. There are, however, studies concerned with preschoolers' learning number concepts (Saxe, Guberman, & Gearhart, 1987) and of junior high school children's developing reading comprehension (Palincsar & Brown, 1984) that support this interpretation of maintenance and generalization. Both studies also underscore the importance of social interaction and transfer of responsibility for perfect performance from the more skilled to the less skilled individual.

Parental Guidance of Children's Memory Performance

Consistent with Vygotsky's theorizing, Wood, Bruner, and Ross (1976) introduced the metaphor of the "scaffold" to describe the role of the ideal teacher in informal learning settings This scaffold serves many of the same functions of a scaffold in building construction, providing support, extending the range of performance, and selectively promoting completion of a task that would not be possible without it. In the learning situation, the teacher selectively intervenes to provide support for the learner, extending available skills, thus permitting the learner to accomplish a task that otherwise would not be possible. Scaffolding is a cooperative venture in which the teacher and learner both contribute to the eventual transfer of responsibility for task accomplishment to the learner. Ultimately, the scaffolding becomes internalized, enabling the learner to accomplish the task independently. Scaffolding, in contrast to shaping or the method of successive approximations (Skinner, 1938), holds the task constant while simplifying the learner's role through graduated interventions by the teacher (Greenfield, 1984). Like shaping, however, scaffolding leads to relatively errorless learning, since the amount of support provided by the teacher is adjusted to help the learner succeed at each point in learning the task. Whether the task is learning language or learning to weave, teachers are often unaware of their contributions to the learning process, contending that learners have mastered the task by themselves (Greenfield).

A relevant, older line of research examined the relationship between maternal-teaching styles and child cognitive competence (Bee, 1967; Bee, Van Egeren, Streissguth, Nyman, & Leckie, 1969; Hess & Shipman, 1965, 1967). Hess and Shipman (1965, 1967) observed mothers as they taught their 4-year-old children to sort toys, copy etch-a-sketch designs, and respond to questions about hypothetical "1st day at school" and discipline situations. Three maternal interaction styles were found that related to children's cognitive performance: Imperative-normative, in which the mother gave little justification for requests or demands; subjective, in which the mother encouraged the child to see his own behavior from another's point of view; and cognitive-rational, in which the mother offered logical justifications for requests and demands. Children whose mothers used the latter two styles were more verbal and performed better on the cognitive tasks. While these findings suggest the importance of maternal interaction styles for children's cognitive development, the aspects of the mother's communications that foster the child's cognitive development were not explored nor was the child's role in eliciting the mother's interactional style.

More recent studies of parental guidance of children's learning indicate that parents are sensitive to children's zone of proximal development (Greenfield, 1984; Rogoff, 1990; Rogoff & Gardner, 1984), engaging them in cognitive tasks, providing appropriate cues and modeling successful performance. Rogoff and Gardner asked mothers to assist their 6- to 9-year-old children in preparing for a memory test on categorization of familiar objects (putting grocery items on mock kitchen shelves, sorting photographs of common household objects), similar to activities performed in the home or school. Mothers established an instructional context by references to what the child already knew ("Let's pretend we're going on a picnic and we'll think about what we need on a picnic."). Effective instruction often required the mother to lead the child through the solution process, involving the child in every step along the way. Mothers provided children with a rationale for the way they approached the task and specific examples of how to organize the items. ("Okay, that'll be an easy way to remember. Here's lunch. Here's fruit."). Eventually, the responsibility for task solution was transferred to the child, and mothers helped the child monitor skills by asking about the accuracy of their classifications and the usefulness of strategies ("Shall we find out if that's right?" "Again, how did we do it?").

The significance of the interactive communication between mother and child is illustrated by a mother-child pair in the Rogoff and Gardner (1984) study. This mother developed a story mnemonic to facilitate her child's recall. At the beginning of story construction, the mother provided a great deal of structure, attempting to involve the child with pauses and pointing to the next visual cue (sorting box). By the end of the story, the child was making significant contributions, working jointly with the mother. The child's understanding was extended through participation in problem solving using the scaffolding constructed by the mother and eliciting parental assistance appropriate to the child's competence level.

Wertsch and Stone (1978) refer to this guided learning process as "proleptic instruction," in which a novice carries out simple parts of a task with the guidance of an expert. Performing the task under supervision helps the learner acquire some of the expert's understanding of the problem and its solution. In this way, metacognitive development is fostered and children become aware of the importance of strategies and self-monitoring in task solution. Mothers typically use questions to guide children in task solution rather than more directive techniques (Wertsch, 1979). Such questions organize and direct the child's activities and also model the important components of metacognition (e.g., "Is that correct?" "What should we do next?"). These metacognitive inquiries are internalized by children who may later be observed actually questioning themselves aloud (Day, French, & Hall, 1985).

There have been only a few studies that have examined both the process of collaboration between children and adults and the effects of the collaboration upon children's subsequent task performance. Of these studies, some have found a positive influence upon children's later independent performance (Ellis & Rogoff, 1982; Radziszewska & Rogoff, 1988; Wood, Wood, & Middleton, 1978), and some have found no effect (Germond, 1986; Kontos, 1983). These contradictory findings suggest that social interaction may have inconsistent, limited benefits dependent upon the specific circumstances in which the interaction occurs. For example, peer interaction may be less advantageous than adult interaction, even if peers are trained in task performance (Rogoff, 1990). Peers may not be able to communicate as much guiding information as adults who have more instructional experience and better verbal skills.

Most of the studies of parent-child interaction in problem-solving situations have focused upon the cognitive benefits for the child and have failed to address what benefits may accrue for the parent (Verdonick, 1988a, 1988b). During their cooperative efforts, the parent must restructure information about the task in ways that will be useful to the child. The parent also must process information at a more explicit level than usual, sometimes verbalizing intentions and strategies that have become so overlearned that they are no longer easy to talk about (e.g., respond to the many why-questions of preschoolers). The parent must evaluate the effectiveness of the communication to the child, modifying the conceptualization of the task according to the child's feedback. The child plays an active role in directing the parent's structuring of and communicating about problem solution, which may lead the parent to develop more effective metacognitive and communicative skills.

Teachers' Influence on Children's Memory Development

Parent-child interactions have not been the only social context of interest for memory development researchers. For a number of years, the influence of the educational environment on the development of memory skills has been acknowledged (Cole, Gay, Glick, & Sharp, 1971; Cole & Scribner, 1977; Sharp, Cole, & Lave, 1979). However, only recently have researchers carefully examined the specific aspects of the school environment that contribute to memory development. One study in particular, conducted by Moely et al. (1986), illustrates the role of the teacher and the social interactive aspect of teaching memory skills. Moely and her colleagues observed grade school (kindergarten through sixth grade) teachers while they were instructing their classes in language arts or mathematics, and the teachers later filled out questionnaires concerning their perceptions of children's use of memory strategies. Teachers of second and third graders made more strategy suggestions than did teachers of kindergartners and first graders, perhaps assuming that the younger children could not profit from memory strategies and also recognizing that the memory demands were greater for first and second graders. Second and third grade teachers also made more strategy suggestions than teachers of the older children, who may already have mastered the strategies.

Moely et al. (1986) also wanted to see if children's learning styles were affected by exposure to teachers holding different orientations toward cognitive instruction. Children from classes where teachers frequently made strategy suggestions were asked to perform several memory tasks, and their performance was compared with children whose teachers rarely made strategy suggestions. Teachers who made more strategy suggestions had children who were better able to verbalize aspects of memory training and task performance than those trained by teachers who did not emphasize cognitive processes. For high achieving children, teachers' suggestions did not make any difference in the maintenance of trained strategies. However, average and low achievers whose teachers often made strategy suggestions were more likely to continue using the trained strategy on the final learning trial than were children whose teachers rarely made such suggestions. These findings clearly demonstrate the relationship between teachers' expectations for cognitive instruction and children's ability to profit from such classroom memory training.

Metacognitive Abilities and Social Interaction

As active participants in the learning situation, children must use their metacognitive skills to benefit from the interactive instruction they experience. When the transfer of responsibility for task solution is abrupt, children must interpret strategies in the context of their existing metacognitive knowledge. Lave (1977) found that when Liberian apprentice tailors were given full responsibility for making a garment, they received brief intense training and were then on their own. When step-by-step transfer is permitted, metacognitive knowledge is not so heavily taxed and can develop along with problem-solving strategies. However, successful learners are capable of dealing with both abrupt and more gradual transitions (Borkowski, Milstead, & Hale, 1988).

Moore and his colleagues (Moore, Mullis, & Mullis, 1986) have demonstrated how children may acquire such metacognitive abilities through interactions with parents during problem solution. Parents instructed their 9-year-old children how to complete a structured block design task, and memory-monitoring behaviors were recorded, with the task repeated 1 year later. Parents used more memory- monitoring instructions to guide the child's task completion during the 1st year than the 2nd, indicating awareness of the child's changing level of expertise. Children also used fewer memory monitoring strategies the 2nd year, suggesting that as they became more proficient in task solution, conscious memory monitoring was no longer necessary.

Social interactions have also been shown to have important implications for the evaluation of metacognitive skills (Cavanaugh & Perlmutter, 1982; Schneider, 1985). Along with traditional metamemory interview questions, Best and Ornstein (1986) used peer tutoring, a social interaction situation, to assess school-age children's metamemory knowledge of organizational strategies following a sort/recall task. Third and sixth graders were first given three trials with either semantically-related or unrelated picture/word lists. During the test phase, all subjects were given two sort/recall trials with different sets of unrelated items to see if the previous experience with related materials would facilitate the use of organization and subsequent recall of the unrelated items. Following the memory task, metamemory was assessed in two ways. First, children were asked standard interview-type metamemory questions (e.g., "What did you do to try to remember the words?"). Second, each child was asked to teach a first grader how to perform the memory task, telling the younger child the strategies they had used to make the task easier. It was assumed that the older children would give more explicit information if the "pupil" was obviously younger. Instructions given to the first grader, as well as the memory performance of these younger children, reflected the older children's differential experience with related versus unrelated materials. In the context of the metamemory-interview questions, the older children gave little strategic information, and there were no significant differences as a function of prior experience with semantically related or unrelated materials. On the other hand, in the context of teaching a younger child the game, the older children stressed the importance of meaning-based organization in their directions, and those who had prior experience with related materials displayed greater awareness of organizational principles than did those who only had experience with unrelated items.

In a subsequent study, Best (in press) found that the presence of a younger child is an important factor in determining the quality of information that older children provide in the teaching task. She used a simulated peer-tutoring assessment, in which children were asked to pretend that the experimenter was a first grader and to explain how to play the "memory game" and what they did to make the game easier. Although the level of strategy information provided in the simulated teaching task instructions was not as great as Best and Ornstein (1986) found when a first grader was actually present to be taught, the pattern of group differences was, nevertheless, the same.

These findings are clarified when the referential communication literature is examined. Shatz and Gelman (1973) found that children will adapt their speech to the appropriate linguistic level of their listener. For example, 4-year-olds will modify their speech when talking to 2-year-olds, using shorter phrases, fewer complex constructions, repetition, and more attention-getting and holding phrases. The differential adjustments that these children make suggest that the speakers are responding to direct feedback from their listeners, such as inattention when the message is too advanced. Research demonstrating that mothers will simplify speech more when a 2-year-old actually is present than when told to talk as if a 2-year-old were present provides additional evidence for the importance of feedback in eliciting more explicit information (Snow, 1972). These studies point to the value of the social context for eliciting more explicit information than usual from children about their understanding of how their memory works.

To briefly summarize, while social aspects of memory development have been researched from several theoretical viewpoints, the current revival of interest in Vygotsky's (1978; 1981) theory has brought the role of social interaction in cognitive growth to the forefront. This renewed interest in social influence on memory development has encouraged cognitive research in naturalistic settings, examining the role of parent-child, teacher-child and peer interactions. It is obvious that other people, particularly parents, have a profound influence upon the development of children's cognitive abilities. Indeed, memory abilities are socially transmitted, socially constrained, socially nurtured, and socially encouraged (Day et al., 1985). The expectations and demands that parents and teachers make help to shape children's memory development. Metacognitive abilities are strengthened and are evaluated more accurately through social interaction. The importance of social interaction for memory performance and development can also be seen with older adults in the context of memory improvement.

Memory Improvement and Social Interaction

Shortly after my mother turned 70, I went to visit her for the weekend. Since there were many friends and relatives that we needed to see and a number of errands we had to run on Saturday, we went in and out of her house many times. On one of those occasions, while absorbed in a

> typical mother and daughter conversation, we went out the front door to my car and discovered that I had locked my keys in her house. I chastised myself for being so forgetful at age 31, but she assured me that I was so busy with my many professional and personal responsibilities that despite the minor forgetfulness I had just displayed, my memory abilities were exceptional.
>
> That afternoon, we went out the back door to her car only to find that she had locked her keys in the house. She immediately berated herself for being so forgetful and told me that she was becoming senile in her old age. "It is so hard getting old and losing your memory," she said. She further elaborated that recently she had been having a hard time remembering names and faces, and she now had to repeat things over and over that she needed to remember. Furthermore, she often had to slow down a conversation so that she could remember the important information, asking many more questions than she had when she was younger. Nothing I could say would convince her that she was still mentally alert, active, and in command of her intellectual faculties and that we both had just demonstrated the same memory failure.

On the surface this story may simply suggest the similarity of cognitive abilities in a mother and her daughter, but with closer inspection the story illustrates a number of issues related to social interaction and memory improvement in older adults. For example, while we both displayed a similar memory failure, my mother's evaluation of her memory deficiency was much more serious than her evaluation of mine. Believing the social stereotype that memory fails with age, she interpreted her memory failure as an indication of her impending cognitive deterioration, and she interpreted mine as an indication of my busy lifestyle. My mother also demonstrated that she had developed several means of improving her memory in social contexts, such as slowing conversations, rehearsing to-be-remembered information, and asking questions. In this section, I will review some of the issues linking memory improvement and social interaction.

Social Interaction and Memory

At the adult level, social interaction or context is assumed to influence memory in two major ways: First, in the context of social situations that actually involve memory tasks and second, through attitudes or stereotypes about memory performance. A number of issues, such as person impressions, affective reactions, person memory, and social judgments, related to these two domains have been investigated by social cognition researchers. These social psychologists, however, have emphasized the social rather than the cognitive aspects of social information processing (Belmore & Hubbard, 1987; Hastie,

1980; Rogers, Kuiper, & Kirker, 1977; Wyer & Srull, 1984, 1986), and none have addressed memory improvement in the social context. Hence, we will not discuss these topics, since they are not directly related to memory improvement.

On the other hand, cognitive psychologists have generally ignored or experimentally controlled many variables from the social realm, such as expectancies, prior attitudes, person impressions, and behavioral decisions (Wyer & Srull, 1986). Without integrating research from both the social and cognitive domains, knowledge of cognitive functioning will continue to be limited to a restricted set of phenomena.

Memory Improvement and Social Interaction

Many memory demands placed upon adults, particularly older adults who have retired from the work force, focus upon social interactions and social obligations. Unlike younger children, adults must remember such diverse things as what meetings they should attend, the errands they promised their spouses they would run, when the dentist appointment is scheduled, what time to pick up the children's car pool, what they discussed with their boss the day before, and how formally one should dress for a local charity gala that is attended every year. From casual conversation to serious discussion to formal points of etiquette, social interactions require adults to garner information that will be needed in the future and to recall relevant details from the past (Herrmann & Searleman, 1990). As a result, adults develop strategies to improve memory performance in the context of social interactions. As shown in the vignette with my mother, as she grew older, she found that slowing conversation permitted more time for encoding, that rehearsing helped her remember conversational details, and that asking questions facilitated recall. All are effective methods for improving memory in the social context. Limiting conversation to one or two topics, referring questions to others (Rabbitt, 1981), and asking others to remember (Intons-Peterson & Fournier, 1986) are additional means by which adults try to simplify conversational memory demands.

To date, the only memory improvement training to address conversational-control techniques, such as those discussed above, was conducted by Herrmann (reported in Herrmann & Searleman, 1990) with college students. In this training, which was part of a college course, students learned strategies to improve the encoding and retrieval of conversational information, such as a person's name when being introduced, and they reported that the training was effective. Similar approaches have been used in rehabilitation programs with brain-damaged individuals who are experiencing memory difficulties with verbal information (Wilson & Moffat, 1984), but conversational- control techniques are usually not central to memory improvement training.

Memory Performance and Interpersonal Evaluations

Improving memory performance in social interactions not only benefits the individual in terms of information that is appropriately recalled but also in terms of evaluations that others make of the person. Gentry and Herrmann (1990) have suggested four ways that memory performance affects interpersonal evaluations:

1. Memory performance affects how the performer of the memory act is perceived, particularly when the performance facilitates or hinders the achievement of goals shared with others. For example, when a person forgets to bring food for a picnic, others evaluate the "forgetter" negatively. If forgetting is a continual problem, the forgetter may be considered irresponsible and may develop a negative "memory reputation." In contrast, when a person remembers to pick up the clothes at the cleaners, the "rememberer" is considered to be responsible, organized, and thoughtful, and a good memory reputation may evolve. Even when a person with a good memory reputation forgets, others assume the person was tired or overburdened with other responsibilities, as my mother assumed I was in the earlier vignette.

2. Memory performance can affect the evaluation of the performer even when the observer has no vested interest in the outcome of the memory performance. The absent-minded professor stereotype is an excellent example of the negative connotations attributed to those who forget. Likewise, stereotypes of those good at remembering lead to positive evaluations, such as photographic memory, memory expert, or genius.

3. Memory performance is often regarded as an indication of the importance of the task or relationship to the memory performer. For example, forgetting your girl friend's birthday, your wedding anniversary, or someone's name is assumed to indicate that you do not care about the relationship or person.

4. Accountability for memory failures is sometimes transferred to others who are considered responsible for the memory performer's behavior. Parents and teachers may be regarded as inadequate instructors if children cannot remember information supposedly taught to them. Such evaluations may lead to the development of stereotypes about memory performance.

Stereotypes and Memory Performance

Before examining the impact of memory-related stereotypes, we must first explore the nature and extent of these beliefs. Herrmann (1989) asked college students to estimate four kinds of memory ability (knowledge, events, intentions, and actions) as a function of a person's age, occupation, and marital roles. Memory ratings were lowest for the child, highest for the young adult and middle-aged person, and low for the senior citizen, who was rated particularly low for remembering intentions and actions. Among the occupations, pilots were rated as having the best memory overall, professors and lawyers were rated highest in knowledge, and policemen were judged to have the best memory for intentions. There were slight variations between husbands and wives, with husbands receiving higher ratings for knowledge and actions and wives receiving higher ratings for events and intentions. Clearly, there are stereotypes about memory abilities based upon social characteristics of the groups being rated, with age accounting for the greatest variation in attributions. Stereotypes about memory performance may have important consequences for people's attitudes when facing memory tasks and for the amount of effort they will expend.

Given the stereotypes about memory changes attributed to age, it is not surprising that forgetfulness in older adults is often viewed as a sign of senility, even though everyone, regardless of age, forgets names or items on shopping lists. Memory failures may be considered inconsequential for younger adults but much more serious for older adults. Using a person perception paradigm, Eber (1989) found that young adults rated memory failures more seriously when they were attributed to a 70-year-old target person than when attributed to a 30-year-old target person. Young adults were more stringent in their ratings, regardless of the previously established seriousness level of the memory failure, suggesting that they used a double standard when judging the seriousness of the memory failure. Older adults, on the other hand, were more lenient with both the younger and older target, rating the seriousness of the memory failure of the young and older target persons the same. In a follow-up study in which the ages of the targets were more strongly emphasized (Eber, Szuchman, & Rothberg, 1990), the double standard used in evaluating memory failures was also found with older adults. Moreover, given identical memory failures, older targets were perceived as having greater mental difficulties than younger targets, and recommendations for memory training were higher for the older targets as well. In contrast, memory failures of the young targets were more frequently attributed to "all the other things going on around [the target and] all the other things on her mind" (Eber et al., p. 239). These findings demonstrate the negative stereotypes in our culture concerning the memory abilities of the elderly, but similar stereotypes also have been found in cultures that generally express high value for the elderly (Noesjirwan, Gault, & Crawford, 1983).

Stereotypes concerning differential memory abilities due to gender have also been investigated recently (Crawford, Herrmann, Holdsworth, Randall, & Robbins, 1989; Herrmann & Crawford, 1990). With both adult and college student samples, gender was strongly related to beliefs about others' memory performance and only weakly related to beliefs about one's own performance. Consistent with other gender-based stereotypes (Williams & Best, 1982), subjects' opinions of their own memory capabilities were not viewed stereotypically. Men and women agree that men are better at remembering directions and previously visited places, while women are better at remembering shopping lists, names, faces, childhood memories, and who said what in conversations.

Finding that gender biases in memory beliefs were pervasive, Herrmann and Crawford (1990) wanted to see the extent to which these beliefs influence memory performance. They found that men performed better on a free recall task when a set of directions to be remembered were given a masculine label (viz., directions for making a workbench), and women performed better when the directions were given a feminine label (viz., directions for making a shirt). In a second experiment, gender-biased labels were provided for directions (viz., making a shirt or making a workbench) and for a shopping list (viz., either a grocery list or hardware store list). Males were strongly affected by the label in the directions task, recalling more of the directions when they had a masculine label, but females were only minimally affected by the label. On the shopping list task, recall was in the gender-biased direction, but the differences were not statistically significant. While it is unclear whether effort expended or greater familiarity with the gender consistent task were responsible for differential recall of gender relevant items, it is clear that gender-biased stereotypes about memory skills and tasks are widespread and can influence memory performance.

Memory Contrivances

Given the negative evaluations that often follow memory failures and the stereotypes about memory performance that exist in our culture, people may use self-presentation and impression management to control the information that is conveyed to others about their memory performance. Gentry and Herrmann (1990) have used the label *memory contrivances* for the distortions and fabrications about memory performance that people use to achieve social goals. These researchers found that college students reported a number of memory contrivances, such as showing off their good memory, excusing someone else's memory failures, or pretending not to remember something unpleasant. Contrivances are used in everyday social interactions to enhance one's own image, to be considerate of someone who has forgotten, or to maintain positive social relationships. Moreover, memory contrivances enhance social interactions and self-presentation, and they demonstrate the social value of competent memory performance. While memory contrivances do not directly contribute to memory improvement, they certainly alter the way that memory performances are evaluated.

Prospective Remembering

Regarding memory performance as an indicator of the importance of social relationships not only has implications for the evaluations that we make of other's memory competence, but it may also be an important aspect of prospective memory. Intentions constructed in conversations between two people involve a·commitment of one to the other to perform some task, such as meeting for lunch on Thursday. The commitment is fulfilled when it is prospectively remembered at the appropriate time, and the suitable action is taken. Whether the intention will be remembered and the appropriate action performed depends upon the quality of the interpersonal relationship that is the basis of the commitment (Meacham, 1988). In a study of prospective remembering by college students, Meacham (Meacham; Meacham & Kushner, 1980) found that tasks of a social nature, such as meeting someone, were more likely to be remembered than personal or object-oriented tasks, such as mailing a letter. It is the social context that causes intentions to remember to have the potential to direct behavior.

Self-Evaluations and Memory Performance

In addition to intentions, our self-evaluations of memory performance also have a critical impact on how we assess a task and how well we perform. We are our own harshest memory critic, reprimanding ourselves when we forget, rarely praising ourselves for remembering, and vigilantly watching for further memory failures. The way we view our failures is greatly influenced by our attitudes and beliefs about our own and other's memory performance. We tend to learn more easily when we believe that we are superior at a task (Rapaport, 1942), generally finding it less effortful than most tasks. Likewise, when we believe that we are poor at a memory task, such as remembering names, we may see no point in trying. Allocation of effort seems to be associated with how much we think we control our memory performance and how we compare our performance to that of others.

Poon (1985) suggests that feeling that one's ability to remember and to retrieve information is not as good as it used to be is a universal complaint among middle-aged and elderly adults. Although such stereotypical thinking about memory and aging may perpetuate a self-fulfilling prophecy, research has found that the relationship between complaints about memory and actual memory performance are not as strongly associated as expected (Cavanaugh, Grady, & Perlmutter, 1983; Kahn, Zarit, Hilbert, & Niederehe, 1975; Poon, 1985). In fact, only 15% of a national sample of persons aged 55 and older said they frequently had problems with forgetting in the past year, while more than 25% said they had never had problems (Cutler & Grams, 1988). Self-reported memory problems did increase with age, but only 23% of those aged 85 and older reported having frequent problems. For this sample, health deterioration and functional and sensory impairments were the best predictors of reported memory problems.

In one of the first studies of memory complaint in the elderly, Kahn et al. (1975) examined the relationship between memory complaint, memory performance, and depression among depressed elderly outpatients and their relatives. Regardless of objective memory performance, depression was related to memory complaint. In a similar study, Popkin, Gallagher, Thompson, and Moore (1982) found that depressed older adults complained more about memory than did nondepressed elderly, even though actual memory performance did not differ. Memory complaints were significantly reduced following remission of depression. While these studies suggest that depression may be an important component in memory complaint, most elderly are not clinically depressed nor are all those who complain about memory problems depressed either.

Scogin (1985) examined the relationship between memory complaint and memory performance among nondepressed older adults with low memory concerns, nondepressed older adults with high memory complaints, and depressed older adults. Depressed older adults and those seeking memory training demonstrated lower relationships between self-reported memory complaints and memory performance than did nondepressed older adults who were not seeking memory training. Healthy community-dwelling older adults who have fewer memory complaints evaluate their memory more accurately than do those who have greater memory concerns (Reige, 1982; Scogin; Zelinski, Gilewski, & Thompson, 1980), and in fact, they may be more accurate in memory appraisals than younger adults. It does appear, however, that older adults with memory complaints have distinct expectations about cognitive abilities and perhaps fears about memory decline with aging. These attitudes, as well as their heightened awareness of memory failures (Cavanaugh, 1989), may be responsible for their high level of memory complaint and their interest in memory training.

Attributions About Memory and Memory Improvement

When attributions about memory performance are internal, the individual is considered responsible for his or her own memory successes and failures. In contrast, when attributions about memory performance are external, responsibility for memory performance is attributed to forces such as chance, luck, task difficulty, or others (Weiner, 1985). Lachman and Jelalian (1984) have shown that older adults are more likely to attribute their memory performance to internal stable factors, whereas younger adults more often make stable external attributions to task difficulty. Compared with younger adults, older adults also are more likely to believe in age-related memory decline (Dixon & Hultsch, 1983).

This attributional difference between younger and older adults may be responsible for memory-training failures with older adults and also may contribute to their high level of memory complaint, even following successful memory instruction (Cavanaugh & Morton, 1988; Cavanaugh, Morton, &

Tilse, 1989). Indeed, older adults who believe that training will result in improved memory demonstrate decreased levels of memory complaint following training participation (Zarit, Cole, & Guider, 1981). Strategy training alone does not address the self-evaluation process that lies at the heart of memory performance. When an older adult is taught a memory strategy and it fails, as it inevitably will do, the technique is abandoned. Social stereotypes about age-related memory declines are incorporated into the failure attributions and are internalized, suggesting that the effort required for using memory strategies is too great. Eventually such attributions become routine and may serve as excuses for not performing well and for minimizing effort in memory tasks (Williams, Denney, & Schadler, 1983). To be effective, strategy training should be coupled with developing realistic self-evaluations and analysis of everyday memory tasks.

Consistent with these notions about the influence of memory expectations on memory improvement, Best, Hamlett, and Davis (in press) conducted a study that compared strategy training with instruction designed to change expectations about memory performance and to breakdown stereotypes about memory deterioration with advancing age. Older adults participated in four training sessions over a 2 week period or in an art discussion control group. An additional evaluation comparison group was tested at the same intervals as the training and control groups. Subjects were administered several memory tasks (e.g., recall of grocery list items, names and faces, prose paragraph, phone numbers, and an unrelated word list) and completed a memory complaint questionnaire before training, immediately following training, and 2 weeks following the completion of training. Memory training improved the memory performance of the elderly but had only minimal effect on memory complaint. In contrast, changing the subjects' expectations about their cognitive capabilities decreased complaints about memory but had little effect on memory performance.

Contrary to our findings, Zarit, Gallagher, and Kramer (1981) found that both memory training and noncognitive personal effectiveness training had similar effects in reducing subjective memory complaint and enhancing memory performance in the elderly. The differential findings of their study and ours may be due to variations in the personal competence interventions used, length of training and testing intervals, and differences in the memory evaluation tasks. Zarit, Gallagher, and Kramer's (1981) personal growth intervention addressed interpersonal skills rather than stereotypes about cognitive aging. Further, memory was assessed repeatedly, providing both memory-training and personal effectiveness subjects with many opportunities for practice on the recall tasks. From examination of both studies, it appears that combining memory skills training and expectancy change would provide the most effective intervention.

Social Interactive Aspects of Memory Training

Several recent reviews of memory-training programs for the elderly (Cavanaugh et al., 1989; Greenberg & Powers, 1987; West, 1989) have suggested that maintenance and generalization of training, which have been weak in most previous research (e.g., Scogin & Bienias, 1988), should be addressed directly. Noncognitive factors, such as expectations about memory performance and beliefs in stereotypes concerning memory deterioration with age, may play an important role in the maintenance and generalization of memory training. Finding out that other older adults in a memory-training group are experiencing similar memory problems may be beneficial in breaking down concerns about age-related memory deterioration and in creating more realistic expectations about memory performance. Research has demonstrated that interpersonal skills training (Zarit, Gallagher, & Kramer, 1981), discussion of memory and personal problems, relaxation training (Schaffer & Poon, 1982), and lectures aimed at developing a positive attitude toward memory and aging (Hill, Sheikh, & Yesavage, 1987) can be as effective as memory strategy training for improving memory performance and decreasing memory concerns. Indeed, noncognitive, social factors may be critical for maintenance and generalization of memory strategy training.

Memory self-evaluation retraining (Cavanaugh et al., 1989), following attribution-retraining methods suggested by the models of Bandura (1982) and Weiner (1985), could be incorporated into memory improvement programs. Such training would address the elderly's memory concerns and make them aware that memory performance is never perfect, not even for younger adults, and that memory unfortunately seems to fail at the most inopportune times. Being comfortable with memory performance and believing that one's own performance is no different from others' may be crucial for maintaining memory competence into older adulthood.

Along with addressing self-evaluations of memory and beliefs in stereotypes about aging, the social interactive and social supportive aspects of memory-training groups should be examined more closely. In the context of such groups, older adults often develop new social contacts and may find a number of social reinforcements for improved memory performance. Group dynamics may create a cohesive, supportive reference group in which self-esteem is increased and improved memory performance is positively reinforced. Token reinforcement for correct memory performance can improve both immediate and remote memory of nursing home residents, suggesting that maintaining and increasing memory demands on the elderly can have positive consequences (Langer, Rodin, Beck, Weinman, & Spitzer, 1979). Memory demands could be introduced into the group dynamics so that members could prompt and reinforce each other for improved memory skills, providing the scaffolding needed to support improved memory performance.

It is interesting to note that with community-dwelling elderly, the majority of memory improvement studies have used group training (e.g., Zarit, Cole, & Guider, 1981; Zarit, Gallagher, & Kramer, 1981) rather than individual instruction, which has been used more frequently with brain-injured patients (e.g., Camp & Schaller, 1989). One successful individualized intervention program that was self-paced and self-administered did include a social support mechanism in which the experimenter telephoned each participant weekly to assess progress and to provide support (Flynn, 1986; Scogin & Bienias, 1988; Scogin, Storandt, & Lott, 1985). Since most programs have used group training, it would be beneficial to compare the effectiveness of the group approach with the individual approach to see what aspects of each were responsible for success. Group training may simply be a matter of convenience for the researcher, but group effects, such as quality and quantity of member interactions and social supports, deserve examination. Moreover, strategies designed to increase maintenance and generalization of memory training could be built on the social support aspect of the group, much like the successful techniques used by Alcoholics Anonymous and Weight Watchers. Of course, such techniques would need to be tailored to the memory domain and concerns of the elderly.

To briefly summarize the adult literature, social interaction, by its very nature, requires memory performance for adequate interaction to occur. Even casual conversation requires participants to remember the thread of a discussion and to recall relevant information to contribute. Each of us has developed a number of techniques for dealing with these demands and for improving our memory abilities in such situations. Memory performance also has implications for evaluations of self and others, with repeated successes and failures contributing to the development of memory reputations and stereotypes about group memory performance. Moreover, elderly adults are generally assumed to have deteriorating memory abilities, and men and women are believed to remember certain types of information better than others. Furthermore, prospective memory is assumed to reflect the value of the social interaction on which it is based. Given the importance of memory reputations and the existence of stereotypes about memory performance, people often use memory contrivances to enhance social interaction and self-presentation.

Memory-training programs have been somewhat successful in improving the memory performance of elderly adults, but maintenance and generalization of these effects have been limited. Addressing memory concerns directly in these programs has successfully reduced memory complaints and has led to more realistic memory performance goals. These may be the keys to improving maintenance and generalization of memory training. Moreover, social support in memory-training programs warrants more thorough investigation and may provide the key for improved maintenance and generalization.

Conclusions

It is obvious from the foregoing discussion that social interaction plays an important role in both memory development and memory improvement. While social interaction has received more attention in the child cognitive development literature, perhaps due to renewed interest in Vygotsky's (1978; 1981) theory, examples of the continuing influence of social factors on memory performance and improvement are evident throughout the age span. Future memory development research should address such areas as children's self-evaluations of memory performance, their attributions about memory, and their stereotypes concerning memory performance. These topics have received only minimal attention in the adult memory improvement literature and would greatly benefit from a developmental perspective. It is apparent that children's attitudes and beliefs could influence their memory performance and development in ways similar to those found with adults.

Similarly, memory improvement research with older adults should address the social interactive mechanisms used by adults to facilitate memory. Certainly everyday adult memory expectations, such as a comparison of job, social, and other memory demands, and the strategies used to meet these expectations should be examined across the course of adulthood. For adults learning new tasks, such as driving a car, working on a new computer program, or meeting colleagues in a new job situation, examination of memory strategies employed and the role of interactions with more skilled peers would benefit from Vygotsky's (1978; 1981) ideas about the importance of social interaction. Indeed, Guttentag (1985) has shown that comparing children's strategy deficiencies and older adults' memory failures provides a useful and parsimonious view of memory functioning across the life span. A blending of questions and concerns from the child memory development and adult memory improvement areas would greatly improve our understanding of how social interaction and memory performance interact throughout the course of development.

References

Ashmead, D.H., & Perlmutter, M. (1980). Infant memory in everyday life. In M. Perlmutter (Ed.), *New directions for child development: Children's memory* (Vol. 10, pp. 1-16). San Francisco: Jossey-Bass.

Bandura, A. (1982). Self-efficacy mechanism in human agency. *American Psychologist*, *37*, 122-147.

Bee, H.L. (1967). Parent-child interaction and distractibility in 9 year old children. *Merrill-Palmer Quarterly*, *13*, 175-190.

Bee, H.L., Van Egeren, L.F., Streissguth, A.P., Nyman, B.A., & Leckie, S.L.

(1969). Social class differences in maternal teaching strategies and speech patterns. *Developmental Psychology*, *1*, 726-734.
Belmont, J.M. (1989). Cognitive strategies and strategic learning: The socio-instructional approach. *American Psychologist*, *44*, 142-148.
Belmore, S.M., & Hubbard, M.L. (1987). The role of advance expectancies in person memory. *Journal of Personality and Social Psychology*, *53*, 61-70.
Best, D.L. (in press). Inducing children to generate mnemonic organizational strategies: An examination of longterm retention and materials. *Developmental Psychology*.
Best, D.L., Hamlett, K.W., & Davis, S.W. (in press). Memory complaint and memory performance in the elderly: The effects of memory-skills training and expectancy change. *Applied Cognitive Psychology*.
Best, D.L., & Ornstein, P.A. (1986). Children's generation and communication of mnemonic organizational strategies. *Developmental Psychology*, *22*, 845-853.
Bird, J.E., & Berman, L.S. (1985). Differing perceptions of mothers, fathers, and children concerning children's academic performance. *The Journal of Psychology*, *119*, 113-124.
Borkowski, J.G., Milstead, M., & Hale, C. (1988). Components of children's metamemory: Implications for strategy generalization. In F.E. Weinert & M. Perlmutter (Eds.), *Memory development: Universal changes and individual differences* (pp. 73-100). Hillsdale, NJ: Erlbaum.
Camp, C.J., & Schaller, J.R. (1989). Epilogue: Spaced-retrieval memory training in an adult day-care center. *Educational Gerontology*, *15*, 641-648.
Carpenter, G.C., Tecce, J.J., Stechler, G., & Friedman, S. (1968). Differential visual behavior to human and humanoid faces in early infancy. *Merrill-Palmer Quarterly*, *14*, 25-46.
Cavanaugh, J.C. (1989). The importance of awareness in memory and aging. In L.W. Poon, D.C. Rubin, & B.A. Wilson (Eds.), *Everyday cognition in adulthood and late life* (pp. 416-436). Cambridge: Cambridge University Press.
Cavanaugh, J.C., Grady, J.G., & Perlmutter, M. (1983). Forgetting and use of memory aids in 20- and 70-year olds' everyday life. *International Journal of Aging and Human Development*, *24*, 271-277.
Cavanaugh, J.C., & Morton, K.R. (1988). Older adults' attributions about everyday memory. In M.M. Gruneberg, P.E. Morris, & R.N. Sykes (Eds.), *Practical aspects of memory: Current research and issues* (Vol. 1, pp. 207-214). Chichester: Wiley.
Cavanaugh, J.C., Morton, K.R., & Tilse, C.S. (1989). A self-evaluation framework for understanding everyday memory aging. In J.D. Sinnott (Ed.), *Everyday problem solving: Theory and applications* (pp. 266-284). New York: Praeger.
Cavanaugh, J.C., & Perlmutter, M. (1982). Metamemory: A critical examination. *Child Development*, *53*, 11-28.
Ceci, S.J., Bronfenbrenner, U., & Baker, J.G. (1988). Memory in context:

The case of prospective remembering. In F.E. Weinert & M. Perlmutter (Eds.), *Memory development: Universal changes and individual differences* (pp. 243- 256). Hillsdale, NJ: Erlbaum.

Cole, M., Gay, J., Glick, J.A., & Sharp, D.W. (1971). *The cultural context of learning and thinking*. New York: Basic Books.

Cole, M., & Scribner, S. (1977). Developmental theories applied to cross-cultural cognitive research. *Annals of the New York Academy of Sciences, 285*, 366-373.

Crawford, M., Herrmann, D.J., Holdsworth, M.J., Randall, E.P., & Robbins, D. (1989). Gender and beliefs about memory. *British Journal of Psychology, 80*, 391-401.

Cutler, S.J., & Grams, A.E. (1988). Correlates of self-reported everyday memory problems. *Journal of Gerontology, 43*, 582-590.

Day, J.D., French, L.A., & Hall, L.K. (1985). Social influences on cognitive development. In D.L. Forrest-Presley, G.E. MacKinnon, & T.G. Waller, (Eds.), *Metacognition, cognition, and human performance: Theoretical perspectives* (Vol. 1, pp. 33-56). New York: Academic Press.

DeCasper, A.J., & Fifer, W.P. (1980). Of human bonding. *Science, 208*, 1174-1176.

Dixon, R.A., & Hultsch, D.F. (1983). Structure and development of metamemory in adulthood. *Journal of Gerontology, 38*, 682-688.

Eber, J.T. (1989). Young and older adults' appraisal of memory failures in young and older adult target persons. *Journal of Gerontology, 44*, 170-175.

Eber, J.T., Szuchman, L.T., & Rothberg, S.T. (1990). Everyday memory failure: Age differences in appraisal and attribution. *Psychology and Aging, 5*, 236-241.

Ellis, S., & Rogoff, B. (1982). The strategies and efficacy of child vs. adult teachers. *Child Development, 53*, 730-735.

Fagan, J.F., III. (1979). The origins of face perception. In M.H. Bornstein & W. Kessen (Eds.), *Psychological development from infancy* (pp. 83-113). Hillsdale, NJ: Erlbaum.

Fivush, R. (1984). Learning about school: The development of kindergartners' school scripts. *Child Development, 55*, 1697-1709.

Fivush, R., Hudson, J., & Nelson, K. (1984). Children's long term memory for novel events: An exploratory study. *Merrill-Palmer Quarterly, 30*, 303-316.

Flynn, T. (1986). *Memory performance, memory complaint, and self-efficacy in older adults*. Unpublished doctoral dissertation, Washington University, St. Louis, MO.

Gentry, M., & Herrmann, D.J. (1990). Memory contrivances in everyday life. *Personality and Social Psychology Bulletin, 16*, 241-253.

Germond, J.L. (1986). *Does maternal assistance influence young children's planning in maze problems?* Unpublished master's thesis, University of Utah, Salt Lake City.

Greenberg, C., & Powers, S.M. (1987). Memory improvement among adult learners. *Educational Gerontologist, 13*, 263-280.

Greenfield, P.M. (1984). A theory of the teacher in the learning activities of everyday life. In B. Rogoff & J. Lave (Eds.), *Everyday cognition* (pp. 117-138). Cambridge, MA: Harvard University Press.

Guttentag, R.E. (1985). Memory and aging: Implications for theories of memory development during childhood. *Developmental Review*, *5*, 56-82.

Hastie, R. (1980). Memory for behavioral information that confirms or contradicts a personality impression. In R. Hastie, T.M. Ostrom, E.B. Ebbesen, R.S. Wyer, D. Hamilton, & D.E. Carlston (Eds.), *Person memory: The cognitive basis of social perception* (pp. 155-177). Hillsdale, NJ: Erlbaum.

Herrmann, D.J. (1989). *Memory improvement*. Gaithersburg, MD: Cognitive Associates.

Herrmann, D.J., & Crawford, M. (1990). *Gender-linked differences in everyday memory performance*. Unpublished manuscript.

Herrmann, D.J., & Searleman, A. (1990). The new multi-modal approach to memory improvement. In G. Bower (Ed.), *Advances in learning and motivation* (pp. 175-205). New York: Academic Press.

Hess, R.D., & Shipman, V.C. (1965). Early experience and the socialization of cognitive modes in children. *Child Development*, *36*, 869-886.

Hess, R.D., & Shipman, V.C. (1967). Cognitive elements in maternal behavior. In J. P. Hill (Ed.), *Minnesota Symposium on Child Psychology* (Vol. 1, pp. 57-81). Minneapolis: University of Minnesota Press.

Hill, R.D., Sheikh, J.I., & Yesavage, J. (1987). The effect of mnemonic training on perceived recall confidence in the elderly. *Experimental Aging Research*, *13*, 185-188.

Intons-Peterson, M., & Fournier, J. (1986). External and internal memory aids: When and how often do we use them? *Journal of Experimental Psychology: General*, *115*, 267-280.

Istomina, Z.M. (1975). The development of voluntary memory in preschool-age children. *Soviet Psychology*, *13*, 5-64.

Kahn, R.L., Zarit, S.H., Hilbert, N.M., & Niederehe, G. (1975). Memory complaint and impairment in the aged: The effects of depression and altered brain function. *Archives of General Psychiatry*, *32*, 1569-1573.

Kontos, S. (1983). Adult-child interaction and the origins of metacognition. *Journal of Educational Research*, *77*, 43-54.

Lachman, M.E., & Jelalian, E. (1984). Self-efficacy and attributions for intellectual performance in young and elderly adults. *Journal of Gerontology*, *39*, 577-582.

Langer, E.J., Rodin, J., Beck, P., Weinman, C., & Spitzer, L. (1979). Environmental determinants of memory improvement in late adulthood. *Journal of Personality and Social Psychology*, *37*, 2002-2013.

Lave, J. (1977). Tailor-made experiments and evaluating the intellectual consequences of apprenticeship training. *Quarterly Newsletter of the Laboratory of Comparative Human Cognition*, *2*, 1-3.

Macfarlane, A. (1978). What a baby knows. *Human Nature*, *1*, 74-81.

Meacham, J.A. (1988). Interpersonal relations and prospective remembering. In M.M. Gruneberg, P.E. Morris, & R.N. Sykes (Eds.), *Practical aspects of memory: Current research and issues* (Vol 1, pp. 354-359). Chichester: Wiley.

Meacham, J.A., & Kushner, S. (1980). Anxiety, prospective remembering, and performance of planned actions. *Journal of General Psychology, 103*, 203-209.

Miller, S.A. (1988). Parents' beliefs about children's cognitive development. *Child Development, 59*, 259-285.

Moely, B.E., Hart, S.S., Santulli, K., Leal, L., Johnson, T., Rao, N., & Burney, L. (1986). How do teachers teach memory skills? *Educational Psychologist, 21*, 55-71.

Moore, J.J., Mullis, R.L., & Mullis, A.K. (1986). Examining metamemory within the context of parent-child interactions. *Psychological Reports, 59*, 39-47.

Nelson, K. (1978). How young children represent knowledge of their world in and out of language. In R. Siegler (Ed.), *Children's thinking: What develops?* Hillsdale, NJ: Erlbaum.

Nelson, K., & Gruendel, J. (1981). Generalized event representations: Basic building blocks of cognitive development. In M. Lamb & A. Brown (Eds.), *Advances in developmental psychology* (Vol. 1, pp. 131-158). Hillsdale, NJ: Erlbaum.

Ninio, A. (1983). Joint book reading as a multiple vocabulary acquisition device. *Developmental Psychology, 19*, 445-451.

Noesjirwan, J., Gault, U., & Crawford, J. (1983). Beliefs about memory in the aged. *Journal of Cross-Cultural Psychology, 14*, 455-468.

Palincsar, A.S., & Brown, A.L. (1984). Reciprocal teaching of comprehension-fostering and comprehension-monitoring activities. *Cognition and Instruction, 1*, 117-175.

Poon, L.W. (1985). Differences in human memory with aging: Nature, causes, and clinical implications. In J.E. Birren & K.W. Schaie (Eds.), *Handbook of the psychology of aging* (2nd ed. pp. 427-462). New York: Van Nostrand Reinhold.

Popkin, S.J., Gallagher, D., Thompson, L.W., & Moore, M. (1982). Memory complaint and performance in normal and depressed older adults. *Experimental Aging Research, 8*, 141-145.

Price, G.G. (1984). Mnemonic support and curriculum selection in teaching by mothers: A conjoint effect. *Child Development, 55*, 659-668.

Rabbitt, P.A. (1981). Talking to the old. *New Society, 55*, 140-141.

Radziszewska, B. & Rogoff, B. (1988). Influence of adult and peer collaborators on the development of children's planning skills. *Developmental Psychology, 24*, 840-848.

Rapaport, D. (1942). *Emotions and memory*. Baltimore, MD: Williams & Wilkins.

Ratner, H.H. (1980). Memory demands and the development of young children's memory. *Child Development, 55*, 2173-2191.

Reige, W.H. (1982). Self-report and tests of memory aging. *Clinical Gerontologist*, *1*, 23-35.

Rogers, T.B., Kuiper, N.A., & Kirker, W.S. (1977). Self-reference and the encoding of personal information. *Journal of Personality and Social Psychology*, *35*, 677-688

Rogoff, B. (1990). *Apprenticeship in thinking: Cognitive development in social context*. New York: Oxford University Press.

Rogoff, B., & Gardner, W. (1984). Adult guidance of cognitive development. In B. Rogoff & J. Lave (Eds.), *Everyday cognition: Its development in social context* (pp. 95-116). Cambridge, MA: Harvard University Press.

Saxe, G.B., Guberman, S.R., & Gearhart, M. (1987). Social processes in early number development. With commentary by R. Belman and by C.M. Massey & B. Rogoff; with reply by G.B. Saxe, S.R. Guberman, & M. Gearhart. *Monographs of the Society for Research in Child Development*, *52* (2, Serial No. 216).

Schaffer, G., & Poon, L.W. (1982). Individual variability in memory training with the elderly. *Educational Gerontology*, *8*, 217-229.

Schneider, W. (1985). Developmental trends in the metamemory-memory behavior relationship: An integrative review. In D.L. Forrest-Pressley, G.E. MacKinnon, & T.G. Waller (Eds.), *Cognition, metacognition, and human performance* (Vol. 1., pp. 57-109). New York: Academic Press.

Scogin, F. (1985). Memory complaints and memory performance: The relationship reexamined. *Journal of Applied Gerontology*, *4*, 79-89.

Scogin, F., & Bienias, J.L. (1988). A three-year follow-up of older adult participants in a memory-skills training program. *Psychology and Aging*, *3*, 334-337.

Scogin, F., Storandt, M., & Lott, L. (1985). Memory-skills training, memory complaint, and depression in older adults. *Journal of Gerontology*, *40*, 562-568.

Sharp, D., Cole, M., & Lave, C. (1979). Education and cognitive development: The evidence from experimental research. *Monographs of the Society for Research in Child Development*, *38* (5, Serial No. 178).

Shatz, M., & Gelman, R. (1973). The development of communication skills: Modifications in the speech of young children as a function of listener. *Monographs of the Society for Research in Child Development*, *38* (5, Serial No. 152).

Skinner, B.F. (1938). *The behavior of organisms*. New York: Appleton-Century-Crofts.

Snow, C. (1972). Mothers' speech to children learning language. *Child Development*, *43*, 549-565.

Somerville, S.C., Wellman, H.M., & Cultice, J.C. (1983). Young children's deliberate reminding. *The Journal of Genetic Psychology*, *143*, 87-96.

Verdonick, F. (1988a). Co-construction cognitive challenges: Their emergence in social exchanges. In J. Valsiner (Ed.), *Child development within culturally structured environments: Social co-construction and environmental guidance in development* (Vol. 2, pp. 111-136). Norwood, NJ: Ablex.

Verdonick, F. (1988b). Reconsidering the context of remembering: The need for a social description of memory processes and their development. In F.E. Weinert & M. Perlmutter (Eds.), *Memory development: Universal changes and individual differences* (pp. 257-271). Hillsdale, NJ: Erlbaum.

Vygotsky, L.S. (1978). *Mind in society: The development of higher psychological processes* (M. Cole, V. John-Steiner, S. Scribner, & E. Souberman, Eds. & Trans.). Cambridge, MA: Harvard University Press.

Vygotsky, L.S. (1981). The genesis of higher mental functions. In J.V. Wertsch (Ed.), *The concept of activity in Soviet psychology* (pp. 144-188). Armonk, NY: Sharpe.

Weiner, B. (1985). An attributional theory of achievement motivation and emotion. *Psychological Review, 92*, 548-573.

Weisberg, J.A., & Paris, S.G. (1986). Young children's remembering in different contexts: A reinterpretation of Istomina's study. *Child Development, 57*, 1123-1129.

Wertsch, J.V. (1979). From social interaction to higher psychological processes: A clarification and application of Vygotsky's theory. *Human Development, 22*, 1-22.

Wertsch, J.V., & Stone, C.A. (1978). Microgenesis as a tool for developmental analysis. *Quarterly Newsletter for the Laboratory of Comparative Human Cognition, 1*, 8-10.

West, R.L. (1989). Planning practical memory training for the aged. In L.W. Poon, D.C. Rubin, & B.A. Wilson (Eds.), *Everyday cognition in adulthood and late life* (pp. 573-597). Cambridge: Cambridge University Press.

Williams, J.E., & Best, D.L. (1982). *Measuring sex stereotypes: A thirty nation study*. Beverly Hills, CA: Sage.

Williams, S.A., Denney, N.W., & Schadler, M. (1983). Elderly adults' perception of their own cognitive development during the adult years. *International Journal of Aging and Human Development, 16*, 147-158.

Wilson, B.A., & Moffat, N. (1984). *Clinical management of memory problems*. Rockville, MD: Aspen Systems.

Wood, D., Bruner, J.S., & Ross, G. (1976). The rôle of tutoring in problem solving. *Journal of Child Psychology and Psychiatry, 17*, 89-100.

Wood, D.J., Wood, H., & Middleton, D. (1978). An evaluation of four face-to-face teaching strategies. *International Journal of Behavioral Development, 2*, 131-147.

Wyer, R.S., & Srull, T.K. (Eds.). (1984). *Handbook of social cognition* (Vols. 1-3). Hillsdale, NJ: Erlbaum.

Wyer, R.S., & Srull, T.K. (1986). Human cognition in its social context. *Psychological Review, 93*, 322-359.

Zarit, S.H., Cole, K.D., & Guider, R.L. (1981). Memory training strategies and subjective complaints of memory in the aged. *The Gerontologist, 21*, 158-164.

Zarit, S.H., Gallagher, D., & Kramer, N. (1981). Memory training in the community aged: Effects of depression, memory complaint, and memory performance. *Educational Gerontology*, *6*, 11-27.

Zelinski, E.M., Gilewski, M.J., & Thompson, L.W. (1980). Do laboratory tests relate to self-assessment of memory ability in the young and old. In L.W. Poon, J.L. Fozard, L.S. Cermack, D. Arenberg, & L.W. Thompson (Eds.), *New directions in memory and aging: Proceedings of the George A. Talland Memorial Conference* (pp. 519-544). Hillsdale, NJ: Erlbaum.

Attention and Memory Improvement

Dana J. Plude

"Attention is the stuff that memory is made of, and memory is accumulated genius" - James Russell Lowell (cited in Aiken, 1896)

One purpose of the present chapter is to question the extent to which memory complaints center on the appropriate mechanism. I contend that a substantial percentage of memory complaints has little to do with memory but rather is due to faulty attentional allocation. This position can be defended on grounds that the human information-processing system is limited in its capacity to process environmental information, thus necessitating selective processing of stimuli available to an observer. Should selective processing be misdirected away from a source of to-be-remembered information, that information will not be encoded into the memory system and will subsequently be unavailable to retrieval efforts, not because of faulty storage or retrieval but instead due to a failure to register the information in the first place. Such a fate may await not only information that is unattended by failure to direct processing resources accordingly but also information that is not fully attended due to its habitual, or automatically processed, nature. In other words, information that is processed automatically is unlikely to be recalled at a later time because of insufficient attentional allocation at initial exposure.

A second purpose of this chapter is to formalize a linkage between attention and memory, which borrows heavily from others' work in mainstream cognitive psychology. This formalization integrates research involving attention, levels of processing, automaticity, and memory and goes further to address their status in aging. The intent is to present a model of information processing that not only accommodates extant findings in the cognitive aging literature but also suggests prescriptions for overcoming attentional impairments that may be mistaken for memory deficits.

The third, and final, purpose of this chapter is to review attention-training programs that have been proposed previously. Unfortunately, there have been no systematic, experimental long-term (or even short-term) follow-ups to these programs to determine their efficacy, thus their implications for memory theory and memory improvement are dubious. Suggestions for rectifying this state of affairs are offered in the concluding section of this chapter.

Two vignettes exemplify the connection between attention and memory as conceptualized in the present chapter and aid in identifying the kinds of "memory" failure to which an attentional analysis seems appropriate. The first vignette involves leaving one's home but worrying if the kitchen stove has been turned off. Being uncertain about the appliance's status, a return trip home is made only to find that, in fact, the stove is shut off. Often this situation is characterized by some sort of self-deprecating remark concerning the inability to remember what has (or has not) been done.

The second vignette involves the inability to recall a recently made acquaintance's name. Recognition verifies that the acquaintance has been introduced, but it fails to yield the acquaintance's name. Again, such apparent retrieval failures are often accompanied by a complaint about faulty memory function. The common thread in both experiences, however, is that a failure to selectively attend to the target information (an act in the former instance, a fact in the latter) may lie at the core of the alleged memory failure.

These two vignettes represent the kinds of memory complaints that are most commonly lodged by older adult audiences to whom I lecture on the topic of memory and aging. Before initiating my lectures, I request members in the audience to list on index cards the kinds of memory problems and interests they have and wish me to address. Of the several hundred responses accumulated to date, by far the highest percentage of complaints concerns remembering facts, and within this domain, remembering people's names is the hands down winner (comprising some 90% of complaints!). The second most common complaint involves remembering whether or not routine activities have been performed (comprising some 20% of the responses overall). I recognize that this sampling is far from representative of the kinds of memory complaints that may be lodged in a clinical setting wherein the incidence of dementing diseases and other disorders of cognition is much larger and in which the degree of memory impairment has far greater significance for everyday functioning. Nevertheless, these data fairly represent the kinds of memory phenomena that are of interest (if not concern) to community-dwelling, senior-citizen-center-attending elderly adults and, I suspect, to other age groups of adults as well. Thus it is the role of attention in remembering (and performing) everyday actions and in the intentional learning of new information that is the focus of the present chapter. I begin by outlining the definition of attention adopted for the present purposes and then turn to a consideration of the link between attention and memory. Having laid this foundation, I next consider age effects on attention and memory and then move on to memory-training programs that address the role of attention. In concluding, I attempt to describe the kind of attention-training research that is needed to move the field forward.

Varieties of Attention

Attention is a multidimensional construct as witnessed by a variety of indicators. For example, a survey of the 13 published volumes of the series entitled *Attention and Performance*, indicates a span of topics ranging from sensory detection to text comprehension. Similarly, Parasuraman and Davies' (1984) text entitled *Varieties of Attention*, comprised no fewer than eight chapters, each devoted to a different aspect of attention. The impressive diversity of attention defies a single encompassing definition. Perhaps that is why William James (1892) observed that "we all know what attention is" and went on to discuss various aspects of attention in his classic text that introduced psychology in America near the turn of the century. Despite its diversity, attention can be conceptualized as comprising three fundamental dimensions: alertness, capacity, and selectivity (e.g., Posner & Boise, 1971). The alertness dimension concerns the ability to maintain concentration over time, such as in a vigilance task in which an observer monitors some repetitive event in order to detect an infrequent target event (e.g., Parasuraman, 1984). The capacity dimension is analogous to the energy available to sustain an electric appliance, such as a computer, with decreasing capacity (an electrical "brown out") yielding progressively poorer performance (e.g., Kahneman, 1973). Finally, the selective dimension of attention concerns the ability to restrict information processing to a relevant source (or sources) of information while ignoring or filtering out irrelevant sources (e.g., Johnston & Dark, 1986). The selective aspect of attention recognizes that humans are limited in their ability to process multiple sources of information simultaneously. James (1892) discussed this limitation in considering the focal nature of attention as: the taking possession by the mind, in clear and vivid form, of one out of what seem several simultaneously possible objects or trains of thought. Focalization, concentration, of consciousness are of its essence. It implies withdrawal from some things in order to deal more effectively with others (pp. 403-404). This conceptualization of the selective aspect of attention forms the cornerstone of intentional memory as it proposes attention as a kind of gatekeeper to consciousness (Reason, 1984b).

Clearly the different dimensions of attention described above are interdependent; however, the focus of the present chapter centers on the selective aspect of attention. Further, I restrict consideration to the relationship between explicit, or intentional, memory and the selective processing of external environmental information, thus excluding that aspect of attention that focuses on internal processes (e.g., thoughts, ideas, emotions) as well as other aspects of attention relating to the other dimensions discussed above.

Having identified selectivity as the relevant dimension of attention, it is important to consider its role in performance and memory. Selective attention is critical for performing optimally in a wide variety of situations, such as driving an automobile and operating precision equipment. Even the simple act of listening to a friend's conversation requires selective attention insofar as that message must be discriminated from the host of other acoustic signals in the environment. In addition to its involvement in performing various everyday activities, selective attention also plays a key role in everyday memory. The ability to recall some desired fact presupposes that the fact is stored in memory. Although it is possible that some facts may be encoded into memory "automatically," that is, without conscious awareness or selective processing, it is more often the case that purposeful memories, those that we intend to remember at some later time, require selective attention in order to be encoded for successful retrieval later on. It is to this linkage between selective attention and explicit memory that discussion now turns.

Attention and Memory

At the outset, it is important to acknowledge that formal linkages between selective attention and memory are generally uncommon in the mainstream cognitive literature. A clear exception to this rule, however, is recent work by Reason (1979, 1984a, 1984b), Harris (1984), and others (see Harris & Morris, 1984, for review) on the topic of absent-mindedness and memory for actions. These efforts have rekindled some of James' (1892) earlier ideas on the attention-memory link. The common thread between the present linkage and these others is that attention is given a central role in the memory process. Indeed, selective attention can be conceived as *executive control* in the memory system, determining which inputs receive priority processing and which are ignored. Selection is a necessary (albeit insufficient) condition for explicit memory storage and (later) retrieval.

The conceptualization of selective attention as executive control relates to the model of memory introduced by Baddeley and associates (e.g., Baddeley, 1976; Baddeley & Hitch, 1974) in which the active part of memory consists of two slave systems (an articulatory loop and a visual-spatial scratch pad) dedicated to an executive control process that oversees the flow of information through the slave systems and other, relatively static components of the memory system (e.g., long-term memory). Although other models of memory also contain a control process of one sort or another (e.g., Atkinson & Shiffrin, 1968; Reason, 1984b), Baddeley's captures the essence of an intentional, consciously allocated, limited capacity process for selectively processing environmental inputs. Further, Wingfield and Stine (1989), among others, have argued for the selective aspect of attention as occupying an early position, that is, prior to memory, in a linear-processing model. Thus, attentional control exerts an early influence on to-be-remembered information by selecting that subset of external environmental information that is to be stored in and later retrieved from the explicit memory system.

Another important element of the attention-memory link is the assumption that executive control can be allotted in a continuous manner to input. That is, some inputs require the full capacity of the executive control to coordinate their progress through the information-processing system, while other inputs require relatively little (if any) of the executive control's capacity for their processing. Although such processing has usually been dichotomized as constituting either effortful or automatic processing, respectively, (e.g., Hasher & Zacks, 1979; Schneider & Shiffrin, 1977) it is probably more accurate to conceive of a continuum of processing with effortful and automatic processing falling at the end points (e.g., Kahneman, 1973). The importance of this assumption for the attention-memory link is apparent in considering the fate of inputs that are processed with relatively little attentional control compared with those that are processed with attentional effort. James recognized this aspect of attention in commenting that "habit diminishes the conscious attention with which our acts are performed" (1892, p. 139). Given that attentional control is necessary for encoding inputs into memory, then the more habitually a given input is processed, the less well that input should be recalled at a later time.

Fisk and Schneider (1984) engineered a laboratory-based study to examine just this relationship. In brief, subjects participated in various conditions that varied in their demand on executive control, with memory for certain words tested subsequent to participating in the different attention tasks. As shown in Figure 9.1, memory for the frequency of occurrence for test words varied directly with attentional involvement: Highest accuracy was found when attention was maximally allocated to the target words, and it was lowest when attention was misdirected from those words. In discussing this pattern of results, Fisk and Schneider (1984) argued that attentional control is necessary for modifying connections in long-term memory (and thereby yielding durable memory traces) and that automatic processing does not modify such connections (and thereby leaves virtually no trace to be detected later). The notion that executive control relates to explicit memory for everyday activities has been investigated by Reason and his associates (Reason, 1979, 1984a, 1984b; Reason & Lucas, 1984). Reason's conceptualization of the attention mechanism differs somewhat from the one outlined above but is similar in exerting its influence early in the sequence of processing by selecting the subset of activated nodes in long-term memory that are relevant for processing. Like Fisk and Schneider, Reason has argued that attentional control is a key determinant of memory performance. Reason has gone further to consider the role of attentional control in absent-mindedness and "slips of actions." Action slips occur when an unintended action is performed in lieu of an intended one, such as going upstairs into one's bedroom rather than into the bathroom to fetch a desired item. According to Reason, the momentary lapse of attentional control allows a routinized action to run itself off in response to some evoking stimulus in the environment. Carrying this logic further, it can be reasoned that memory for actions that are performed automatically should be poor, due to the withdrawal of executive control from their execution. For example, memory for turning off the kitchen stove, an action that may be performed automatically, should be quite poor, as exemplified in one of the vignettes introduced earlier.

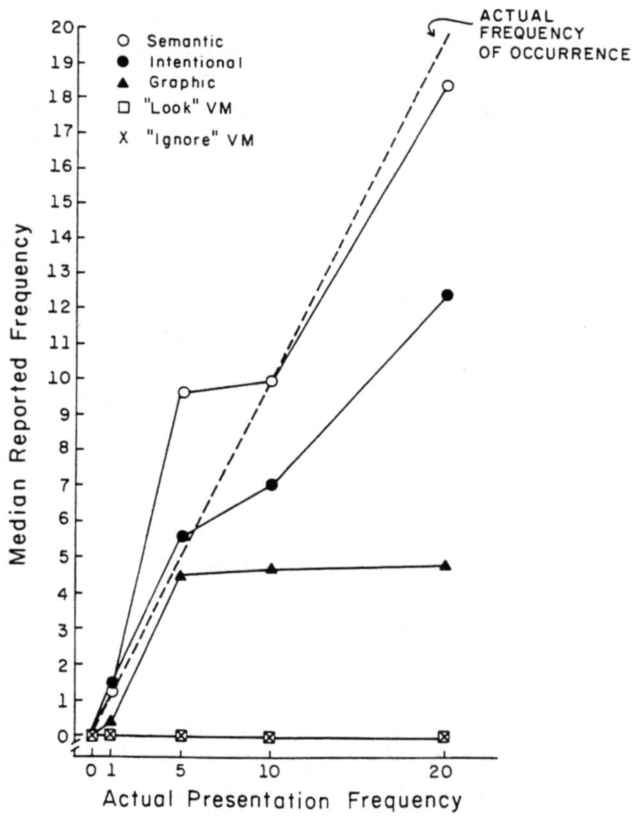

Figure 9.1. Word repetition estimates (ordinate) as a function of actual repetition rate (abscissa) for various levels of attention (VM = variably mapped). From "Memory as a Function of Attention, Level of Processing, and Automatization" by A.D. Fisk and W. Schneider, 1984, *Journal of Experimental Psychology: Learning, Memory, and Cognition, 10*, pp. 181-197. Copyright by the American Psychological Association. Reprinted by permission.

Although Reason's work is unique in addressing the attention-memory link explicitly in regard to everyday memory and performance, the applicability of various laboratory-based findings to everyday situations is readily apparent. Indeed, many investigators have explicitly linked empirical findings to aspects of performance in everyday life. For example, automobile driving has served as a popular topic for articulating the fundamental principles of selective attention (see, for example, Schneider & Shiffrin, 1977; Shiffrin & Schneider, 1977). The basic premise is that early on in learning to drive, much attention must be devoted selectivity to the component actions that constitute this complex task, such as finding the appropriate gear, coordinating accelerator and clutch in a standard shift car, and monitoring patterns of traffic activity. As component parts are automatized via consistent practice, less demand is placed on selective attention that frees the limited capacity processing system for engaging in other activities, such as carrying on a conversation with a passenger and the like. This reduction in attention demand with consistent practice generalizes beyond the laboratory and characterizes the development of skill in almost any domain (see Hoyer, 1985; Salthouse, 1984). The benefit of acquired automaticity is clear cut: Information processing is expedient and effortless. However, there is a cost of automatic performance as well: Habitual acts are resistant to modification and as such, may interfere with performance when the automatized activities are no longer appropriate. This latter scenario is exemplified when attempting to drive an unfamiliar car, especially if it is a foreign car in which the driver/passenger layout is reversed! Thus, automatization is a mixed blessing with regard to everyday performance.

The same conclusion applies to automatization with regard to everyday memory: It is a mixed blessing. As noted before, laboratory-based research has shown that memory for automatic performance is poorer than memory for effortful performance (e.g., Fisk & Schneider, 1984). Thus, the cost of automatization is a decreased memory for habitual acts that have been performed. Of course, the benefit of automatization has to do with the economy of habitual acts: They needn't be remembered (consciously) in order to be performed. It is important to recognize that attending to habitual acts not only disrupts those acts (as discussed by James, 1892) but also should yield a more durable memory trace for later retrieval (Reason, 1984b). Thus, disrupting automatic processing should be an effective means by which to reduce slips of action and bolster memory performance.

One way to account for the different patterns of recall for automatic versus effortful activities appeals to a "levels of processing" approach to memory (Craik & Lockhart, 1972; Craik & Tulving, 1975). In brief, this approach envisions memory as a by-product of the analysis performed on information encountered in the environment: A shallow level of analysis, that is, attending to physical features of a stimulus, yields an ephemeral memory trace, whereas a deep (semantic) level of analysis, that is, attending to the meaning of a stimulus, yields a durable memory trace. Executive control might be represented in the levels of processing framework by stipulating it as the mechanism that engages the encoding processes activated during initial orienting to selected inputs. In this view, automatic processing requires little, if any, executive control and thus would be expected to yield labile memory traces. Increasing the involvement of executive control, as required under effortful processing, would be expected to prompt a meaningful level of analysis that yields stable and enduring memory traces.

Aging, Attention, and Memory

As is the case in the mainstream cognitive literature, cognitive-aging research on selective attention (see Plude, 1990) and on explicit memory for facts and actions (see Kausler, 1985) has taken quite separate paths. Despite this divergence, there is a tendency in recent times to integrate the two bodies of research (e.g., Backman, 1989; Plude & Murphy, in press) in order to yield a comprehensive picture of cognitive aging. The present analysis follows this recent trend.

The assessment of selective attention involves comparing patterns of performance trade-offs in various conditions that place different demands on selective processing. Considerable cognitive-aging research has been devoted to this enterprise with the magnitude of age effects depending on an impressive variety of factors all of which concern the complexity of the task being performed in conjunction with the level of skill and/or practice of the individual. In a nutshell, it is commonly found that age decrements in performance increase proportionally with the complexity of the task being performed. We have demonstrated this pattern of age effects in various studies involving "visual search," in which an individual searches for a specific target (usually an alphanumeric character) in a visual display that varies in the number of nontargets (other characters), with performance assessed on both speed and accuracy of target identification (see Plude & Hoyer, 1985, for review). In such a task, age decrements increase with increasing emphasis on selective attention. Data from a recent experiment (Plude & Doussard-Roosevelt, 1989) are illustrative of this point and are summarized in the upper half of Figure 9.2. Note that the demand on selective attention increases from the left to the right panel of the figure. This kind of outcome is often visualized in a graph that plots the performance of older adults (typically in their 60s) against the performance of young adults (typically in their 20s) with the relationship being described in large part by a linear function with a slope somewhere in the vicinity of 1.5 to 2.0 or so (e.g., Cerella, 1985, 1990; Salthouse, 1985). The lower half of Figure 9.2 depicts this "complexity" relationship for the visual search data given in the upper half of the figure and indicates that the complexity of a task is a critical determinant of age decrement. Thus as the task imposes greater demand on the performance of young adults (i.e., increments in response time along the abscissa), the elderly exhibit a proportionally greater demand on performance (i.e., increments in response time along the ordinate). Such complexity effects (Birren, 1965) can be accounted for by an age reduction in the selectivity of attention (e.g., Plude, 1990; Plude & Doussard-Roosevelt, 1990).

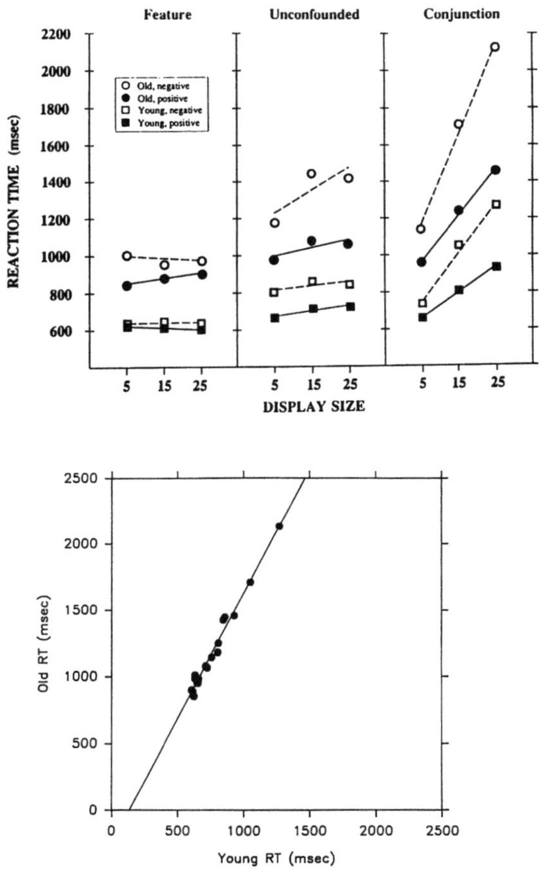

Figure 9.2. Age differences in visual search as a function of the demand on selective attention (upper figure) and as a function of task complexity (lower figure). (Note the lower figure replots the data shown in the upper figure).

In addition to the voluminous literature on age effects on selective attention, there also has been considerable research devoted to age effects on explicit memory within the levels of processing framework (see, for example, Craik & Byrd, 1982; Craik & Simon, 1980). In general, it has been found that elderly adults tend to engage a more shallow level of analysis compared with younger adults, which impairs the older adult's performance in laboratory-based memory tasks. Craik and his associates have ascribed these findings to an age reduction in attentional resources supporting the encoding process. The greater degree of "environmental support" required by the elderly to produce a level of memory performance commensurate with young adults has been taken as further evidence of diminished selectivity with increasing adulthood age (e.g., Backman, 1989). It is noteworthy that matching the level of analysis with the level of retrieval cues enhances the older adult's ability to recall information but does not eradicate the age deficit in memory test performance (e.g., Smith, 1980).

These two independent lines of investigation implicate age decrements in executive control as playing a central role in the alleged memory difficulties of elderly adults. Although I am aware of no research that has explicitly linked selective attention with memory performance in the elderly, the connection would seem to have adequate face validity to justify further scrutiny. Indeed, Graf, Tuokko, and Gallie (1990) recently argued with similar logic in accounting for the memory and performance deficits associated with Alzheimer's disease. Their main thesis was that attentional dysfunctions accompanying this and other forms of dementia provide a parsimonious explanation of a wide variety of deficits (including memory impairments) in demented elderly adults. Moreover, Guttentag (1985) presented a cogent argument in favor of an attention-based account of memory changes across the entire lifespan, although his argument focused on *attentional capacity* rather than its selective allocation. Nonetheless, even in the absence of the much needed experimental work on the selective attention-explicit memory link, there is sufficient basis for evaluating past memory-training programs that have emphasized an attentional training component.

Before moving to a consideration of attention training as a means by which to improve memory performance, it is important to briefly review research on expertise and the acquisition of skill as it relates to performance among elderly adults (e.g., Charness, 1989). This digression is important for establishing the trainability of elderly adults in light of the potential compensatory benefits of such training. Performance in skilled domains, such as typing (Salthouse, 1984) and chess (Charness, 1985), shows relatively little age impairment compared with performance in nonskilled domains. The acquisition of skill depends in large part on consistent practice, which reduces the demand on selective attention (Schneider & Shiffrin, 1977), which, in turn attenuates age decrements in performance (Hoyer & Plude, 1980, 1982). With regard to age differences in attention, it has been shown that consistent practice in a visual search task reduces or eliminates age decrements in performance (e.g., Madden & Nebes, 1980; Plude & Hoyer, 1981). Recent evidence suggests, however, that aging may compromise certain aspects of the consistent practice effect such that after extensive practice, age decrements remain (see Fisk, McGee, & Giambra, 1988). This may indicate that the ability to acquire expert levels of skill is impaired in later life. Nevertheless, it appears that previously acquired skill remains intact well into the late adulthood years and as such, provides a means by which the elderly can compensate for cognitive decrements (Charness, 1989). Further, that older adults exhibit benefit from consistent mapping procedures versus varied mapping procedures (despite their apparent inability to achieve full automaticity) bodes well for the success of attentional training programs intended to compensate for memory impairments.

Attention Training

Returning to the two vignettes introduced at the beginning of this chapter, we might question how to optimize the older adult's memory of habitual acts and recent acquaintances. Two suggestions derive from our review of selective attention research. In order to remember having performed an automatized act, the actor should endeavor to de-automatize it. This recommendation is based on the inverse relationship between automaticity (or habit) and memory described previously. One means by which to accomplish this, quite simply, is to speak aloud when committing the act: "I am turning off the stove now." In addition to disrupting the automated behavior (Reason, 1984b) this sort of overt statement forces attention to be devoted to the performance of the task, increasing the likelihood that it will be recalled later on. It is worth noting that the attention-attracting utility of such self-directed speech forms the cornerstone of "cognitive-behavioral therapy," which often has proven useful in modifying undesired (habitual?) behavior in clinical/intervention situations (e.g., Meichenbaum, 1977).

In order to increase the probability of retrieving a previously encountered fact, such as remembering a recent acquaintance's name, Cermak (1976) suggested four steps, the first of which has direct relevance to the present discussion. Cermak recommended that upon meeting a new acquaintance the following steps should be followed: (a.) Pay attention, (b.) repeat the name, (c.) elaborate on the name, and (d.) test yourself in the absence of the target person. Each of these steps involves devoting some attention to the act of remembering the new acquaintance. The 1st step clearly implicates selective attention by emphasizing the importance of attending to the relevant aspect of the environment, that is, the person's name.

Both of these recommendations hinge on a common theme: Information must be attended to be remembered. The central question remains, though, how to train attention to work in the service of memory. Many writers have suggested a variety of ways to train attention, but I could not find a single shred of evidence that any of these techniques has been investigated scientifically with reasonable follow-up work to determine their efficacy. Let me review several of the prescriptions I was able to find before suggesting the kind of work that I believe is necessary to advance attentional training beyond idle speculation.

Cermak (1976) certainly was not the first author to suggest that focused attention is a necessary prerequisite to adequate memory function. The earliest reference that I found was a volume written by Catherine Aiken who proffered that "the art of attentive listening...is more rare than of fluent speech" (1896, p. 46). Aiken placed emphasis squarely on "concentrated attention" and devoted nearly her entire text to describing various exercises intended to sharpen the ability to concentrate attention. One such exercise consisted of the following computations (to be performed mentally):

> Multiply 9 times 8, multiply by 32, subtract 4, add 200, square root, divide by 5, subtract 1/2, square it, multiply by 11, subtract 9, multiply by 25, add 1400, multiply by 10, cube root, add 8, divide by 4, cube it, multiply by 2, give the answer, 3456, in Roman numerals. (Aiken, 1896, pp. 56-67, Exercise 10)

According to Aiken, practicing this sort of exercise each day yields impressive gains in concentrated attention. She recommends that we "set aside 20 minutes every morning for mental training...[because] a boy will whittle his stick faster and easier with a sharp knife than with a dull one...and not begrudge the time spent at the grindstone" (Aiken, 1896, pp. 62-63). Although Aiken describes the impressive gains made by her students after undergoing this kind of intensive training, there are (not surprisingly) no formal statistics presented, nor are data even described! We are asked to take her word that "all that is embraced in the expression 'a good memory' [is]...attention"(Aiken, 1896, p. 74).

Another early entrant in the memory-training literature is Kleiser (1918) who also emphasized the power of "concentration." According to Kleiser, concentration involves "bringing your best mental powers to bear steadily and persistently upon a chosen subject" (1918, p. 3). He recognized that the ability to do so depends largely upon one's interest in the chosen subject and in this sense reflects James' (1892) idea that attentión varies directly with one's intrinsic interest in a topic. James suggested that "there is no such thing as voluntary attention sustained for more than a few seconds at a time... sustained voluntary attention is a repetition of successive efforts" (1892, p. 224). Kleiser seems sensitive to this notion, but like Aiken before him, there is no explicit recognition of, nor reference to, psychological writings (either by James or others) of the time. Nevertheless, Kleiser prescribes an eight step program for developing concentration:

1. Check every tendency to wander from your chosen subject.
2. Bring mental pressure to bear upon your chosen subject.
3. Learn to think in a straight line.
4. Enforce a difficult task on yourself each day.
5. Seek the best conditions for your work in concentration.
6. Have stated periods of rest from your mental work.

7. Cultivate sincerity, definiteness, and vigor of thought.
8. Form the habit of selective thinking.

Kleiser goes on to describe what might be called a "topic a day" lesson plan for training concentration, which essentially amounts to identifying a single topic that should be the focus of thinking for that particular day. Although there are (again) no formal data presented on this attention-training program, nor any statistical analyses of its merit, Kleiser's plan bears striking similarity to attention-training programs which arrived on the scene considerably after the "Cognitive Renaissance" of the mid-1960s.

Two of these more modern entrants have clear ties with the experimental cognitive psychology of the day (Cermak, 1976; West, 1985), and two others have more uncertain connections (Minninger & Dugan, 1988; Nideffer & Sharpe, 1978). Let me review very briefly the two nonexperimentally based recent entries first.

Nideffer and Sharpe (1978) introduced what they coined "attention control training (ACT)," which was derived in large measure from the first author's instruction in martial arts. According to this training program (which is described in three ACTs), "attention control is nothing more than being able to voluntarily direct your attention, to concentrate in ways that are consistent with the demands placed on you by your home, family, and job" (Nideffer & Sharpe, 1978, p. 21). The program recognizes that attention may either be focused or broad and directed toward internal or external events but like its predecessors, makes no explicit connection with the cognitive psychology of the time. The training program emphasizes the role of "centering," which is the ability to focus concentration on a single idea or input. The authors claim that complete centering renders the individual impervious to pain and capable of resisting the strongest of physical assaults. (In one section, they describe how the totally centered individual cannot be toppled by someone even twice his size!) However, the connection between this capability and later memory and retrieval is difficult to fathom. Again, like its predecessors, this program offers no data (nor analyses) of its short-term or long-term efficacy.

The other recent attention-training program having nonexperimental roots was introduced by Minninger and Dugan (1988). It is noteworthy for addressing the two aspects of memory/attention central to the present chapter. In Chapter 6 of their prescription on how to "make your mind work for you," the authors address selective attention with instructions on how to activate curiosity and imagination in service of better memory. They argue that the ability to remember new information rests largely on one's ability to pay attention to the information and relate it in creative ways to what one knows already. These notions have clear connections with principles of modern cognitive psychology, but there is no explicit recognition of it provided by the authors. Similarly, in Chapter 9, the authors discuss how to break old habits, but here the focus is more on habits of thinking (e.g., procrastination, compulsive ideation, etc.) rather than on memory for habitual acts, and the authors' prescriptions involve a behavioral shaping program for modifying unwanted habits.

In sum, these two relatively recent attention-training programs are not grounded in the principles of modern experimental cognitive psychology and as such, do not make explicit connections with the attention-memory link outlined above, despite their consideration of attention as an important component in remembering. In contrast to these programs are those that are embedded within cognitive psychology--or at least have their roots squarely planted in that literature--and to which discussion now turns. One might have suspected that these more recent entries, having the benefit of solid empirical research on attention, would constitute radical modifications beyond the attention-training programs introduced near the turn of the century. However, it would seem that little has changed as exemplified in the attention-training prescriptions offered by Laird Cermak (1976) and Robin West (1985).

Cermak (1976) suggested various means by which to enhance the selective aspect of attention, what he termed "focusing on material we want in our memory." He emphasized two parts of the puzzle, focusing on relevant information and detecting the relevant aspects of it. Although this program benefits from a more precise vernacular associated with the experimental cognitive psychology of the day, his prescriptions for honing attentional selectivity strike a familiar chord. For example, Cermak suggested that distractions should be minimized and that concentrated attention should be attempted for only relatively brief periods of time due to its effortful nature (see Kleiser's Points 6 and 7). Similar to the turn-of-the-century entrants, Cermak cites no empirical data (nor supportive analyses) to support his recommendations, though like his earlier counterparts, his prescriptions have intuitive appeal.

Of all the attention-training programs reviewed in this chapter, Robin West's (1985) is the only one explicitly tailored to elderly adults. West's contribution is unique not only in this regard but also in its explicit treatment of extant research in both mainstream experimental psychology and in cognitive aging. West is singular in integrating principles taken from these literatures into her training program as well as in providing a detailed appendix with source references. Having acknowledged the strong empirical base of West's work, let me turn to her prescriptions for attention training. West identifies two objects of attention that are consistent with the central themes of the present chapter: habitual acts and to-be-learned facts. She proposes that memory for habitual acts can be improved by increasing attentiveness. The prescription for increasing attentiveness involves: (a.) becoming more observant of one's own behavior, (b.) attending to behavior that is performed automatically, and (c.) remaining attentive in spite of interruptions. West proposes that memory for to-be-learned facts can be improved by increasing concentration. The prescription for increasing one's ability to concentrate involves: (a.) capturing attention, (b.) holding place during interruptions, (c.) eliminating distractions (both external and internal), (d.) setting deadlines, (e.) limiting the time period of concentration, (f.) establishing priorities, and (g.) increasing motivation.

Despite the fact that these prescriptions are grounded in experimental cognitive psychology and despite their intuitive appeal, West (1985) offers no evidence that these training procedures actually produce changes in memory performance. Among the few reference citations for this attention-training battery, West cites the text on managing clinical memory disorders edited by Wilson and Moffat (1984). In that volume, the contribution by Wood (1984) is most relevant in that it addresses the management of attention disorders in brain-injured subjects. However, at its outset, the author acknowledges that what are offered are ideas and suggestions rather than hard data on the efficacy of attention-training procedures! This is not to say that Wood's contribution is insubstantial. Indeed, it is quite the contrary. Like West's integration of mainstream experimental work with prescriptions for the elderly, Wood couches his suggestions firmly in current cognitive theory. He argues that "attentional retraining" has three-fold importance: (a.) efficient processing is the cornerstone of adequate memory and behavior, (b.) typical memory-training programs may not include important components of attentional behavior (e.g., short-term attention span and distractibility), and (c.) such training provides a point of departure for further development both of training techniques and their underlying rationale. Nevertheless, it is sad commentary that the efficacy of such attention training has been left unassessed.

Clearly, what is sorely lacking in nearly a century's worth of speculation on the centrality of attention to memory function is a comprehensive assessment of the efficacy of attention-training programs. Given the advances in recent years in various recording instruments and methodologies (e.g., Reason & Lucas, 1984), it is now possible to determine adequate baseline measures of attention/memory function against which to compare performance during and subsequent to attention training. There remain, of course, substantial obstacles to determining time on task, the nature and frequency of feedback, and other components of self-monitored performance, but the need for even the roughest assessment of attention-training efficacy offsets the limitations accompanying whatever compromises (methodological and otherwise) that might be made in engineering such a follow-up study. Whereas Wood (1984) recommended a multisystems approach that recognizes various aspects of the attention construct for the clinical management of attention disorders, I recommend a more focused approach that centers on the selective aspect of attention because of its centrality to memory function, not only in elderly adults but in all age groups. Indeed, the centrality of selective attention may generalize across species as suggested by Aiken (1896) in a quotation attributed to Sir Charles Darwin:

> "When an animal trainer desires to select monkeys for training, he will take a number of them, range them about him, and then attempt to attract their

attention by various performances. Those whose attention cannot be secured are cast out as unfit for training." (p. 15)

If nothing else, formulating an attention-training evaluation program focusing on selective attention provides a reasonable starting point for evaluating the efficacy of attention-training programs. Further, this starting point would begin to fill the void currently standing between attention-training programs and theories of memory and memory improvement.

Endnote 1

Preparation of this chapter was facilitated by National Institute on Aging Grant #1R01-AG08060.

I wish to thank Doug Herrmann for his many discussions of the ideas put forth in this chapter as well as for his generosity in sharing with me many antiquated references contained in his personal library. Alas, the shortcomings of the present work cannot be attributed to him; that is a burden I alone must shoulder.

References

Aiken, C. (1896). *Methods of mind training: Concentrated attention and memory*. New York: Harper & Brothers.

Atkinson, R.C., & Shiffrin, R.M. (1968). Human memory: A proposed system and its control processes. In K.W. Spence & J.T. Spence (Eds.), *Advances in the psychology of learning and motivation research and theory* (Vol. 2, pp. 89-195). New York: Academic Press.

Backman, L. (1989). Varieties of memory compensation by older adults in episodic remembering. In L.W. Poon, D.C. Rubin, & B.A. Wilson (Eds.), *Everyday cognition in adulthood and late life* (pp. 509-544). Cambridge: Cambridge University Press.

Baddeley, A. (1976). *The psychology of memory*. New York: Basic Books.

Baddeley, A., & Hitch, G. (1974). Working memory. In G.H. Bower (Ed.), *The psychology of learning and motivation* (Vol. 8, pp. 47-90). New York: Academic Press.

Birren, J.E. (1965). Age changes in speed of behavior: Its central nature and physiological correlates. In A.T. Welford & J.E. Birren (Eds.), *Behavior, aging and the nervous system* (pp. 191-216). Springfield, IL: Charles C. Thomas.

Cerella, J. (1985). Information processing rates in the elderly. *Psychological Bulletin*, *98*, 67-83.

Cerella, J. (1990). Aging and information processing rate. In J.E. Birren &

K.W. Schaie (Eds.), *Handbook of the psychology of aging* (3rd ed., pp. 201-221). New York: Van Nostrand Reinhold.

Cermak, L.S. (1976). *Improving your memory*. New York: McGraw-Hill.

Charness, N. (1985). Aging and problem-solving performance. In N. Charness (Ed.), *Aging and human performance* (pp. 225-259). London: Wiley.

Charness, N. (1989). Age and expertise: Responding to Talland's challenge. In L.W. Poon, D.C. Rubin, & B.A. Wilson (Eds.), *Everyday cognition in adulthood and late life* (pp. 437-456). Cambridge: Cambridge University Press.

Craik, F.I.M., & Byrd, M. (1982). Aging and cognitive deficits: The role of attentional resources. In F.I.M. Craik & S.E. Trehub (Eds.), *Aging and cognitive processes* (pp. 191-211). New York: Plenum.

Craik, F.I.M., & Lockhart, R.S. (1972). Levels of processing: A framework for memory research. *Journal of Verbal Learning and Verbal Behavior*, *11*, 671-684.

Craik, F.I.M., & Simon, E. (1980). Age differences in memory: The roles of attention and depth of processing. In L.W. Poon, J.L. Fozard, L.S. Cermak, D. Arenberg, & L.W. Thompson (Eds.), *New directions in memory and aging* (pp. 95-112). Hillsdale, NJ: Erlbaum.

Craik, F.I.M., & Tulving, E. (1975). Depth of processing and the retention of words in episodic memory. *Journal of Experimental Psychology: General*, *104*, 268-294.

Fisk, A.D., McGee, N.D., & Giambra, L. (1988). The influence of age on consistent and varied semantic-category search performance. *Psychology and Aging*, *3*, 323-333.

Fisk, A.D., & Schneider, W. (1984). Memory as a function of attention, level of processing, and automatization. *Journal of Experimental Psychology: Learning, Memory, and Cognition*, *10*, 181-197.

Graf, P., Tuokko, H., & Gallie, K. (1990). Attentional deficits in Alzheimer's disease and related dementias. In J.E. Enns (Ed.), *The development of attention: Research and theory* (pp. 527-544). Amsterdam: Elsevier.

Guttentag, R.E. (1985). Memory and aging: Implications for theories of memory development during childhood. *Developmental Review*, *5*, 56-82.

Harris, J.E. (1984). Remembering to do things: A forgotten topic. In J.E. Harris & P.E. Morris (Eds.), *Everyday memory, actions, and absent-mindedness* (pp. 71-92). London: Academic Press.

Harris, J.E., & Morris, P.E. (1984). *Everyday memory, actions, and absent-mindedness*. London: Academic Press.

Hasher, L., & Zacks, R.T. (1979). Automatic and effortful processes in memory. *Journal of Experimental Psychology: General*, *108*, 356-388.

Hoyer, W.J. (1985). Aging and the development of expert cognition. In T.M. Shlechter & M.P. Toglia (Eds.), *New directions in cognitive science* (pp. 69-87). Norwood, NJ: Ablex.

Hoyer, W.J., & Plude, D.J. (1980). Attentional and perceptual processes in the study of cognitive aging. In L.W. Poon (Ed.), *Aging in the 1980's: Psychological issues* (pp. 227-238). Washington, DC: American Psychological Association.

Hoyer, W.J., & Plude, D.J. (1982). Aging and the allocation of attentional resources in visual information processing. In R. Sekuler, D. Kline, & K. Dismukes (Eds.), *Aging and human visual function* (pp. 245-263). New York: Alan R. Liss.

James, W. (1892). *Psychology (Briefer Course)*. New York: Holt.

Johnston, W.A., & Dark, V.J. (1986). Selective attention. *Annual Review of Psychology*, *37*, 43-75.

Kahneman, D. (1973). *Attention and effort*. Hillsdale, NJ: Erlbaum.

Kausler, D.H. (1985). Episodic memory: Memorizing performance. In N. Charness (Ed.), *Aging and human performance* (pp. 102-141). London: Wiley.

Kleiser, G. (1918). *How to improve mental power*. New York: Funk and Wagnalls.

Madden, D.J., & Nebes, R.D. (1980). Aging and the development of automaticity in visual search. *Developmental Psychology*, *16*, 377-384.

Meichenbaum, D. (1977). *Cognitive-behavior modification: An integrative approach*. New York: Plenum Press.

Minninger, J., & Dugan, E. (1988). *Make your mind work for you*. Emmaus, PA: Rodale Press.

Nideffer, R.M., & Sharpe, R.C. (1978). *A.C.T.: Attention control training*. New York: Simon & Schuster.

Parasuraman, R. (1984). Sustained attention in detection and discrimination. In R. Parasuraman & D.R. Davies (Eds.), *Varieties of attention* (pp. 243-271). Orlando, FL: Academic Press.

Parasuraman, R., & Davies, D.R. (Eds.). (1984). *Varieties of attention*. Orlando, FL: Academic Press.

Plude, D.J. (1990). Aging, feature integration, and visual selective attention. In J.E. Enns (Ed.), *The development of attention: Research and theory* (pp. 467-487). Amsterdam: Elsevier.

Plude, D.J., & Doussard-Roosevelt, J.A. (1989). Aging, selective attention, and feature integration. *Psychology & Aging*, *4*, 98-105.

Plude, D.J., & Doussard-Roosevelt, J.A. (1990). Aging and attention: Selectivity, capacity and arousal. In E.A. Lovelace (Ed.), *Aging and cognition* (pp. 97-133). Amsterdam: Elsevier.

Plude, D.J., & Hoyer, W.J. (1981). Adult age differences in visual search as a function of stimulus mapping and information load. *Journal of Gerontology*, *36*, 598-604.

Plude, D.J., & Hoyer, W.J. (1985). Attention and performance: Identifying and localizing age deficits. In N. Charness (Ed.), *Aging and human performance* (pp. 47-99). London: Wiley.

Plude, D. J., & Murphy, L.J. (in press). Attention and everyday memory. In R.L. West & J.D. Sinnott (Eds.), *Everyday memory and aging: Current research and methodology*. New York: Springer-Verlag.

Posner, M.I., & Boise, S.J. (1971). Components of attention. *Psychological Review, 78*, 391-408.

Reason, J. (1979). Actions not as planned: The price of automatization. In G. Underwood & R. Stevens (Eds.), *Aspects of consciousness* (Vol. 1, pp. 67-89). London: Academic Press.

Reason, J. (1984a). Absent-mindedness and cognitive control. In J.E. Harris & P.E. Morris (Eds.), *Everyday memory, actions, and absent-mindedness* (pp. 113-132). London: Academic Press.

Reason, J. (1984b). Lapses of attention in everyday life. In R. Parasuraman & D.R. Davies (Eds.), *Varieties of attention* (pp. 515-549). New York: Academic Press.

Reason, J., & Lucas, D. (1984). Using cognitive diaries to investigate naturally occurring memory blocks. In J.E. Harris & P.E. Morris (Eds.), *Everyday memory, actions, and absent-mindedness* (pp. 53-70). London: Academic Press.

Salthouse, T.A. (1984). Effects of age and skill in typing. *Journal of Experimental Psychology: General, 113*, 345-371.

Salthouse, T.A. (1985). Speed of behavior and its implications for cognition. In J.E. Birren & K.W. Schaie (Eds.), *Handbook of the psychology of aging*, (2nd ed., pp. 400-426). New York: Van Nostrand Reinhold.

Schneider, W., & Shiffrin, R.M. (1977). Controlled and automatic human information processing: I. Detection, search, and attention. *Psychological Review, 84*, 1-66.

Shiffrin, R.M., & Schneider, W. (1977). Controlled and automatic human information processing: II. Perceptual learning, automatic attending, and a general theory. *Psychological Review, 84*, 127-190.

Smith, A.D. (1980). Age differences in encoding, storage, and retrieval. In L.W. Poon, J.L. Fozard, L.S. Cermak, D. Arenberg, & L.W. Thompson (Eds.), *New directions in memory and aging* (pp. 23-45). Hillsdale, NJ: Erlbaum.

West, R. (1985). *Memory fitness over 40*. Gainesville, FL: Triad.

Wilson, B.A., & Moffat, N. (1984), *Clinical management of memory problems*. Rockville, MD: Aspen.

Wingfield, A., & Stine, L. (1989). Modeling memory processes: Research and theory on memory and aging. In G.C. Gilmore, P.J. Whitehouse, & M.L. Wykle (Eds.), *Memory, aging, and dementia* (pp. 4-40). New York: Springer-Verlag.

Wood, R.I. (1984). Management of attention disorders following brain injury. In B.A. Wilson & N. Moffat (Eds.), *Clinical management of memory problems* (pp. 148-170). Rockville, MD: Aspen.

Memory in Context: A Case Study of "Bubbles P.," A Gifted but Uneven Memorizer

Stephen J. Ceci, Michelle DeSimone, and Sarah Johnson

It is commonly believed by laypersons that memory is a singular, "trait-like" attribute, one which operates with a uniform efficiency across most of the life course. Some individuals are thought to be endowed with excellent "all-around" memories whereas others are seen as pervasively forgetful. Friends are classified as "having a great memory" or as "totally absent-minded" as though such labels reflect something as enduring and transcontextual about them as their social security numbers.

Scientific support for this lay view of a singular memory system comes from both psychometric and information-processing analyses. Concerning the former, the most widely used individual intelligence tests (the Wechsler series) and occupational screening batteries (the General Aptitude Test Battery) contain one or more subtests designed to assess memory, for example, Digit Span and Coding. It would be of little use if such subtests told us only about a person's memory for digits presented auditorially at a 1-second rate or for symbol-number correspondences of visually presented materials. The presumption, of course, is that such tests tell us something of interest about other forms of remembering, too. Because the memory system is seen as singular and operable at the same level of efficiency in all domains, any single test of memory is considered to be a test of all memory. In addition to these common assessments of memory found on IQ and employment tests, numerous other memory tests have been developed by psychometric researchers and are used for a variety of neuropsychological assessment and vocational advising purposes (e.g., the Johnson O'Connor Vocational Aptitude Battery, the Halstead-Reitan Neuropsychological Profile). Again, the presumption by those who develop and administer these tests is that there is something that exists within the individual that is called their memory and that although this may be comprised of different components, all of them operate with equivalent efficiency across task and stimulus domains. If this were not the case, then these test developers would need to assess memory in various contexts and with different types of stimuli and paradigms before any inference could be drawn about one's memory. It would be of little use to purveyors and consumers of memory tests if mnemonic aptitude was shown to be labile and dependent on aspects of the testing context, including the materials and procedures employed.

Factor analytic studies of information-processing tasks provide another source of support for the view that memory is a singular entity that operates on diverse material and procedures with uniform efficiency. In this literature, one finds the existence of a "memory factor" that appears invariant across tasks and samples. Countless factorists have reported a memory factor in their solutions, even though they use different tasks, materials, and samples (Horn, Donaldson, & Engstrom, 1981; Humphreys, 1962). In addition, this memory factor has been validated as an important source of cognitive differences among subjects. For example, Hunt (1985) has found that high verbal college students differ from low verbal college students (those from the top and bottom quartiles of the Verbal SATs) in their retrieval speed of overlearned lexical codes from long-term memory. This memory difference is thought to be a source of a wide range of cognitive differences between high and low verbal subjects. Similar processing differences have been found in developmental studies, in which younger children generally require more time to access the contents of their memories than older children (Kail, 1990). Again, it would be of little interest if cognitivists limited their conclusions about high and low verbal subjects' access speeds (or about age differences in encoding rates) to the specific task materials and procedures that comprised their studies. The presumption, of course, is that these tasks reflect the efficiency of a singular memory system and therefore provide a benchmark for all forms of remembering.

From Singularity to Modularity

Recently, it has been suggested that the memory system is comprised of many modules and self-contained subsystems (e.g., explicit vs. implicit systems) that have evolved to handle different types of material, modalities, levels of conscious awareness, and semantic representations (e.g., Reber, 1990; Tulving, 1989). According to this view, someone can be good at remembering one type of material but not another, a finding supported by Wilding and Valentine's (1988) data on memory across domains. In their study, they found that individuals who were good at one type of memory task (e.g., facial recognition) were often unremarkable at others (e.g., digit span). If memory in one context does not predict memory in another context, what are the implications for the way memory is assessed and for efforts to improve it? Below we provide some tentative answers.

In this chapter we shall argue that memory does *not* operate with uniform efficiency across stimulus and task domains. Being good at remembering one thing often has no implication for remembering other things. Efforts to improve memory must, therefore, focus on task specific methods and processes, a suggestion advanced by Herrmann and his colleagues in recent years (Herrmann, Rea, & Andrzejewski, 1988).

The Contextual Nature of the Memory System

A major achievement of the cognitive science revolution has been to succeed in describing memory at a reduced level of understanding, that is, at the level of molecules and synaptic connections that sum impulses and information arriving from various input sites in the neuroarchitecture. However, this focus on the operation of isolated parts of the memory system may miss an essential feature of "memorial compensation." Instances of this compensation can be seen in the case of individuals who suffer from deficits in visual memory, but who, whenever possible, offset these deficits through a reliance on auditory coding. (That is, it is possible to code stimuli in either modality, and a stimulus that would normally be coded visually can also be coded auditorially, or vice versa.) Thus, the efficiency of operation of the social, biological, and cognitive systems are differentiated by aspects of the remembering context, such as encoding modality. Without taking into account the context of remembering, one is hard-pressed to explain many everyday memory phenomena, such as the classic Reicher-Wheeler effect. This effect, wherein words can be recognized faster than the letters that comprise them, has been interpreted as an instance in which context influences the operation of components (Ankrum & Palmer, 1989).

The Minds of Experts: A Window to the Normal World

In this paper, we extend the view that memory is context specific by focusing on an individual with an exceptional memory. The study of individuals with exceptional memories has occupied a venerable niche in 20th century psychology ever since the reports by Binet and Muller of the mental calculators Diamandi, Ruckel, and Inaudi (see Brown & Deffenbacher, 1985). Although these men were best known for their mental calculations, they also exhibited exceptional memories. For instance, Inaudi had a digit span that Binet reported to be 42 digits, and Ruckel could commit 60 digits to memory in approximately 4 minutes. Brown and Deffenbacher have reviewed this early work, describing several individuals who seem to have been overshadowed by the best known study of a mnemonist, Luria's subject named Sherashevski, or simply S (Luria, 1968). We will come back to S and the others later.

We acknowledge at the outset the many interpretative hazards of relying on the performance of exceptional individuals to make claims about the way memory operates in the general population. However, used in conjunction with more systematic research with representative samples, studies of expertise can shed light on normal cognitive development (e.g., Chi, Glaser, & Rees, 1982). This is exactly the approach we have taken in our own work, with the study of experts supplementing, rather than replacing, our work with larger, more representative samples.

The Study of S

Luria (1968) met S in the 1920s and studied him for almost 30 years. S, who came from Soviet Georgia, had studied music and worked briefly as a journalist before becoming a professional mnemonist. By any standard, S's memory was truly exceptional. He claimed to perceive colors and synesthesia associated with words, and he could vividly recall dialogues verbatim, even after many years. Fifteen years after presentation, he could spontaneously recall tables of random digits and lists of nonsense syllables. Luria reported that S found it so difficult to forget names, faces, and certain other types of information that he suffered from some emotional difficulties because of it. Accounts of S's peculiar form of memory can still be found in many texts on memory.

The Study of A.C. Aitken

In the early 1960s the British psychologist, I.M.L. Hunter, conducted a series of interviews and tests with the scholar, A.C. Aitken (Hunter, 1962). Aitken, a professor of mathematics, had extraordinary recall for mathematical and numerical material, English and Latin verse, and autobiographical events. When asked by Hunter to recall a list of 25 unrelated words he'd been tested on 27 years earlier, Aitken was able to recall all 25 in their proper order within the space of several hours. Exceptional as this might be, Aitken really excelled at recalling material that had meaning and interest for him. Hunter concluded that Aitken's ability to discern properties and patterns of materials that interested him enabled him to organize information into complex conceptual maps.

The Study of VP

Since Luria's detailed description of S (1968), four additional mnemonists have been systematically studied. Hunt and Love (1972) studied VP, a Seattle man who could play up to seven games of chess simultaneously while blindfolded, and who could play up to 60 correspondence games without consulting written records. VP had been a graduate student in history at the University of Washington, although he did not complete his degree. On tests of digit recall, he reached a span of approximately 16 digits after five practice trials.[1] VP reported that he did this by associating the digits with meaningful information. Like Luria's S, he was able to correctly reproduce a 48-digit matrix after 6 minutes of study.

On tests of verbal recall, VP was equally exceptional. One indication of his verbal prowess was his memory of the verbs and nouns in Bartlett's famous story *The War of the Ghosts*. Hunt and Love (1972) compared his recall of this material with that of the best control subject they had studied (a computer science graduate student). Six weeks following the presentation of *The War of the Ghosts*, the best control subject recalled 31% of its verbs and 33% of its nouns. In contrast, VP recalled 57% and 61% of the nouns and verbs, respectively.

The Study of SF and DD

In the past decade, the Skilled Memory Project at Carnegie-Mellon University has produced two men capable of impressive feats of memory, SF and DD. Both of these men were successful track and cross-country athletes on the intercollegiate level. Both learned through extensive practice how to transform digits into meaningful track records, using a combination of ample track knowledge and some personal mnemonics. Although DD's digit span at his first session was exactly average for college students (number of digits = 8), he was able to increase it to 106 digits after 4.5 years of training (Staszewski, 1989). He learned much of his method from his predecessor in the Skill Training Project, SF, who could recall more than 80 digits himself.

The Study of Rajan

The fourth modern study of a mnemonist is an ongoing project at the Universities of Minnesota and Kansas State (Fox, 1989; Thompson, Cowan, Frieman, Mahadevan, & Vogl, 1990; Thompson, Mahadevan, Frieman, Vogl, & Cowan, 1990). The mnemonist, "Rajan," has been studied for nearly a decade and has provided data on the long-term recall of materials encountered over 9 years ago. Rajan is an Indian man who attended graduate school in biopsychology. His IQ is described as "comparable to that of a typical US student at a good college" (Fox, 1990). Rajan has been reported to be able to memorize huge strings of digits, provided he is given ample time to commit the material to memory. For example, he has been able to report the value of *pi* to the 31,811th place! "Tests of Rajan's recall of random digit matrices, ranging in size from 4 x 4 to 16 x 16, reveal virtually no forgetting. It makes no difference if he is tested for an entire matrix or a single row, column, or diagonal. Furthermore, it does not matter if the testing is immediate or weeks later, or if the original presentation is visual or auditory" (Fox, 1989). When it comes to remembering digits, Rajan is indeed exceptional, and yet, his memory for other types of materials has been unremarkable, prompting his examiners to conclude that his memory performance is content or material specific. Indeed, Rajan is reported to achieve dramatically different levels of proficiency, depending upon the type of material to be learned (Fox, 1989; Thompson, Cowan, Frieman, Mahadevan, & Vogl, 1990).

The Case of Bubbles P.

We begin our own study by providing some background information about our subject, Bubbles P. Following this, we shall describe his performance on various psychometric and information-processing tasks we administered to him in an effort to better understand his mnemonic talent.

Background

Bubbles P. is a 33-year-old man who is married and lives in the Philadelphia area. He is a professional gambler and at the time of this study, earned whatever living he did from playing craps at both legal and illegal gaming clubs. When he is broke, Bubbles deals cards for money in illegal poker games and has occasionally worked in a liquor store owned by a relative. Although he claimed to have invented three gambling innovations (one of which was a telephone-wagering system that used credit cards and transmitted the lottery information over phone lines), it was apparent that none of these discoveries had brought Bubbles any sizeable wealth, despite his investment of substantial sums of money to obtain formal patents and to create engineering designs for them.

Bubbles was seen for a total of approximately 25 hours to complete the formal and informal assessment and video demonstrations that formed the basis of the conclusions we reach in this paper. To begin with, we tested Bubbles' ability to recall digits backward, something that we had been told he could do at an exceptional level.[2] Initially, we presented a series of digits at a 1-second rate and asked for immediate recall backward. Bubbles had no difficulty recalling between 15 and 20 digits backward, if tested immediately after the presentation of the final digit. His performance was equally good at presentation rates as fast as 250 milliseconds per digit. However, Bubbles could not recall digits if they were presented faster than this speed. He claimed that he needed time to organize the digits, and 250 milliseconds appeared to be his lower limit. The interpolation of a 30-second distractor task involving mental arithmetic reduced Bubbles' performance, on average, to 10 digits backward, which, while still exceptional by any standard, represents a significant decrement. The use of a visual distractor task that required Bubbles to keep track of a series of shapes in a preordained sequence also reduced his ability to recall digits backward to, on average, 12 digits.

Next, we asked Bubbles to recall the digits forward. He could do this at the same level as he could recall digits backward, that is, he could recall 15 to 20 digits forward. If asked to recall digits forward and then backward, he could also do this at the same level. It did not seem to matter to him in the slightest to be asked to recall the digits in one order, and then to recall them in reverse order. He volunteered to recall the digits in any order, including starting in the middle of the series and recalling first to the left, then to the right. Systematic testing confirmed he could do this, usually at an errorless rate, up to a maximum of 20 digits. Finally, Bubbles was able to recall any digit in the string if cued with its serial position, for example, "give me the 11th number from the left." It took him several seconds to do this, as he appeared to mentally count digits, rather than to have an immediate spatial readout.

The average number of forward digits that an adult can recall is seven (eight for college students), if the digits are presented too quickly to be recoded into meaningful chunks (Miller, 1956). The average number of digits that an adult can recall backward is only four. By such standards, Bubbles is indeed statistically exceptional. Moreover, he appears to be quite flexible, recalling digits in any order requested even if the request is made after he has already studied them. His memory remains exceptional even when auditory and visual distractor tasks are used and even when the rate of presentation is as fast as 250 milliseconds.

Unexpected recall tests of digit strings 30 minutes after their initial recall were almost always fruitless. However, when Bubbles was asked to retain the digits for later recall, he was usually able to do this at his original level. For example, on 19 out of 24 of these delayed trials, Bubbles was able to correctly recall the original string of 18 digits with, on average, one reversal of a contiguous pair of digits per string. Based on the Johnson-O'Connor test of digit recall, Bubbles' ability to recall digits forward and backward places him squarely in the top .001% of the population of adults. Our next question is, "How does he do this?"

In the few cases of exceptional memories that have been systematically studied, a variety of mnemonics and recoding tricks have been reported. VP (Hunt & Love, 1972), for example, used a number of recoding tricks, as did Staszewski's (1989) track runner. "The mnemonics were devices for recoding by row; for example, storing a row as a date, then asking himself what he was doing on that day" (Hunt & Love, 1972, p. 246).

We quickly ruled out any obvious tricks or recoding strategies for Bubbles, other than his self-reported attempt to segregate the stream of digits into groups of two, three, or four when they were first presented to him (e.g., chunking the string 361839702428655910473 into the following triads: 361, 839,

702, 428, 655, 910, 473). Although we are unable to verify his claim that he has read only two books in his life--one being a self-help manual to stop smoking--it is unlikely from what we know about him that he has ever read any books on memory training. None of his performances belied the use of published mnemonics. This study of his ability to recall digits backward is the first time that such a skill has been systematically evaluated in the scientific literature. This unusual skill would seem to require additional mental resources over what is needed to recall digits forward. To probe Bubbles' ability to recall digits backward, we administered a series of information-processing tasks that were developed by ourselves and others to help isolate various processing stages.

Word-Number Paired Associates Test

After Hunt and Love's study of VP (1972), we gave Bubbles several short-term and long-term serial recall tasks, among them the continuous paired associate task (Atkinson & Shiffrin, 1968). This task entails presenting a series of consonant-vowel-consonant (CVC) nonsense syllables that are paired with different double digits (e.g., CUH-95). Following lags of various lengths of intervening pairs of CVC-digits, we probed the digits that were associated with a particular CVC by presenting the CVC. Study time for each CVC-digit pair was self-paced, though Bubbles seldom required more than a few seconds to store it. Unlike VP, Bubbles did not perform well on this task. Using the Hunt and Love control subjects' data, we found that Bubbles was slightly poorer than the typical college student at all lags we tested. The information-processing parameters we derived form his performance suggest that Bubbles engages in serial searches through short term memory and then long term memory; his latency to report is a linear function of the length of the intervening lag (and, by inference, a function of the increasing memory load created by the accumulating pairs).

Face and Word Recognition Tests

In order to assess Bubbles' other forms of memory, we gave him the Warrington face recognition test and the Warrington word recognition test. In the former task the subject is shown 50 black and white photographs and asked to remember them. Immediately following the presentation of the final photograph, subjects are presented 50 pairs of photographs and instructed that one out of each pair of photos was already seen by them. Bubbles did this task in a most peculiar fashion. Although the manual specifies administering the test at a 3-second rate for each photograph, Bubbles preferred a much faster rate of presentation. He correctly recognized 45 out of 50 of these photographs, placing him around the 75 percentile for his age group. He reported that he was good as "reading" faces because this was something that a poker or gin player must do well if he hopes to succeed.

Spatial Readout Memory

Several mnemonists were reportedly highly visual. Hunt and Love's (1972) VP had near eidetic imagery, as did Luria's (1968) S. These individuals were able to create exact spatial replicas of the digit matrices and then read them out from memory. While Bubbles appears to have this same type of spatial memory, it seems to be confined to numerical material as well as materials that can be transformed into numbers, such as playing cards (as discussed later). We gave him 14 trials of a computer game called *Repeat* in which the object is to reproduce a series of blinking lights in the exact order that they were illuminated. Although there are no norms for this task, we administered it to six adults, including four secretaries and two maintenance men. The mean for this group was 6, which represented the highest number of blinking lights presented in a series that they could reliably recall in three repeated trials. Bubbles' memory for the sequence of blinking lights was average for this group, despite his claim that he once reproduced a series of 20.

Luria's Digit Matrix Test

Next, Bubbles was given the classic matrix that Luria (1968) gave to S; Hunt and Love (1972) gave to VP; and Gordon, Valentine, and Wilding (1984) gave to their subject, TE. This matrix is shown in Table 10.1. We were especially interested in this task because of Bubbles' proficiency with numbers, and because it is one of the few tasks that allowed a direct comparison of him with well-known mnemonists. As can be seen in Table 10.2, Bubbles was indeed exceptional on this task but not in the same ways that S and VP had been. Bubbles required just over 7 minutes to study the 50-digit matrix before attempting to recall it. This was slightly longer than VP but much longer than S. Yet, once Bubbles had studied the matrix, he was able to recall it far faster than either of the other mnemonists. In particular, he was able to immediately identify specific numbers when cued by pointing to their corresponding empty cells in a blank matrix, and he was able to recall columns up and down far faster than either of the other mnemonists.

Table 10.1. Luria's 50-Digit Matrix.

6	6	8	0
5	4	3	2
1	6	8	4
7	9	3	5
4	2	3	7
3	8	9	1
1	0	0	2
3	4	5	1
2	7	6	8
1	9	2	6
2	9	6	7
5	5	2	0
X	0	1	X

Table 10.2. Comparison of Mnemonists' Time (in Seconds) Needed to Study and Recall Luria's Matrix of Digits.

	VP	*S*	*Bubbles P.*	*TE*	*Rajan**
Study time	390	180**	424	390	54
7 x 7 matrix					84
Recall					
Matrix forward	41.5	40	47/16	41.5	
Third column	58.1	80	50.6	58.1	11.3
Second column					
top to bottom	39.4	25	35.5	39.4	12.8
bottom to top	39.7	30	18	39.7	--
Matrix backward		--	--	27.2	--

**We report Rajan's performance on a 6 x 6 matrix, except where noted.*
***Approximate*

Table 10.2 shows two times for Bubbles to recall the entire matrix forward; the first time was longer, due to a misunderstanding. We asked him to point to each empty cell and say the digit that had corresponded to it in a slow enough rate that the cameraman could focus on it. So although it took him 47 seconds to recall the entire matrix this way, he was immediately able to recall it in only 16 seconds when unconstrained. The rapidity with which he could recall digits in any location, compared to the long time required by S and VP (c.f. Luria, 1968; Hunt & Love, 1972) strongly suggests that Bubbles had a spatial code that enabled him to read out digits in any location. This interpretation is supported by his own self-report; he claimed to "see" the matrix vividly. In contrast, the fact that S and VP required longer to recall a specific column than they took to recall the entire matrix suggests that they had verbally coded the digits and therefore needed to serially search through the entire matrix to locate specific digits.

It is curious that Bubbles did so much better on this task than he did on the word-digit association task. Of course, this task did not require any linguistic coding, and this may have been the stumbling block for Bubbles on the word-digit association task.

Playing Card Matrix Test

Next, we asked Bubbles to memorize a deck of cards (51 cards, actually, due to a missing card that went undetected until test time). The cards were arrayed in one of two formats: either five rows of nine cards each and the remaining six cards in the sixth row, or else seven rows of seven cards each and the remaining three cards (when a 52-card deck was used) in the eighth row. This exercise proved to be very interesting for several reasons that will be explained below.

First, although the 51-card matrix was similar to the 50-digit matrix, Bubbles spent less time studying it to achieve equivalent levels of recall. Immediately following studying the playing cards, he recalled the entire matrix backward and then forward without error. When asked to supply three specific cards that had corresponded to empty cells that he imagined (in other words, no empty matrix was supplied), he did so without error and usually within 3 seconds. This stands in stark contrast to his longer time requirement to specify digits.

Since the testing of Bubbles has occurred over a period of several months, we thought it might be interesting to re-present a playing card matrix to him that he had not seen in 6 weeks. When he entered the room and saw the matrix of playing cards he immediately exclaimed, "This is the same matrix I saw the last time!" When asked how he could tell, he said that the bottom row was the same as well the top left corner of cards. He was instructed to study it and inform us when he had committed it to memory. He did this in just over 3 minutes. This represented a savings of over 3 minutes from his average study time, based on a half dozen similar matrices. He claimed not to have thought about this particular playing card matrix since recalling it 6 weeks earlier, and he had not been given any encouragement to rehearse and retain it when it was first presented along with several others in a series of tests. In a postexperimental interview, Bubbles insisted that he had not thought about the matrix in the intervening 6 weeks. He claimed that the bottom row "jumped out" at him, signaling it was a matrix he had seen before. It was quite surprising to witness this behavior, because it came at the end of approximately 3 hours of testing, during which he had seen many digits and playing cards. He was asked if he could recall the other matrix he had been shown (approximately 30 minutes earlier), and he at first said that he could not. Then he immediately began to recall the bottom row and the top row and a few other cards.

Word Memory Tasks

We gave Bubbles two types of word memory tasks. One was visually presented words that were presented with the instructions to evaluate each one as to whether it conjured pleasant or unpleasant feelings. (This was the Warrington Recognition Memory Test.) Bubbles examined 50 words and then immediately recognized the old words from their foils with perfect accuracy. When presented with 50 words auditorially, however, Bubbles was unable to recall more than 12 words on either trial. This is distinctly average performance.

Measures of General Intelligence

On the Wechsler Adult Intelligence Scale (WAIS), Bubbles scored in the average range. His profile was fairly even except for the Mental Arithmetic (scaled score of 13) and the Digits Frontward and Digits Backward, both of which he scored "off the scale," obtaining the highest scaled scores possible. All remaining IQ subtests were between 8 (Information and Vocabulary) and 12 (Picture Arrangement) scaled scores. Thus, Bubbles is *roughly* in the average range for all types of skills tapped by this test except for arithmetic and digit memory, for which his score is off the chart. On the Raven's Progressive Matrices (Raven, 1958), Bubbles scored slightly above average, and on the Differential Aptitude Test, his performance was in the low average range. Taken together, these results indicate that Bubbles is a man with a fairly average psychometric profile, who scored exceptionally well on digit memory and math and was poorest on measures of verbal ability. In contrast, the other two mnemonists who have been given comparable types of assessment (Staszewski's track runner DD and Hunt and Love's VP) scored well above average on such measures (VP's short form WAIS score was 136; Hunt & Love, 1972). Historically, however, many mnemonists have been reported to have low psychometric profiles (Brown & Deffenbacher, 1985).

A Contextualist Account of Memory

In contrast to the presumed singularity of memory, our case study, along with more systematic research we have been carrying out with representative samples of children and adults, suggests that memory is extremely context sensitive. Being good at remembering one kind of material has little implication for being good at remembering another kind: Recalling dance steps, for example, has no implication for recalling digits, and therefore, there is no correlation between them. In a sense, the case of memory is but a special instance of the more general case of context specificity in all of cognition. All forms of cognitive performance--from the most basic processes involved in encoding and scanning to the more molar forms of problem solving--are responsive to contextual alterations. Elsewhere we have reviewed the findings that support this statement, and have concluded that:

> The root metaphors that imbue positivist world views of science might be described, in general, as the "world as a machine" and, in the particular topic under discussion, as the "mind as a telephone switchboard or a digital computer." Contextualism, on the other hand, has as its dominant metaphor the ever-changing sociohistorical, cultural, and social milieu in which cognition unfolds. It is manifestly a non-mechanistic world view even though it accepts that regularities of nature can be identified amidst the swirling tides of change. Jaeger and Rosnow (1988) make a crucial distinction between contextualism on the one hand and situationalism and interactionism, on the other. In the latter two approaches context is viewed as something adjunctive to the act, whereas contextualist accounts elevate context to a constituent of the act. Situationalism and interactionism, they note...regard context as a synonym for "environmental stimuli" that determine a behavioral response. For contextualists, the context is an integral part of human actions, to be sure. An act cannot be said to have an identity apart from the context that constitutes it; neither can a context be said to exist independently of the act to which it refers. (Ceci, 1990, p. 155)

Thus, a contextualist perspective on individual differences in memory has certain characteristic features. It emphasizes the ecological dependency of structures that support remembering, as well as their plurality and spontaneity. Individuals participate in the construction of their own memory development by virtue of altering their contexts and being altered by them (Ceci & Bronfenbrenner, 1991). An implication of such a world view is that those of us who study individual differences in memory need to be sensitive to what our experiments are doing to our subjects and, consequently, what strategies they are adopting to surmount our efforts, a point also made by Jaeger and Rosnow (1988).

As one example of how this approach can lead to a different, more "restless" view of the human memory system, consider some recent findings that we reported at a scientific meeting. Subjects were asked to identify simple stimuli that were tachistoscopically presented at brief durations, followed by (a variable) interstimulus interval (ISI) and a patterned mask. Encoding of simple stimuli, of course, is one of the most basic and earliest components of the human memory system. What gets remembered must have first gotten encoded, at least at some level. A great deal of the psychometric thinking hinges on individual differences in encoding efficiency, with some individuals being seen as faster than others, and some researchers have reported that the heritabilities for encoding activity are quite high (see Ceci, 1990 for review). Subjects in our experiment encoded each type of stimulus (e.g., letters, digits, shapes, words, sounds) until the ISI became too brief for them to identify the stimuli. We then asked whether a rank ordering of an individual's encoding speed with one type of stimulus material (e.g., digits) was related to a rank ordering for the same individual with other types of stimuli (e.g., letters). The answer was negative. Being good at encoding one type of stimulus carried no implication for being good at encoding other types, and encoding speed was not related in any clear way to SAT scores. What distinguished those who were good at encoding a particular type of material was the knowledge they possessed about it. Even though all subjects were highly familiar with digits, some subjects represented a *9* as simply greater than 8 and less than 10, and as an odd number. Others represented it in additional characteristics, such as cardinality, roots, and so forth (Ceci & Cornelius, 1989). The more elaborate one's representation of a stimulus, the faster one encoded it. Subjects who had musical training and whose families sang a lot were usually better at auditory encoding than subjects without extensive musical training. Subjects with extensive baseball experience (including several minor league players) were faster at encoding dynamic shapes (twisting balls that were masked) than subjects without such training. If something as simple as identifying well-known, highly familiar letters, shapes, and digits can be differentiated by the context, then imagine how labile more complex mnemonic processes must be.

Getting back to Bubbles P., we see the extreme context-dependency of his memory in the fact that he excels primarily, though not exclusively, when the material to be remembered is of a numerical nature (including playing cards). We find it interesting that both Staszewski (1989) and the researchers who have studied Rajan (Fox, 1989; Thompson, Cowan, Frieman, Mahadevan, & Vogl, 1990) have also concluded that exceptional memory is highly context specific. Even Hunt and Love (1972) reported that VP was unable to recognize the face of Hunt's wife following several social encounters with her, thus calling into question the pervasiveness of his superiority.

A debate has taken place about the nature of exceptional memory, with Ericsson and his colleagues (Ericsson & Chase 1982; Ericsson & Faivre, 1988) forcefully arguing that it is due to the same mechanisms that are responsible for normal memory--only more of them. This "commonality" view is challenged by people like Neisser (1982) who asked, "Are these [exceptional memory] talents simply the upper extremes of continuous distributions of ability, or are the distributions bimodal?" (p. 379).

If memory is to be conceptualized in terms of a singular commonality system that is involved in all forms of storage and reproduction, then clearly we must allow for its efficiency to be differentiated by the context in which the task occurs. Here we use *context* rather promiscuously, to refer not only to aspects of the physical setting in which the task occurs but also to the way that the material presented to the subject is represented in long-term memory. It is not enough to insure that all subjects are familiar with the material (i.e., can recognize and name it); they must be shown to represent it in memory in equivalently elaborate ways. On the basis of the data presented here, we cannot rule out the commonality hypothesis, but we can say that it is insufficient to account for the full range of behavior we have reported. Consider that each of the mnemonists studied differed in the feats they could perform and in the tasks that interfered with them. For example, although VP's and Rajan's memories were unfettered by distractor tasks (Hunt & Love, 1972; Thompson, Cowan, Frieman, Mahadevan, & Vogel, 1990), Bubbles' memory was seriously undermined by them. These men differed in how spatially they encoded nonnumerical material, as well as in their verbal prowess. The only unifying theme among the mnemonists studied is that they all had pockets of exceptional talent that had definite boundaries.

Whatever the implication of this case study for adult mnemonic performance, it is congruent with what we take to be a growing trend in the field of memory development. We are referring to the belief among those who study children's unfolding memory that the processes that regulate their memory are fundamentally context dependent. Elsewhere, we have concluded that:

> There is a "new look" in memory development research, and it is decidedly contextual. The crux of the current view, in fact, is that memory processes cannot be adequately understood or evaluated acontextually: To think about memory without considering the contexts that lead children to remember is akin to thinking about smiles independently of the faces on which they appear. Different contexts not only evoke different strategies to aid recall, but they also differentially shape an individual's perception of the recall task itself. Depending on the context in which remembering takes place, children may recall everything or nothing; their level of performance speaks as much to the power of context as to their native mnemonic capacity. (Ceci & DeSimone, in press)

The potency of context in shaping performance on memory tasks and the consequent necessity of considering context in evaluating such performance, have been vividly illustrated by the studies of exceptional memory discussed in this chapter. It follows that in attempting to improve memory, consideration of the domain in which remembering occurs is essential. It is our contention that future attempts to bolster individuals' performance will meet with the greatest success if they are directed at tasks within well-defined contexts, as opposed to being directed at improving performance on the wide variety of tasks encompassed by the term memory.

Endnote 1

Portions of this research were supported by grants to S. J. Ceci from the National Institutes of Health, DHHS #5RO1HD22839 and KO4HD00801.

Endnote 2

Various procedures to assess digit recall have been used by different investigators, and the differences can at times be important to keep in mind. For instance, Hunt and Love used a 1 second interval between the onset of a digit and the onset of the following digit. Strings of n-length digits were presented to VP, as long as he could recall that length twice in a row. Given success at n length twice in a row, a string of $n+1$ length would be presented. Thus, digit span is operationalized as the longest string that VP could recall perfectly twice in a row. In contrast, Staszewski operationalized digit span as the longest string length that DD could correctly recall in at least half of the trials.

Endnote 3

We became aware of Bubbles' ability to recall digits backward while we were studying other gamblers. One of them informed us about Bubbles' ability to recall long strings of digits backward, as well as write backward with his nondominant (left) hand.

References

Ankrum, C., & Palmer, J. (1989, November). *The perception and memory of objects and their parts*. Paper presented at the annual meeting of the Psychonomic Society, Atlanta, GA.

Atkinson, R.C., & Shiffrin, R.M. (1968). Human memory: A proposed system and its control processes. In K. Spence & J.T. Spence (Eds.), *The*

Psychology of Learning and Motivation (Vol. 2, pp. 89-195). New York: Academic Press.

Brown, E., & Deffenbacher, K. (1985). Forgotten mnemonists. *Journal of the History of the Behavioral Sciences, 11*, 342-349.

Ceci, S.J. (1990). *On intelligence...more or less: A bioecological treatise on intellectual development*. Englewood Cliffs, NJ: Prentice Hall.

Ceci, S.J., & Bronfenbrenner, U. (1991). On the demise of everyday memory: "The rumors of my death are much exaggerated" (Mark Twain). *American Psychologist, 46*, 27-36.

Ceci, S.J., & Cornelius, S.W. (1989, May). *A psychological perspective on intellectual development*. Paper presented at the biennial meeting of the Society for Research in Child Development, Kansas City, MO.

Ceci, S.J., & DeSimone, M.D. (in press). Memory, cognition, and learning: Developmental and ecological considerations. In I. Rapin & S. Segalowitz (Eds.), *Handbook of neuropsychology*. Holland: Elsevier.

Chi, M.T.H., Glaser, R., & Rees, E. (1982). Expertise in problem solving. In R.J. Sternberg (Ed.), *Advances in the psychology of human intelligence* (Vol. 1, pp. 7-75). Hillsdale, NJ: Erlbaum.

Ericsson, K.A., & Chase, W.G. (1982). Exceptional memory. *American Scientist, 70*, 607-615.

Ericsson, K.A., & Faivre, I.A. (1988). What's exceptional about exceptional abilities? In L. Obler & D. Fein (Eds.), *The exceptional brain* (pp. 436-473). New York: The Guilford Press.

Fox, P.W. (1989). *Exceptional memory, variability of performance, and the "common processes" view*. Paper presented at the meeting of the Midwestern Psychological Association, Chicago.

Fox, P.W. (1990, April). *A case study of exceptional memory: Educational implications for understanding the unexceptional*. Paper presented at the annual meeting of the American Education Research Association, Boston.

Gordon, P., Valentine, E., & Wilding, J. (1984). One man's memory: A study of a mnemonist. *British Journal of Psychology, 75*, 1-14.

Herrmann, D.J., Rea, A., & Andrzejewski, S. (1988). The need for a new approach to memory training. In M.M. Gruneberg, P.E. Morris, & R.N. Sykes (Eds.), *Practical aspects of memory: Current research and issues* (Vol. 2, pp. 415-420). Chichester: Wiley.

Horn, J.L., Donaldson, G., & Engstrom, R. (1981). Apprehension, memory, and fluid decline in adulthood. *Research on Aging, 3*, 33-84.

Humphreys, L. (1962). The organization of human abilities. *American Psychologist, 17*, 475-583.

Hunt, E. (1985). Verbal ability. In R.J. Sternberg (Ed.), *Human abilities: An information processing approach* (pp. 31-58). San Francisco: W.H. Freeman & Sons.

Hunt, E., & Love, T. (1972). How good can memory be? In A.W. Melton & E. Martin (Eds.), *Coding processes in human memory* (pp. 237-260). Washington, DC: Winston.

Hunter, I.M.L. (1962). An exceptional talent for calculative thinking. *British Journal of Psychology, 53*, 243-258.
Jaeger, M.E., & Rosnow, R.L. (1988). Contextualism and its implications for inquiry. *British Journal of Psychology, 79*, 63-75.
Kail, R.V. (1990). *The development of memory in children (3rd ed.)*. New York: W.H. Freeman and Company.
Luria, A.R. (1968). *The mind of a mnemonist*. New York: Basic Books.
Miller, G.A. (1956). The magical number seven, plus or minus two: Some limits on our capacity for information processing. *Psychological Review, 63*, 81-97.
Neisser, U. (1982). *Memory observed*. San Francisco: W.H. Freeman.
Raven, J.C. (1958). *Advanced progressive matrices 1 and 2*. New York: The Psychological Corp.
Reber, A. (1990). *The evolution of the cognitive unconscious*. Manuscript submitted for publication.
Staszewski, J.J. (1989). Exceptional memory: The influence of practice and knowledge on the development of elaborative encoding strategies. In W. Schneider & F.E. Weinert (Eds.), *Interactions among aptitudes, strategies, and knowledge in cognitive performance* (pp. 252-285). New York: Springer-Verlag.
Thompson, C.P., Cowan, T., Frieman, J., Mahadevan, R., & Vogl, R. (1990). *Rajan: A study of a memorist*. Manuscript submitted for publication.
Thompson, C.P., Mahadevan, R., Frieman, J., Vogl, R., & Cowan, T. (1990). *Portrait of a skilled memorist*. Paper presented at the European Society for Cognitive Psychology, Como, Italy.
Tulving, E.E. (1989). Remembering and knowing the past. *American Psychologist, 77*, 361-367.
Wilding, J., & Valentine, E. (1988). Searching for superior memories. In M.M. Gruneberg, P.E. Morris, & R.N. Sykes (Eds.), *Practical aspects of memory: Current research and issues* (Vol. 1, pp. 472-477). Chichester: Wiley.

Improving Memory Through Practice

David G. Payne and Michael J. Wenger

This chapter is concerned with the manner in which practice performing various memory tasks influences subsequent performance. Although memory practice involves learning, simply calling the beneficial effects of memory practice "learning" does little to enhance our understanding of these effects, because the standard definition of learning (i.e., "the relatively permanent change in behavior that results from experience") provides us with little information regarding (a) the extent to which changes in memory behavior generalize across tasks, (b) the role that the nature of the experience plays in producing the observed changes, and (c) the structure or processes that change as a result of practice. These three issues must be addressed in order to provide a proper theoretical interpretation of practice effects in memory and constitute the focus of the present chapter.

The remainder of this chapter is organized as follows. The first section briefly reviews several major historical trends in the experimental study of practice effects in memory and describes some of the main empirical and theoretical controversies. As Singley and Anderson (1989) have noted, early studies of transfer of training often were not designed to determine the nature or cause of the change in the learners' performance; rather, these studies were designed to show that positive transfer had occurred as a consequence of practice. However, this early work identifies several important issues in practice and transfer research, and our intent in presenting this brief historical sketch is to provide the reader with a historical perspective from which to evaluate the more recent research on memory practice effects.

The second section reviews several robust and illustrative findings that have emerged from studies of item-specific practice (i.e., repeated study and/or test opportunities with the same items). This section focuses on encoding and retrieval variables and will demonstrate that several factors identified in laboratory research as important determinants of memory performance are key variables affecting the efficacy of practice effects in real-world memory tasks.

The third section of the chapter considers a recent theory that has been provided to account for what may be called "expert memory" or "the rapid and efficient utilization of memory in some knowledge domain to perform at an expert level" (Chase & Ericsson, 1981, p. 141). The subjects in these studies have devoted hundreds of hours to becoming proficient at one or more memory tasks, either as a result of participating in a laboratory study (e.g., Ericsson, Chase, & Faloon, 1980) or through repeatedly performing the memory task as part of their everyday activities (e.g., Ericsson & Polson, 1988a; 1988b). These demonstrations have served to (a) illustrate the impressive levels of memory performance that can be obtained with extensive practice, (b) provide information concerning the generality of observed memory practice effects, and (c) provide the empirical data base from which theoretical explications of skilled memory have been developed.

The concluding section presents some thoughts on and prescriptions for future empirical and theoretical work on memory practice effects. This section also presents several issues that must be taken into account as practitioners endeavor to use the results of empirical and theoretical investigations of memory practice effects in their efforts to produce memory improvements in real-world tasks.

A word of caution is in order regarding the scope of this chapter. The research and theorizing on what are typically called "practice effects" is voluminous, and consequently, several rather arbitrary decisions were made in order to keep the present review manageable. First, we focus on tasks in which the primary demand is memorial. That is, even though many tasks, such as analogical problem solving (e.g., Gick & Holyoak, 1980, 1983; Hayes & Simon, 1977) or text editing (e.g., Kay & Black, 1985; Singley & Anderson, 1985) necessarily involve accessing memory, successful performance in these tasks relies heavily on a number of cognitive processes other than retention and retrieval. Second, we restrict our attention to practice effects in memory tasks involving verbal, numerical, and/or pictorial information, thus eliminating studies of practice effects in the areas of motor memory and what is sometimes called procedural memory. Third, we have excluded studies of the impact of instruction in memory strategies and studies on the efficacy of classical mnemonic techniques. (See the chapter by Pressley and El-Dinary, this volume, for a review of the effect of strategy instruction.) Finally, we have made no attempt to provide a comprehensive survey of the memory skills of mnemonists, since the extant case studies of mnemonists suffer from little, if any, control over the practice conditions that lead to the development of expertise.

Historical Trends in the Study of Practice Effects

The study of practice effects in memory has had a long and diverse history in psychology, education, and other related disciplines. Consider first the efforts of basic research scientists. As Tolman (1938) pointed out, much of the research conducted during the early part of this century was designed to test theoretical accounts of learning such as Thorndike's (1898) law of effect or law of exercise. These early statements contained clear reference to the role of repetition in altering performance, and considerable research efforts were directed towards identifying the specific conditions of practice that were likely to improve subsequent performance.

Practice effects were also of concern to researchers interested in real-world applications. Educators have long been interested in developing curricula that might (a) facilitate the acquisition of new knowledge and (b) promote the development of effective learning strategies. During the early part of this century, numerous American educational practices were based upon the (often untested) assumption that learning materials, such as Latin, would somehow facilitate the development of the memory skills needed to master other content areas. This was known as the doctrine of formal discipline and a number of researchers supported this notion (e.g., Angell, 1908; Pillsbury, 1908; Wallin, 1910; Woodrow, 1927).

The doctrine of formal discipline was taken to task by Thorndike (e.g., Thorndike, 1903, 1922), who conducted a systematic program of research intended to test the notion of generalized transfer. Across numerous studies spanning several decades, Thorndike found very little evidence for the notion that mental skills or "faculties" were positively affected by prior training in other tasks (but see Singley & Anderson 1989, pp. 4-5). These results led Thorndike to conclude that, contrary to the doctrine of formal discipline, most transfer seen in memory and problem-solving tasks is very much task- and material-specific: "Any special school training has a much narrower influence upon the mind as a whole than has commonly been supposed" (Thorndike, 1906, p. 246).

In place of the doctrine of formal discipline, Thorndike (1906) proposed the theory of identical elements. The strong version of this theory maintained that training in a task would transfer to another task if and only if the two tasks shared common stimulus-response associations. If the two tasks shared stimulus-response associations, then any strengthening of these associations that occurred during the training task would benefit performance on the subsequent transfer task.

Several conclusions can be drawn from this brief review of the early experimental work on practice effects. One of the central issues in this early work was whether or not transfer between two nonidentical tasks could be shown. A related issue concerned the necessary and sufficient conditions for obtaining transfer. On the one hand, the doctrine of formal discipline suggested that the effects of practice would generalize across cognitive tasks.

On the other hand, Thorndike's (1906) theory of identical elements assumed that only identical stimulus-response associations would transfer. The issue of specificity of transfer was never adequately resolved; later researchers working within the verbal learning tradition also faced the task of providing an answer to this question. For example, Postman (1969) offered a working definition of transfer that emphasized acquired associations, rather than cognitive processes and memorial representations. This focus on associations is, of course, consistent with the behaviorist paradigm that was dominant during the 1930s, 1940s, and 1950s. The important point to note, however, is that the early experimentalists and the verbal learning workers struggled with the issue of specificity within their respective explanatory frameworks. This issue still begs a resolution, and development of an adequate explanation of practice effects is critically dependent on this resolution.

While practice effects and the specificity of transfer were central topics for experimental psychologists (as well as educational researchers) during the early part of the century, in more recent times, learning phenomena have fallen from favor. George Mandler (1985) has summarized this turn of events quite succinctly:

> Until the 1950s, learning and motivation were the reigning king and queen of American psychology. It is sometimes difficult to comprehend their demise in the ensuing 30 years, but cognitive psychologists were either preoccupied with the steady state organism or unsure how to handle the problem of cognitive change until they understood what it is that changes during learning. (p. 108)

This decline in interest in learning and transfer seems to have been due to the ascendancy of the human information-processing paradigm (see Lachman, Lachman, & Butterfield, 1979, pp. 41-46). Yet, as we will show later (particularly in our discussion of skilled memory theory), learning and transfer have seen revived interest within the last decade.

One of the positive outcomes of the emphasis on the steady state organism was that psychologists developed rather elaborate models of the human cognitive system. These models can now serve as the basis for exploring in more detail the manner in which practice-effects impact the learners' cognitive system. Another positive outcome of this emphasis was that the laboratory memory research conducted during this period identified several variables (e.g., distribution of practice, levels of processing, organization) that have a large impact on memory performance.

Encoding Practice: The Spacing Effect

There is a long line of research documenting the effectiveness of distributed (or spaced) practice as an important encoding variable. Nearly a century ago,

Jost (1897; cited in Hintzman, 1974) inferred from Ebbinghaus' (1885/1964) data that learning is improved if practice is spread out in time rather than massed together. In the early 1900s, researchers examined the effects of varying the amount of practice per day (cf., Woodworth, 1938). During the 1940s and 1950s, studies investigated the effects of varying the length of the rest interval(s) between successive study trials. Central topics during the 1970s and 1980s were (a) the effects of the length of the interitem interval and (b) the nature of activities between repetitions of items within a single list. The vast majority of these studies supported the conclusion that spaced practice produced better memory than massed practice. (For reviews, see Baddeley, 1990; Crowder, 1976; Hintzman, 1974). Basic research on the spacing effect continues today with studies examining a variety of empirical and theoretical issues (e.g., Greene, 1989; Perruchet, 1989). However, despite the strong empirical support for the utility of the spacing effect, to date there has been little application of this finding (see Dempster, 1988). We turn our attention now to illustrative investigations of the spacing effect.

In a prototypical laboratory study, Zeichmeister and Shaughnessy (1980) presented subjects with common nouns to study. Some of the items appeared only once, but other items were repeated, either massed together or spaced throughout the list. For some of the list items, subjects were asked to estimate the likelihood that they would be able to later recall the items. For the repeated items, these ratings were always made after the second presentation of the item. After list presentation, subjects were given a free recall test for their memory of the list items.

Results showed that, not surprisingly, subjects rated the repeated items as more likely to be recalled than the single items. More importantly, subjects rated the massed presentation items as more likely to be recalled than the spaced items. However, this prediction for the massed and spaced items runs counter to the results of the free recall test, which showed that recall was better with the spaced practice than the massed practice.

The tendency to think that massed presentations are effective is reflected in the manner in which subjects typically rehearse items in a list-learning experiment. In a recent study (Grosofsky & Payne, 1989), we presented subjects with items to remember and asked subjects to rehearse the items aloud. Audio recordings showed that subjects frequently repeated the same items together over and over, a strategy analogous to massed presentation. This tendency may also account for the fact that most people report that when they are given new information to learn (e.g., telephone numbers, people's names), they go about attempting to memorize this information by repeating the information silently to themselves; in other words, they use massed practice. To summarize, these findings indicate that, left to their own devices, students will (a) show a spacing effect in recall, (b) underestimate the efficacy of spacing presentations, and (c) not employ spacing of practice.

Spacing has also been studied using list-learning tasks that more closely approximate an educational task. For example, Dempster (1987) examined whether spaced or massed presentations were more effective in a vocabulary-learning task. Subjects were presented with unfamiliar words and their meanings in either a massed or a spaced condition (Experiments 3 & 4). Memory for the meanings was tested by presenting the vocabulary words and asking the subjects to provide the meaning. In two experiments, the spaced presentations yielded a significant improvement in performance relative to the massed condition. Furthermore, the size of the improvement was considerable, ranging from 23% to 102% across the various conditions.

The spacing effect has also been demonstrated with units larger than words or word meanings. For example, when sentences are presented for study multiple times, there is also a spacing effect (e.g., Rothkopf & Coke, 1963). One important boundary condition for producing the spacing effect with sentences is that the repetitions must be identical. Dellarosa and Bourne (1985) found that the spacing effect was either attenuated or eliminated completely when the second presentation of the sentence was changed by varying either the surface structure of the sentence or the person speaking the sentence. Similar results were obtained by Glover and Corkill (1987) using paragraphs. It thus seems that, at least for sentences and paragraphs, the manner in which the items are re-presented plays a major role in determining the presence or absence of the spacing effect.

Landauer and Ross (1977) compared subjects' memory for seven-digit telephone numbers under two conditions, a control condition in which subjects were instructed to study the items, using whatever strategies they would normally employ and an experimental condition in which subjects were instructed to use spaced repetitions. After a 2-week retention interval, the experimental subjects showed significantly better recall than the control subjects. An interesting corollary finding was that subjects' confidence in their incorrect answers was higher in the control condition than the experimental condition, suggesting that the spaced practice improved memory and did not lead to a false sense of confidence. This result is perhaps understandable in light of Zeichmeister and Shaughnessy's (1980) finding that subjects underestimate the efficacy of spaced presentations.

Atkinson (1972) employed a variant of the spacing principle in a study comparing different procedures for teaching second-language vocabulary. Subjects were exposed to German-English pairs under four conditions. In the baseline condition, the item pairs were presented in a random order on each trial. In the learner-controlled condition, the items to be re-presented were determined by the subject, while in two experimenter-controlled conditions, items were re-presented in an order that depended upon the learners' response history. For present purposes, the important finding was that, relative to the baseline condition, there was a large and significant improvement in recall in each of the experimental conditions. This result suggests that the order in which items are rehearsed can affect memory performance.

The spacing principle is known to apply over longer intervals as well. Bloom and Shuell (1981) compared memory of French vocabulary items studied using either spaced practice (three 10 minute sessions, completed on 3 successive days) or massed practice (all three sessions completed within a single 30-minute session). When memory was assessed on a delayed recall test, the spaced condition showed a sizeable (35%) advantage over the massed practice condition; similar results have been reported more recently by Dempster (1987). In addition, Glenberg and Lehman (1980) have demonstrated that spacing repetitions in list-learning over 1 day or 1 week can improve performance dramatically. Taken together, the results of these studies indicate that learning and retention of single words, as well as foreign vocabulary items, are aided by spacing the practice sessions.

Spaced practice has also been shown to improve retention of text, lecture, and other educational materials. Reder and Anderson (1982) had subjects read information derived from introductory texts in several fields (e.g., ecology, photography) under either a massed or distributed (i.e., spaced) presentation format. They found that spacing produced a significant improvement in subjects' retention of the main points of the passages. Di Vesta and Smith (1979) examined students' retention of the main points of a lecture. Within the lecture, there were discussion periods that were either interspersed throughout the lecture, period (spaced practice) or massed at either the beginning or end of the lecture. Here again, spacing facilitated retention of the main points. Smith and Rothkopf (1984) have also examined the effects of spacing materials in an educational setting. In this case, the "materials" consisted of four lectures on statistics that were presented either all on the same day or spaced across 4 days. Note that in this study, the target knowledge that was assessed on the final memory test was not simply repeated verbatim in the four lectures; rather the lectures were separate presentations. Nonetheless, the topics of the lectures were similar, and this provided some overlap. Smith and Rothkopf reported significantly better recall with the spaced lectures than the massed lectures. (Note that this result appears to be somewhat at odds with the findings of Dellarosa and Bourne [1985] and Glover and Corkill [1987] who found that varying the surface form of sentences or paragraphs reduced or eliminated the spacing effect. There are many differences in the materials and procedures used in these studies, and it is impossible at this point to identify the factor[s] responsible for producing the observed results.) In another study, Rea and Modigliani (1985) compared students' memory of spelling lists and multiplication facts learned under either massed or distributed practice. When performance was assessed on a delayed recall test, there was a clear advantage for spaced practice.

Finally, it appears that the spacing effect reflects a fairly general memory process. There are two lines of evidence that support this claim. First, when memory is assessed with a free recall measure, the spacing effect is unaffected by whether learning is intentional or unintentional (e.g., Greene, 1989). Second, Cornell (1980) has reported evidence of a spacing effect in recognition memory in infants 5 to 6 months of age. This finding suggests that the spacing effect reflects a basic aspect of the human memory system, that is, one that is not necessarily dependent upon subjects employing strategic encoding processes.

Taken together, these studies demonstrate clearly that practice in encoding material can be greatly improved by spacing the practice sessions. The spacing effect has been obtained with a wide range of learners, materials, encoding conditions, retention intervals, and memory tasks. It is thus safe to conclude that spacing represents a very potent encoding variable that could potentially be used to improve memory performance. Note, however, that even relatively sophisticated subjects (i.e., college students) do not spontaneously employ distributed practice. One question that remains unanswered is whether subjects would employ spacing as a general strategy if they were given training in the use of this strategy. If so, this would speak to the general issue of the specificity of memory skills.

Retrieval Practice

Item-specific improvement in memory performance has also been demonstrated in investigations of the effects of repeated retrieval practice. In an important early study, Ballard (1913) presented schoolchildren with lines of poetry to memorize and then gave them repeated tests with no intervening study opportunities. Two main findings to emerge from this research were that (a) the *amount* of information recalled increases across tests, and (b) the *rate* with which the information is recalled also increases across tests. While there were several subsequent replications of this effect, there were also numerous failures, and the phenomenon was largely ignored until the early 1970s (see Payne, 1987, for a review).

However, in 1974, Erdelyi and Becker reported that memory for pictorial information improves across repeated tests, whereas memory for verbal materials remains constant. Erdelyi and Becker coined the term "hypermnesia" to refer to the increase in net recall levels they obtained with the pictorial items. Subsequent research on the hypermnesia phenomenon has delineated several factors that contribute to the observed improvement in net recall levels across repeated tests.

Roediger and Payne (1982) asked whether hypermnesia was attributable to changes in the memory trace that occurred over time (e.g., consolidation) or whether hypermnesia depended upon repeated testing. When they compared performance of groups that had had the same length retention interval but a different number of prior tests, they found that performance levels varied directly with the number of prior tests, suggesting that the process of administering repeated tests somehow facilitated subsequent performance. More specifically, they found that, as Ballard (1913) had demonstrated, the rate of recalling items increases with increasing test experience, suggesting that the act of recalling items increases the accessibility of these items.

Further investigations of hypermnesia have indicated that the phenomenon is both robust and explicable in terms of the processes operating at the time of retrieval. These studies have demonstrated that (a) the gain in items recalled across the repeated tests is attributable to additional time to retrieve target items (Payne, 1986; Roediger, Payne, Gillespie, & Lean, 1982; Roediger & Thorpe, 1978), (b) the hypermnesic effect for verbal items is obtained with recall tests but not recognition tests (Payne & Roediger, 1987; but see Erdelyi & Stein, 1981), and (c) the improvement in net recall of verbal items across successive tests does not appear to be due to subjects adopting a more lenient response criterion, since the hypermnesic effect is obtained even when response criterion is held constant by forcing subjects to produce the same number of items on each test (e.g., Erdelyi & Becker, 1974; see also Erdelyi, Finks, & Feigin-Pfau, 1989; Roediger & Payne, 1985; Roediger, Srinivas, & Waddill, 1989).

The results of these studies indicate that practice in retrieving items does confer a direct benefit upon later recall of these items. There is also evidence that there is an indirect benefit of retrieval practice for nonrecalled items in the sense that the speed-up of retrieval of recalled items allows subjects to spend more time searching memory for unrecalled target items. One question that has not been addressed in the studies reviewed thus far is whether this improvement in memory performance generalizes across materials or tasks.

There is some evidence that suggests that the benefits of retrieval are specific to the target items and do not generalize to other items. For example, Roediger et al. (1982, Experiment 3) asked subjects to recall items from common categories on three successive trials. Subjects who recalled items from the same category showed significant improvements across trials, whereas subjects who recalled items from different categories showed no improvement across trials. Herrmann, Buschke, and Gall (1987) have replicated and extended this basic pattern of results. However, they provided subjects with much more retrieval practice than did Roediger et al. In the Herrmann et al. study, up to 42 different categories (Experiment 3) were used to examine whether there would be an improvement that would generalize across items. Their results provided no support for the notion of the development of generalized retrieval skill.

One possible limitation of the retrieval practice studies of Roediger et al. (1982) and Herrmann et al. (1987) is that they employed only semantic memory tasks. Brown-Su and Payne (1988) reported a series of experiments in which subjects were given practice in either episodic (list learning and recall) or semantic (category recall) memory tasks. They found no improvement when subjects were tested with a semantic transfer task (recalling items from a new category), replicating Roediger et al. (1982) and Herrmann et al. However, they did observe positive transfer to an episodic memory task (studying and recalling a list of words). It is possible that in order to obtain a generalized retrieval practice effect, subjects must be given the opportunity to encode the items in a manner that is consistent with the retrieval strategies they have developed. This conjecture is consistent with results obtained within the expert memory paradigm developed by Chase and Ericsson (1982) and described later in this chapter.

One other line of research that has examined the effects of various types of retrieval processes is the work by Geiselman, Fisher, MacKinnon, and Holland (1985; see also Adams, 1985), who investigated the "cognitive interview" as a means to improve eyewitness memory. This approach involves instructing an eyewitness to attempt to recall information using a variety of retrieval strategies including varying the order in which the event is recalled and attempting to reinstate the emotional context surrounding the event. The cognitive interview has proven to be a useful technique for improving subjects' memory performance. One question that has not yet been adequately addressed in this line of research is the extent to which practice in using the retrieval strategies acquired in the cognitive interview will enhance memory performance when the person is not explicitly instructed to use the strategy.

To summarize the work on retrieval practice, there is considerable evidence that such practice produces sizeable improvements in subjects' ability to recall the practiced items. There is mixed evidence as to whether retrieval practice generalizes to new items or across tasks.

Combined Encoding and Retrieval Practice

The concepts of encoding practice (i.e., spacing) and retrieval practice have been combined as a memory improvement technique by Landauer and Bjork (1978). Landauer and Bjork were interested in the types of real-world situations in which an item is presented once, and the learner must decide how to rehearse that item in order to remember it (e.g., remember the name of a newly introduced stranger). Landauer and Bjork noted that people's tendency to try to remember a person's name by rehearsing it over and over in succession is equivalent to massed practice which, based on the spacing effect research, can be assumed to be a less-than-optimal procedure.

Landauer and Bjork (1978) demonstrated that a procedure they called *expanding rehearsal* produced the best retention. With this procedure, initial recall attempts occur soon after the items have been presented in order to ensure that the learner can retrieve them. However, retrieving the item serves as a re-presentation of the item, and in order for these re-presentations to be maximally effective, they should be spaced in time. Thus, with the expanding rehearsal procedure, after the initial short retention interval, the time between successive retrieval attempts is increased. Landauer and Bjork reported that in a laboratory study with college students, the expanding rehearsal procedure produced very good memory performance. This procedure effectively integrates encoding and retrieval processes and has potential as an effective learning tool.

Extensive Practice and the Development of Expert Memory Skills

The research on memory practice effects that we have considered thus far indicates that, at least as far as item-specific effects are concerned, one can improve memory performance by (among other things) encoding practice (e.g., the spacing effect), retrieval practice (e.g., hypermnesia), and combined encoding and retrieval practice (e.g., expanded rehearsal). One consistent aspect of this research is that the amount of practice given to subjects has been rather limited. Evidence from many research areas indicates that to become an "expert" at a task may require hundreds or thousands of hours of practice (Newell & Rosenbloom, 1981). In this section, we consider research on memory practice in which subjects are given very extensive practice.

Normal adults' performance on memory span tasks falls into the relatively narrow range of about 7 $\pm$ 2 items, and this consistency of memory span performance has been taken as evidence indicating that the capacity of working memory represents a severe limitation in cognitive skills. There are, however, reports of individuals with normal memory abilities who have been able to significantly increase their memory span through practice. For example, Miller (1956) reported that Sidney Smith was able to recall up to 40 binary digits in order, by recoding the items into an octal code. Miller argued that recoding represented an important process whereby the limitations of short-term memory could be by-passed.

Skilled Memory Theory

More recently, Chase and Ericsson (1981) examined the development of memory skill by giving a single subject extensive practice in a memory span task. Their subject, SF, began the experiment with average memory ability, as indexed by his performance on a digit span task. However, after over 250 hours of practice spread across 25 months, SF increased his digit span performance from 7 digits to over 80 digits. Chase and Ericsson (1981) examined in detail the development of SF's memory skill from normal levels to expert level. It was this detailed examination of the development of memory skill that led to the formulation of the skilled memory theory (Chase & Ericsson, 1981; Ericsson, 1985). (A detailed evaluation of the theory is beyond the scope of this chapter; what follows is a summary of the key features of the theory.)

According to the skilled memory theory, practice has no effect upon the capacity of STM; this capacity is assumed to be fixed at approximately three to four units (cf. Broadbent, 1975). Rather, the exceptional memory performance demonstrated by experts is assumed to be attributable to improved skill at encoding information into and retrieving it from LTM. Skilled memory is thus portrayed as a complex skill that is acquired and elaborated through practice.

The basic procedure used by Chase and Ericsson (1981) to study the development of memory skill was to present random digits to SF, one per second, and then to ask for an ordered recall of the digits. If the digits were recalled correctly and in correct order, the length of the succeeding sequence was increased by one digit; if the digits were recalled out of sequence, the succeeding sequence was decreased by one digit. After each trial, the experimenters asked SF to report his thought processes during the trial. At the end of each session, they asked SF to recall as much of the material as he could from all of the trials. Thus, in their initial study, Chase and Ericsson obtained quantitative data on SF's recall performance and verbal protocol data on his cognitive processes.

Chase and Ericsson (1982) described how memory experts utilize STM and LTM in conjunction to increase their performance on episodic memory tasks. This coordination of STM and LTM involves three principles of skilled memory, which we will refer to as the mnemonic encoding, retrieval structure, and speed-up principles.

The Mnemonic Encoding Principle

The mnemonic encoding principle states that memory experts encode information in terms of an existing knowledge base. There are several lines of evidence that support this principle. First, studies of mnemonists (e.g., Chase & Ericsson, 1981, 1982; Ericsson, 1985; Ericsson & Polson, 1988a; Staszewski, 1988) have revealed that these individuals use preexisting knowledge, or learned patterns, when encoding new information. Second, studies of experts in a variety of domains (e.g., chess: Chase & Simon, 1973a, 1973b; computer programming: McKeithen, Reitman, Reuter, & Hirtle, 1981; Shneiderman, 1976) indicate that these individuals encode brief presentations of materials in the domain of interest in an organized fashion, and when materials are presented that are not consistent with the experts' knowledge, then the encoding processes are impaired.

Chase and Ericsson (1981, 1982) reported that SF was an accomplished long distance runner, and his familiarity with running times allowed SF to develop a mnemonic encoding strategy for the digit span. Over the first 4 days of the investigation, SF reported using a simple phonemic encoding of the digits, rehearsing the list until the recall test. However, from day 5 onward, he adopted a successively refined semantic organization of digits in terms of running times and hierarchical groupings of running times.

While it was apparent that SF was using a mnemonic encoding strategy with a hierarchical organization, it was not clear whether SF was holding the semantic codes in STM. Consequently, Chase and Ericsson (1981) conducted a series of rehearsal suppression experiments to investigate this question. SF's verbal protocols indicated that he held the last items presented in a rehearsal buffer. In the first of the rehearsal suppression experiments, SF recited the alphabet during the interval between the presentation of the last item and the beginning of the recall test. Predictably, this resulted in an initial loss of the items SF held in the rehearsal buffer; however, SF was able to modify the organization of his encoding to reduce the number of items held in the rehearsal buffer. Second, a set of visual suppression procedures (used to test whether SF's mnemonic strategy relied on any visual-spatial coding component) produced no interference. Third, a concurrent chanting task (see Baddeley & Hitch, 1974) produced no interference. Finally, a letter-shadowing task inserted in the 1-second pauses between presentation of digit groups (as predicted from previous protocols) produced a 35% decrement in SF's performance. Chase and Ericsson concluded:

> The contents of short-term memory were (1) the most recent one, two, or three ungrouped digits in a phonemic code; (2) the previous group of three or four digits (it is not clear how these grouped items are coded); and (3) all the semantic information associated with the active mnemonic coding of the previous group. (1981 p. 158)

The Retrieval Structure Principle

According to this principle, memory experts use specialized and organized structures for encoding information into and retrieving information from LTM. Chase and Ericsson (1981) characterized it initially as follows: "A retrieval structure is a long-term memory structure that is used to make associations with the material to be remembered. In effect, it serves the function of storing retrieval cues in addressable locations without having to use short-term memory" (p. 169). Note the logical interdependence of the retrieval structure and the mnemonic encoding strategy, particularly in the case of SF, who relied on mnemonic grouping of the presented digits and a logical organization of the encoded adjacent groups. Roediger (1980) has shown that one of the advantages of the classical mnemonic techniques (e.g., the method of loci) is that the technique provides a means to order recall; this same advantage accrues in the skilled memory theory through the use of a retrieval structure.

While it was apparent that the initial development of SF's mnemonic encoding included some hierarchical organization, later verbal protocols indicated an increasingly hierarchical organization. SF's final level of performance indicated (from verbal protocol evidence) that three features of any group were needed to locate that group within the hierarchy, indicating a three-level retrieval structure. In addition, analysis of the prosodic features of SF's recall were almost in perfect agreement with a grouping analysis based on the verbal protocols Chase & Ericsson, 1981).

The Speed-Up Principle

This principle asserts that, with practice, the speed with which a person can encode and retrieve is increased. Evidence consistent with this principle is the fact that experts with limited study time can encode much more information than novices, but only when the information is presented in a manner consistent with the organized knowledge structures of the learner (e.g., Chase & Simon, 1973a, 1973b). The notion of a speed-up in memory skill is also consistent with the speed-up observed in many other skill domains (Newell & Rosenbloom, 1981).

Chase and Ericsson (1981) report three lines of evidence supporting speed-up in SF's performance. First, all the major changes to the encoding strategy occurred within the first 100 hours of practice; yet SF continued to improve his performance. Second, with increasing practice, the pauses between groups of presented digits (in conditions in which SF was able to control presentation rate) steadily decreased. Finally, absolute encoding times for groups of digits fell below 1 second, approaching the range of STM operations.

In order to further the theoretical and empirical development that they had accomplished in their work with SF, Chase and Ericsson (1982) enlisted a second runner, DD, and trained him in the use of SF's system. For the most part, DD's performance paralleled SF's, with differences occurring in the specifics of mnemonic encoding and therefore retrieval structures and in the degree of the practice effect.

Chase and Ericsson (1982) report that DD used a mnemonic encoding strategy that was virtually identical to SF's. However, they did observe differences, these being traced to the types of races that DD specialized in. In particular, it appears that, when possible, DD would code digits in terms of 1/4-mile performance, whereas SF would code in terms of 1/2-mile running times. DD's use of a retrieval structure mirrored SF's; DD appeared to use a three-level hierarchy for running times, and he appeared to search systematically from the shortest times (encoded as 1/4-mile times), to the longest times (encoded as marathon performances), to ages, years, and larger patterns.

Although DD's and SF's performances were quite similar in terms of mnemonic encoding and retrieval structure, they did show a notable difference in terms of speed-up of encoding with practice. While SF, in situations where he could control presentation rate, showed a dramatic decrease in terms of latency between encoded groups of digits, DD showed only a slight decrease. While Chase and Ericsson (1982) offer no explanation for this difference, visual inspection of their data (p. 21, Figure 5) does reveal some items of interest that might help us understand the difference.

First, for lists composed of between 25 and 30 digits, presented early in the experimental program (Day 69 for SF, Day 73 for DD), DD shows much smaller latencies (approximately 2 seconds) than SF (approximately 4.5 seconds) (Chase & Ericsson, 1982). Second, with lists of the same size, presented midway through the experimental program (Day 160 for SF, Day 195 for DD), SF and DD show similar latencies (approximately 1.5 seconds for SF, approximately 1.8 seconds for DD). Finally, with lists of 50 digits, presented late in the experimental program (day 200 for SF, day 286 for DD), SF's encoding time (approximately 1.2 seconds) is smaller than DD's (approximately 2.0 seconds). Thus, while it is true that SF did show much more dramatic improvements with practice (with respect to encoding latencies), it is also true that DD's performance was closer to skilled levels earlier in the experimental program. In sum, SF may, because of individual differences, have had more "room" for improvement.

Before moving on to examine tests and extensions of the skilled memory theory, it seems worthwhile to comment on two aspects of the methodology employed by Chase and Ericsson: The use of verbal protocols and the use of a single-subject design (1981). Verbal protocols have, for a major part of this century, been eschewed by experimentalists as less than rigorous (Fiske, 1980) and have been adopted and used without proper methodological controls by a number of workers investigating the usability of computer software (see Wenger & Spyridakis, 1989, for a review). However, as Chase and Ericsson (1981) demonstrate, the verbal protocol contains a wealth of data that can explain the individual patterns that come to light as an individual acquires memory skill. Later studies (e.g., Ericcson & Oliver, 1989; Ericsson & Polson, 1988a, 1988b; Staszewski, 1988) reinforce this conclusion.

Skilled memory theory, as should be evident from the preceding discussions, relies heavily on observations of the meaningful associations that subjects make between the stimuli and prior knowledge (e.g., SF's relating randomly presented digits to patterns of running times). Thus, Ericsson and Oliver (1989) argue that the best information on mnemonic encoding and the use of retrieval structures comes from the verbal reports of the individual's cognitive behavior. However, caution must be exercised in the use of verbal protocols to reveal mental processes. Ericsson and Simon (1984) have observed that the quality of experimental data is often compromised in coding and analysis. They advocate making theoretical commitments explicit and weak, deriving coding schemes from the problem environment rather than the behavior of subjects, and maintaining constant encoding across protocols.

The second aspect of the methodology used to reveal aspects of the skilled memory theory is the use of single subjects. Single subject designs have been disavowed in some circles due to subjective and evaluative abuses and the difficulty in separating serendipitous individual differences from patterned responses to experimental stimuli (Mace & Kratochwill, 1986). However, when used with the proper experimental controls (see Kazdin, 1982), single subject designs can allow for the intensive examination of the acquisition and performance of patterns of interest by an experimental subject.

Tests of Skilled Memory Theory: Expert Memory for Menu Orders

Chase and Ericsson (1982) and Ericsson and Polson (1988a, 1988b) report a set of laboratory studies of a waiter who evidenced expert skills for menu orders. The waiter (JC) was tested on randomly generated orders composed of a meat dish cooked to a specified temperature, a starch, and a salad with a choice of salad dressings. Each experimental presentation consisted of orders from tables of three, five, or eight people.

Ericsson and Polson (1988a, 1988b) describe multiple levels of organization for JC's mnemonic encoding of orders. First, he appeared to organize his rehearsal of orders into groups of four. Second, he represented the orders in terms of a matrix composed of food categories and individual orders. In addition, he used within-category encodings (such as the first letter of the salad dressings), interactive representations of the order and characteristics of the person ordering, and spatial organization of the orders at the table (clockwise). Ericsson and Polson note that JC was able to reliably encode orders in two conditions (within-order and within-category) with no difference in overall study time. He was also able to encode orders presented in varied sequence (not strictly clockwise) with no decrement in performance for tables of three or five people. However, he did show a decrement for tables of eight people; Ericsson and Polson suggest that this effect is due to the fact that JC had to encode two units of four orders presented out of sequence.

Regarding the issue of specificity of practice effects, an important aspect of JC's performance concerned his memory for nondinner lists. JC's category retrieval structure appeared to generalize to lists composed of items either isomorphic or partially isomorphic to the structures used for restaurant orders. JC rapidly increased his study times for each of these lists across experimental sessions to the degree that his performance on these lists was equivalent to his early performance with the randomly generated restaurant orders. This result indicates transfer beyond the surface items used to acquire memory skill and thus represents some degree of generality. On the other hand, when JC was presented with lists that did not correspond to the dinner order structure, his performance was comparable to that of novices (Ericsson & Polson, 1988a, 1988b). This reveals that there are limits in the generality of JC's memory skills.

Tests of Skilled Memory Theory: Expert Mental Calculation

Staszewski (1988) investigated the applicability of the skilled memory theory to the domain of expert mental calculation, the skill that allows individuals to solve complex multiplication problems quickly and accurately. Specifically, Staszewski was interested in exploring the notion that expert performance results from an increase in working memory capacity due to efficient encoding and retrieval of information from LTM.

Two undergraduates (JA and GG) of normal intelligence (as reflected by GPAs and SAT scores) were given extended training on a mental multiplication algorithm used by an individual who evidenced expert level skill (AB). Each of the subjects was given practice for 45 minutes per day, 3 to 5 days a week. Over the duration of the investigation, JA accumulated 175 hours of practice (over a 3- year period) and GG accumulated 300 hours of practice (over a 4-year period). Following Chase and Ericsson (1981), Staszewski (1988) collected both performance data and verbal protocols.

Staszewski (1988) reported that the mnemonic encoding patterns used by each of the subjects resembled the pattern recognition capabilities of experts in other domains (Chase & Simon, 1973a, 1973b; McKeithen et al., 1981). That is, the subjects were able to discover and recognize repeating patterns of multiplicands and partial products which allowed them to accrue improvements to performance on top of those improvements resulting from increasingly skilled use of the multiplication algorithm.

Evidence for the use of retrieval structures was found in the organized representation of partial products apparent in both subjects' verbal protocols. In addition, the verbal protocols and tests of serial recall of presented items (conducted at the end of trials) showed evidence of hierarchical organization. Analysis of errors in the verbal protocol data showed that the same retrieval structure could accommodate both correctly and incorrectly retrieved items, suggesting that the structure is independent of the contents. Analysis of the pause boundaries of the serial recall of all presented items agreed with the boundaries suggested by the organization observed in the verbal protocols.

Finally, evidence for speed-up was found by the fit between the observed data and a power function (see Newell & Rosenbloom, 1981). The power function provided an acceptable fit to the data in all cases except for smaller problem sizes.

Conclusions

The data that have been reviewed indicate clearly that memory can be improved through practice. The present chapter concentrated on several types of item-specific improvements that are observed with relatively little practice and more general improvements that seem to require considerable practice. To summarize these improvements, it is worth revisiting the major points set out in the introduction.

First, we stated that it is important to examine the extent to which changes in memory behavior generalize across tasks. The studies reviewed have demonstrated that it is possible to move from the laboratory to real-world application. However, use of the methods examined and developed in the laboratory does not occur spontaneously and importantly, does not show great generality. Related to this issue is the issue of motivation. Studies of dramatic improvements in memory skill (e.g., SF) have relied on extensive, disciplined practice over an extended period. Importantly, several other subjects quit the experiment after several weeks, and these subjects did not show large improvements in memory span. It is thus unclear whether similar benefits could be obtained in less-well-controlled contexts. Thus, these issues invite additional exploration.

Second, we stated that it was necessary to examine the role that the nature of the practice experience plays in producing observed changes. Relative to this issue, we reviewed the literature on the spacing effect and found that the spacing effect has been obtained in a range of tasks with various materials, subjects, retention intervals, and memory measures. However, to date, there has been relatively little application of this general procedure (cf. Dempster, 1988).

Third, we stated that it was necessary to examine the structure or processes that change as a result of practice, and it was in regards to this issue, that we reviewed the development and tests of the skilled memory theory. The studies reviewed show that this theory holds great promise and that there is a wealth of data available to examine. However, the extant data is somewhat limited in terms of the range of tasks that have been examined.

Thus, this review suggests a number of avenues for exploration. First, we have the skilled memory theory available as a working theoretical base; thus, basic tests and extensions of the theory should be explored. In addition to the theoretical base, the skilled memory theory also shows the promise of using verbal protocols and intensive single subject designs to reveal processes. Second, investigations involving extensive practice seem to be called for. Finally, a wider range of tasks and materials than previously employed should be used.

References

Adams, L.T. (1985). Improving memory: Can retrieval strategies help? *Human Learning: Journal of Practical Research and Applications*, *4*, 281-297.

Angell, J.R. (1908). The doctrine of formal discipline in the light of the principles of general psychology. *Educational Review*, *36*, 1-14.

Atkinson, R.C. (1972). Optimizing the learning of a second-language vocabulary. *Journal of Experimental Psychology*, *96*, 124-129.

Baddeley, A. (1990). *Human memory: Theory and practice*. Boston, MA: Allyn and Bacon.

Baddeley, A.D., & Hitch, G. (1974). Working memory. In G.H. Bower (Ed.), *The psychology of learning and motivation* (Vol. 8, pp. 47-90). New York: Academic Press.

Ballard, P.B. (1913). Obliviscence and reminiscence. *British Journal of Psychology Monograph Supplements*, *1*, 1-82.

Bloom, K.C., & Shuell, T.J. (1981). Effects of massed and distributed practice on the learning and retention of second-language vocabulary. *Journal of Educational Research*, *74*, 245-248.

Broadbent, D.E. (1975). The magical number seven after fifteen years. In A. Kennedy & A. Wilkes (Eds.), *Studies in long-term memory* (pp. 3-18). New York: Wiley.

Brown-Su, A., & Payne D.G. (1988, March). *Memory as a skill: Encoding and retrieval practice effects*. Paper presented at the annual meeting of the Eastern Psychological Association.

Chase, W.G., & Ericsson, K.A. (1981). Skilled memory. In J.R. Anderson (Ed.), *Cognitive skills and their acquisition* (pp. 141-189). Hillsdale, NJ: Erlbaum.

Chase, W.G., & Ericsson, K.A. (1982). Skill and working memory. *The Psychology of Learning and Motivation*, *16*, 1-58.

Chase, W.G., & Simon, H.A. (1973a). Perception in chess. *Cognitive Psychology*, *4*, 55-81.

Chase, W.G., & Simon, H.A. (1973b). The mind's eye in chess. In W.G. Chase (Ed.), *Visual information processing* (pp. 215-281). New York: Academic Press.

Cornell, E. H. (1980). Distributed study facilitates infants' delayed recognition memory. *Memory and Cognition*, *8*, 539-542.

Crowder, R.G. (1976). *Principles of learning and memory*. Hillsdale, NJ: Erlbaum.

Dellarosa, D., & Bourne, L.E. (1985). Surface form and the spacing effect. In R.L. Solso (Ed.), *Theories in cognitive psychology: The Loyola Symposium* (pp. 123-144). Hillsdale, NJ: Erlbaum.

Dempster, F.N. (1987). Effects of variable encoding and the spaced presentations on vocabulary learning. *Journal of Educational Research*, *79*, 162-170.

Dempster, F.N. (1988). The spacing effect: A case study in the failure to apply the results. *American Psychologist*, *43*, 627-634.

Di Vesta, F.J., & Smith, P.A. (1979). The pausing principle: Increasing the efficiency of memory for ongoing events. *Contemporary Educational Psychology*, *4*, 288-296.

Ebbinghaus, H. (1964). *Memory: A contribution to experimental psychology* (H.A. Ruger & C.E. Bussenius, Trans.). New York: Dover. (Original work published 1964).

Erdelyi, M.H., & Becker, J. (1974). Hypermnesia for pictures: Incremental memory for pictures but not words in multiple recall trials. *Cognitive Psychology*, *6*, 159-171.

Erdelyi, M.H., Finks, J., & Feigin-Pfau, M.B. (1989). The effect of response bias on recall performance, with some observations on processing bias. *Journal of Experimental Psychology: General*, *118*, 245-254.

Erdelyi, M.H., & Stein, J.B. (1981). Recognition hypermnesia: The growth of recognition memory (d') over time with repeated testing. *Journal of Experimental Psychology: Human Learning and Memory*, *4*, 275-289.

Ericsson, K.A. (1985). Memory skill. *Canadian Journal of Psychology, 39*, 188-231.
Ericsson, K.A., Chase, W., & Faloon, S. (1980). Acquisition of a memory skill. *Science, 208*, 1181-1182.
Ericsson, K.A., & Oliver, W.A. (1989). A methodology for assessing the detailed structure of memory skills. In A.M. Colley & J.R. Beech (Eds.), *Acquisition and performance of cognitive skills* (pp. 193-214). New York: Wiley.
Ericsson, K.A., & Polson, P.G. (1988a). A cognitive analysis of exceptional memory for restaurant orders. In M.T.H. Chi, R. Glaser, & M.J. Farr (Eds.), *The nature of expertise* (pp. 23-70). Hillsdale, NJ: Erlbaum.
Ericsson, K.A., & Polson, P.G. (1988b). An experimental analysis of the mechanisms of a memory skill. *Journal of Experimental Psychology: Learning, Memory, and Cognition, 14*, 305-316.
Ericsson, K.A., & Simon, H.A. (1984). *Protocol analysis: Verbal reports as data*. Cambridge, MA: MIT Press.
Fiske, D.W. (1980). When are verbal reports veridical? *New Directions for Methodology of Social and Behavioral Science, 4*, 59-66.
Geiselman, R.E., Fisher, R.P., MacKinnon, D.P., & Holland, H.L. (1985). Eyewitness enhancement in the police interview: Cognitive retrieval mnemonics versus hypnosis. *Journal of Applied Psychology, 70*, 401-412.
Gick, M.L., & Holyoak, K.J. (1980). Analogical problem solving. *Cognitive Psychology, 12*, 306-355.
Gick, M.L., & Holyoak, K.J. (1983). Schema induction and analogical transfer. *Cognitive Psychology, 15*, 1-38.
Glenberg, A.L., & Lehman, T.S. (1980). Spacing repetitions over 1 week. *Memory & Cognition, 8*, 528-538.
Glover, J.A., & Corkill, A.J. (1987). Influence of paraphrased repetitions on the spacing effect. *Journal of Educational Psychology, 79*, 198-199.
Greene, R.L. (1989). Spacing effects in memory: Evidence for a two-process account. *Journal of Experimental Psychology: Learning, Memory, and Cognition, 15*, 371-377.
Grosofsky, A., & Payne, D.G. (1989). *A direct test of the selective displaced rehearsal hypothesis of the generation effect*. Paper presented at the meeting of the Midwestern Psychological Association.
Hayes, J.R., & Simon, H.A. (1977). Psychological differences among problem isomorphs. In J. Castellan, D.B. Pisoni, & G. Potts (Eds.), *Cognitive theory* (Vol. 2). Hillsdale, NJ: Erlbaum.
Herrmann, D.J., Buschke, H., & Gall, M.B. (1987). Improving retrieval. *Applied Cognitive Psychology, 1*, 27-33.
Hintzman, D.L. (1974). Theoretical implications of the spacing effect. In R.L. Solso (Ed.), *Theories in cognitive psychology: The Loyola Symposium* (pp. 77-97). Potomac, MD: Erlbaum.
Jost, A. (1897). Die assoziationstestigkeit in ihrer Abhangigkeit der Verteilung

der Wiederholungen. *Z Psychology*, *14*, 436-472.

Kay, D.S., & Black, J.B. (1985). The evolution of knowledge representations with increasing expertise using systems [Summary]. *Proceedings of the Seventh Annual Conference of the Cognitive Science Society*, Boston, MA.

Kazdin, A.E. (1982). *Single case research designs: Methods for clinical and applied settings*. New York: Oxford.

Lachman, R., Lachman, J., & Butterfield, E.C. (1979). *Cognitive psychology and information processing: An introduction*. Hillsdale, NJ: Erlbaum.

Landauer, T.K., & Bjork, R.A. (1978). Optimal rehearsal patterns and name learning. In M.M. Gruneberg, P.E. Morris, & R.N. Sykes (Eds.), *Practical aspects of memory* (pp. 625-632). London: Academic Press.

Landauer, T.K., & Ross, B.H. (1977). Can simple instructions to use special practice improve ability to remember a fact?: An experimental test using telephone numbers. *Bulletin of the Psychonomic Society*, *10*, 215-218.

Mace, F.C., & Kratochwill, T.R. (1986). The individual subject in behavior analysis research. In J. Valsiner (Ed.), *The individual subject and scientific psychology* (pp. 153-180). New York: Plenum.

Mandler, G. (1985). *Cognitive psychology: An essay in cognitive science*. Hillsdale, NJ: Erlbaum.

McKeithen, K.B., Reitman, J.S., Rueter, H.H., & Hirtle, S.C. (1981). Knowledge organization and skill differences in computer programmers. *Cognitive Psychology*, *13*, 307-325.

Miller, G.A. (1956). The magical number seven, plus or minus two: Some limits on our capacity for processing information. *Psychological Review*, *63*, 81-97.

Newell, A., & Rosenbloom, S. (1981). Mechanisms of skill acquisition and the law of practice. In J.R. Anderson (Ed.), *Cognitive skills and their acquisition* (pp. 1-51). Hillsdale, NJ: Erlbaum.

Payne, D.G. (1986). Hypermnesia for pictures and words: Testing the recall level hypothesis. *Journal of Experimental Psychology: Learning, Memory, and Cognition*, *12*, 16-29.

Payne, D.G. (1987). Hypermnesia and reminiscence in recall: A historical and empirical review. *Psychological Bulletin*, *101*, 5-27.

Payne, D.G., & Roediger, H.L. (1987). Hypermnesia occurs in recall but not in recognition. *American Journal of Psychology*, *100*, 145-165.

Perruchet, P. (1989). The effect of spaced practice on explicit and implicit memory. *British Journal of Psychology*, *80*, 113-130.

Pillsbury, W.B. (1908). The effects of training on memory. *Educational Review*, *36*, 15-27.

Postman, L. (1969). Experimental analysis of learning to learn. In G.H. Bower & J.T. Spence (Eds.), *The psychology of learning and motivation* (Vol. 3, pp. 241-296). New York: Academic Press.

Rea, C.P., & Modigliani, V. (1985). The effect of expanded versus massed practice on the retention of multiplication facts and spelling lists. *Human Learning: Journal of Practical Research and Applications*, *4*, 11-18.

Reder, L.M., & Anderson, J.R. (1982). Effects of spacing and embellishment for the main points of a text. *Memory & Cognition*, *10*, 97-102.
Roediger, H.L. (1980). The effectiveness of four mnemonics in ordering recall. *Journal of Experimental Psychology: Human Learning and Memory*, *6*, 558-567.
Roediger, H.L., & Payne, D.G. (1982). Hypermnesia: The role of repeated testing. *Journal of Experimental Psychology: Learning, Memory, and Cognition*, *8*, 66-72.
Roediger, H.L., & Payne, D.G. (1985). Recall criterion does not affect recall level or hypermnesia: A puzzle for generate/recognize theories. *Memory & Cognition*, *13*, 1-7.
Roediger, H.L., Payne, D.G., Gillespie, G.L., & Lean, D.S. (1982). Hypermnesia as determined by level of recall. *Journal of Verbal Learning and Verbal Behavior*, *21*, 635-655.
Roediger, H.L., Srinivas, K., & Waddill, P. (1989). How much does guessing influence recall? Comment on Erdelyi, Finks, and Feigin-Pfau. *Journal of Experimental Psychology: General*, *118*, 255-257.
Roediger, H.L., & Thorpe, L.A. (1978). The role of recall time in producing hypermnesia. *Memory & Cognition*, *6*, 296-305.
Rothkopf, E.Z., & Coke, E.U. (1963). Repetition interval and rehearsal method in learning equivalences from written sentences. *Journal of Verbal Learning and Verbal Behavior*, *2*, 406-416.
Shneiderman, B. (1976). Exploratory experiments in programmer behavior. *International Journal of Computer and Information Sciences*, *5*, 123-143.
Singley, M.K., & Anderson, J.R. (1985). The transfer of text-editing skill. *Journal of Man-Machine Studies*, *22*, 403-423.
Singley, M.K., & Anderson, J.R. (1989). *The transfer of cognitive skill*. Cambridge, MA: Harvard University Press.
Smith, S.M., & Rothkopf, E.Z. (1984). Contextual enhancement and distribution of practice in the classroom. *Cognition and Instruction*, *1*, 341-358.
Staszewski, J.J. (1988). Skilled memory and expert calculation. In M.T.H. Chi, R. Glaser, & M.J. Farr (Eds.), *The nature of expertise* (pp. 71-128). Hillsdale, NJ: Earlbaum.
Thorndike, E.L. (1898). Animal intelligence: An experimental study of the associative processes in animals. *Psychological Review Monographs*, *2* (8, Pt.).
Thorndike, E.L. (1903). *Educational psychology*. New York: Lemke & Buechner.
Thorndike, E.L. (1906). *Principles of teaching*. New York: A. G. Seiler.
Thorndike, E.L. (1922). The effect of changed data upon reasoning. *Journal of Educational Psychology*, *15*, 1-22.
Tolman, E.C. (1938). The determiners of behavior at a choice point. *Psychological Review*, *45*, 1-41.

Wallin, J.F.W. (1910). The doctrine of formal discipline. *Journal of Educational Psychology*, *1*, 168-171.

Wenger, M.J., & Spyridakis, J.H. (1989). The relevance of reliability and validity to usability testing. *IEEE Transactions on Professional Communication*, *32*, 265-271.

Woodrow, H. (1927). The effect of the type of training upon transference. *Journal of Educational Psychology*, *18*, 159-172.

Woodworth, R.S. (1938). *Experimental psychology*. New York: Henry Holt.

Zeichmeister, E.B., & Shaughnessy, J.J. (1980). When you know that you know and when you think that you know but you don't. *Bulletin of the Psychonomic Society*, *15*, 41-44.

Memory Improvement in Context: Implications for the Development of Memory Improvement Theory

Cathy L. McEvoy

Memory improvement, both as an academic and a commercial pursuit, has a mixed history. On the one hand, the classic mnemonic devices, notably the method of loci and imagery, are well documented in their effectiveness and appear in probably every introductory psychology text ever published. Students faced with large bodies of seemingly incomprehensible information sometimes rely on mnemonic techniques to organize and remember the various facts. Many business people, politicians, and college professors intentionally memorize the names of clients, constituents, and students, using classic as well as personalized memory improvement techniques. Recent studies indicate that older adults can learn to improve their performance on various cognitive tasks (see Willis, 1990), and schoolchildren benefit from strategy training in their academic endeavors (Pressley & El-Dinary, this volume).

On the other hand, there is a substantial literature that suggests that mnemonic techniques are used only infrequently by most people and that training individuals in their use does not often generalize to improved day-to-day memory performance. Even memory researchers and college professors who teach about the classic mnemonics report using them only infrequently, if at all (Park, Smith, & Cavanaugh, 1990). Instead, writing notes appears to be the technique of choice (Intons-Peterson & Fournier, 1986). Older adults can be taught the classic mnemonics, and their effectiveness can be demonstrated on laboratory tasks but with no reported decreases in everyday forgetfulness (Scogin, Storandt, & Lott, 1985; Zarit, Cole, & Guider, 1981). Memory improvement books, tapes, and courses are popular sellers despite the lack of evidence regarding their effectiveness. Concern about poor memory performance appears to be ubiquitous; successful attempts at memory improvement appear to be much more rare.

In an earlier chapter of this volume, Herrmann and Searleman reviewed the history of memory improvement activities and the theoretical orientations that have driven these activities. One interesting aspect of their review is that it illustrates the unidimensional nature of most of these theories. Memory performance and by implication, memory improvement was viewed as the result of a single or a small number of processes, operating in isolation from much of the surrounding environment. Different models emphasized different processes, including biological, motivational, and associative functions; but no model incorporated all of the processes emphasized in its various predecessors. Herrmann and Searleman concluded their chapter with a discussion of the multimodal theory of memory improvement, in which both the internal and external environment of the learner play a role in remembering. The findings reported in this volume, as well as other data from memory improvement research, suggest that the best framework for explaining and predicting memory improvement will come from multidimensional approaches (Herrmann & Searleman, 1990; Poon, 1980; Wilson, 1987). Memory improvement, like memory performance in general, is the end product of a collection of factors. In order to develop a useful theory of memory improvement, we should consider the separate and interactive influences of the tasks, individuals, and environments for which memory improvement is a goal. However, before we discuss a theory of memory improvement, there are several aspects of memory performance in general that should be mentioned.

Practical Factors that Affect Memory

Memory improvement techniques act upon the same factors that affect baseline or preimproved memory performance. This is an obvious point but an important one for the development of a model of memory improvement. Zacks and Hasher (this volume) discussed the implications of many factors that influence memory and that have been studied both in the laboratory and in the field. I will concentrate on some of the factors that are generally referred to as practical or applied aspects of memory. The study of such factors has burgeoned over the past 10 to 15 years, as demonstrated by the success of two international conferences on practical aspects of memory (Gruneberg, Morris, & Sykes, 1978, 1988) and the journal, *Applied Cognitive Psychology*. Although we know quite a lot about many of the practical factors that affect memory, we still don't know enough. Our lack of knowledge is on two levels: We don't fully know the parameters of the applied phenomena, and we don't know enough about the underlying mechanisms of the phenomena.

Perhaps because the study of applied memory is still in its early developmental stage, most of the research has been devoted to identifying phenomena and exploring their parameters, rather than studying underlying mechanisms. At the phenomena level, we have many interesting findings and also much conflicting data. For example, depression negatively affects memory performance but only in some tasks and with certain types of materials (Bower & Cohen, 1982; Hertel & Hardin, 1990). Although learning strategies can greatly increase performance, subsequent use of the strategies occurs in some cases but not in others (Best & Ornstein, 1986; Borkowski, Milstead, & Hale, 1988; Willis & Nesselroade, 1990). Psychopharmacological agents that have been advanced as possible treatments for memory loss sometimes help, sometimes hinder, and sometimes have no effect at all (Satlin & Cole, 1988; Weingartner & Herrmann, this volume; Wenk, 1989). These phenomena and several more are discussed in the earlier chapters of this volume, and it has become clear that many of them are interactive. For example, Hertzog (this volume) points out that use of memory strategies interacts with the user's metamemory, both about the effectiveness of the strategy and the user's evaluation of his memory skills. Payne and Wenger (this volume) note that the beneficial effects of practice depend on the type of practice and the context in which it is employed.

Memory is a complex process, and we should be mindful of the factors that may interact with the phenomena we wish to study. One area in which this has already proven to be critical is research on emotional state and memory. Researchers in this area are aware of the potential cognitive influences of psychotropic medications used by their depressed subjects. The cognitive psychologist cannot manipulate these medications but must take them into consideration when collecting and interpreting data. However, the extent to which this is a problem for the study of memory and depression may depend on the type of antidepressant drug used. Recent findings suggest that antidepressant effects on memory may be limited to those drugs that have a sedative component (Curran, Sakulsriprong, & Lader, 1988; Curran, Shine, & Lader, 1986; Siegfried & O'Connolly, 1986). Studies of depression and memory must also consider the frequent cooccurrence of depression and anxiety. Although this confounding was routinely ignored in the past, attention is now being focused on the differences between depression and anxiety in the ways that they affect memory and other cognitive processes (Greenberg & Beck, 1989; Hertel, this volume; Ingram, Kendall, Smith, Donnell, & Ronan, 1987; Thomas-Robe, 1990).

As we gain more knowledge about the effects of depression and anxiety and various medications on memory, we may be able to develop categories of memory tasks that are sensitive to each factor, which can then be used to evaluate the effectiveness of memory improvement procedures. Weingartner and Herrmann (this volume) mentioned the beginnings of a memory task taxonomy when they discussed the task specificity of each of the memory-enhancing drugs being considered. Similarly, the research on depression has identified tasks that show depressive effects and tasks that do not. Much recent effort has been directed toward developing taxonomies of tasks that are differentially affected by maturation, both in childhood development and in aging. Cognitive neuropsychological research is attempting to identify tasks in which performance is impaired by neurological disorders and tasks in which performance is spared. Not only does this knowledge allow us to narrow down the range of possible measures for evaluating memory improvement techniques, but a careful task analysis may provide insight into the underlying cognitive mechanisms affected by mood state, drugs, maturation, dementia, and so forth.

Underlying Mechanisms for Memory Phenomena

In addition to having a fuller picture of the factors that affect memory, we should also strive toward a better understanding of the underlying mechanisms responsible for the memory phenomena we wish to improve. Attempts to develop memory improvement techniques and theory will be poorly served if we ignore the mechanisms responsible for producing baseline memory performance. Without an understanding of these mechanisms, we can apply various techniques in a hit-or-miss fashion, but we will have difficulty developing a comprehensive theory to guide our applications. For example, we know that time of day affects cognitive performance. Although some progress has been made toward understanding the connection between time of day and cognition (Humphreys & Revelle, 1984; Matthews, Jones, & Chamberlain, 1989; Petros, Beckwith, & Anderson, 1990), the basic mechanisms that produce these effects are not well understood. At the present time, we are limited to making recommendations about when different tasks should be performed, based on findings such as better performance in English instruction in afternoon classes relative to morning classes (Davis, 1987). However, we can offer little advice on how to improve performance in English classes that must be taught in the morning, because we do not fully understand the mechanism producing time-of-day effects.

One underlying mechanism that may have considerable implications for memory improvement is attention. Few researchers in memory would argue with the statement that attention plays an important role in most memory tasks (Fisk & Schneider, 1984; Hasher & Zacks, 1979; Reason, 1984). However, the mechanism by which attention affects memory is still under study, and there are almost no data in the literature which indicate that improving a person's capacity to pay attention has a facilitating effect on memory (see review by Plude, this volume). In fact, there is only mixed evidence that attention training has a positive effect on attention (Benedict & Harris, 1989; Butler & Namerow, 1988; Ben-Yishay, Piasetsky, & Rattok, 1987; Sohlberg & Mateer, 1987). Despite the lack of evidence that improving attention improves memory, most memory improvement books list "paying attention" as the primary step toward better remembering (Cermak, 1976; West, 1985). Loftus advises her readers that "Probably the most important thing a person can do to improve memory is learn how to pay attention" (1980, p. 178).

The advice to pay attention in order to improve memory seems logical, particularly for some special populations, such as older adults who may be experiencing decreases in both attentional factors (Cerella, 1990; Plude, 1990; but see Giambra & Quilter, 1988) and in memory performance. The connection between attention and age decline in cognitive performance is dramatically illustrated in recent work by Stankov (1988). In his study, declines in measures of fluid intelligence as a function of age were virtually eliminated when measures of attention were partialled out from the age-intelligence correlation. While it is not possible to attribute causality for the age decline in fluid intelligence to changes in attention from these data, they do suggest a strong link between the two. Clearly, we need carefully controlled studies that explore this link to determine whether there is a causal connection and if so, to determine whether we can bring about changes in attention that result in improvement of memory and other cognitive abilities. The dearth of research on improvement of attention and any possible effects it may have on memory is not entirely surprising. Until we fully understand the mechanisms by which attention can be concentrated, directed, selected, divided, or switched; progress in improving attention will be slow. Nonetheless, because attention may be critical to remembering, it is important that we continue to study its underlying mechanisms and means of improvement for the elderly, children with attention deficit disorders, brain-injured patients, and so forth.

The issue of underlying mechanisms is also critical to the problem of poor generalization of memory improvement techniques across tasks. Much has been said about the lack of generalization from the training situation to new experiences, and many explanations have been proposed for this problem. As a result of the generalization problem, many successful memory improvement programs concentrate on teaching specific techniques for specific problems, rather than teaching more general techniques that theoretically transcend tasks but in practice often do not (e.g., Herrmann & Searleman, 1990; Leirer, Morrow, Pariante, & Sheikh, 1988; McEvoy & Moon, 1988). The specific training approach has been successful with several different types of subjects (college students, elderly, etc.), but the goal of developing a comprehensive theory of memory improvement urges us to continue searching for general, as well as specific, principles. This is not to suggest that people can be taught a single technique, such as imagery, and be expected to use this tool to solve all of their memory problems. We already know that this does not work, because people fail to see the relevance of the technique beyond the training context, and more importantly, because the technique frequently is not relevant. However, many memory tasks do share some components, and as a result, they should be amenable to some common memory improvement techniques.

One example of common components includes the tasks of remembering to keep an appointment, remembering to return books to the library before the due date, and remembering to buy a gift for an upcoming birthday. The shared component in all three of these tasks is the use of "prospective memory," or remembering to do something in the future (Ceci &

Bronfenbrenner, 1985; Dobbs & Rule, 1987; Einstein & McDaniel, 1990; Meacham & Leiman, 1982). Prospective memory relies upon an underlying mechanism that Craik (1986) describes as the self-initiation of retrieval cues. Problems of prospective memory occur when the self-initiation of internal cues fails, and external cues are either not present or not sufficiently salient. These problems are perhaps most easily addressed by increasing the availability of external cues or by improving the salience of cues that are already available. Although each task requires different behaviors and takes place in different locations, the essential problem for all three tasks is that of cuing the initiation of the behavior. One general technique can be applied to the cuing of all three tasks, namely making notations regarding the dates and times for each task on a central calendar. This simple technique makes available an external cue, and its usefulness is supported by the fact that notes and calendars are among the most frequently used external memory aids (Cavanaugh, Grady, & Perlmutter, 1983; Intons-Peterson & Fournier, 1986). It should be noted, however, that the effectiveness of this technique is only as good as the salience of the calendar or other external cue. Unless the person makes a habit of consulting the calendar on a very regular basis, it will not serve as an effective external cue for prospective memory tasks. This problem is well demonstrated by the average college professor, who seldom forgets committee meetings that are recorded on her office desk calendar but routinely forgets birthdays that are recorded on the low-salience calendar at home.

The above example suggests that general techniques can be used when tasks share common underlying components, but context-specific techniques may still be relevant. Making notations on a calendar is a general technique that applies to a large number of prospective memory tasks. Remembering to consult the calendar on a regular basis is more context specific. Most of us consult our desk calendar at least once a day, perhaps because it provides needed information every day, whereas the calendar at home provides needed information far less frequently. Thus, the general technique of making notations on a calendar must be combined with context-specific techniques that prompt a person to actually consult the calendar. A complete program of memory improvement may include techniques that generalize from situation to situation, but the implementation of those techniques will probably require context-specific training.

The What of Memory Improvement

As researchers continue to explore the practical applications of memory in the field and the underlying mechanisms of memory phenomena in the laboratory, work will continue on the development of a comprehensive theory of memory improvement. Toward this goal, we should first consider two questions: What is memory improvement, and whose memory are we trying to improve? With regard to the first question, I think we are in error if we conceptualize memory improvement as a singular endeavor. Just as there is no single behavior or mechanism that we can call memory, there is no single process that we can call memory improvement. As I read the contributions of the other authors in this book, I noticed that they were talking about a variety of memory tasks in a variety of contexts, using many different measures of memory performance. These differences are critical when we talk about memory improvement. We have long known that the optimal learning conditions for a recognition test are different from the optimal learning conditions for a recall test, even when all others variables are held constant. When we go beyond laboratory studies of recognition and recall and actually try to improve everyday memory performance, these effects are magnified. Improvement of memory for textbook material may be a main goal for students, whereas improvement of memory for the steps involved in preparing a cold lunch may be a goal for a dementing patient. Both involve processes that come under the rubric of memory, and in both cases we wish to improve the effectiveness of those processes, but we rely upon different techniques to address those processes.

What, then, is memory improvement? At first glance the easiest way to define memory improvement is through an outcome measure--if memory performance reliably changes for the better, we have observed memory improvement. However, this definition is insufficient. Memory performance may reliably change for the better due to maturation processes, in the absence of any intention to change that performance. Thus memory improvement is not simply an end product; it is an intervention designed to produce the end product of better memory performance. These interventions might be initiated by the subject himself, or by a teacher, spouse, or other caregiver. Although most interventions are initiated by the person who is the subject of improvement, this is not always the case. For many cognitively impaired populations, a hallmark problem is poor self-initiation of behaviors leading to recall. Posting a reminder on a mentally retarded child's bathroom mirror to cue her to brush her teeth every morning can be a memory improvement technique, even though she may not have initiated the posting of the reminder.

Many people would argue that only internal techniques, such as mnemonic devices, can be classified as memory improvement interventions, because external aids replace the act of remembering. Writing one's grocery list on a sheet of paper and taking it to the store, some would argue, does not improve memory for the items on the list; it eliminates the need for memory of the items. This argument has some legitimacy. However, the goal of memory improvement in everyday life is to increase the probability of accomplishing a task that is dependent, at least in part, on remembering aspects of the task. When a grocery list is developed, the goal is not so much to "memorize" the items on the list, as it is to obtain all the items and bring them back home. Writing a list may improve unprompted recall of the items on the list (Intons-Peterson & Newsome, this volume), but this recall is not necessary to accomplish the task, unless the list is lost. Although many external memory aids produce no improvement in recall in the absence of the aids, they do improve performance on the parts of the task that rely upon remembering something, and for this reason, I have chosen to classify external memory aids in the domain of memory improvement.

It can also be argued that interventions that are supportive of remembering but not directly involved in remembering are not technically part of memory improvement. Examples of supportive interventions include increasing memory self-efficacy; decreasing negative mood states, such as depression and anxiety; enlisting the social context for remembering; eliminating environmental interference; improving health and diet; and so forth. Technically, these are not direct memory improvement interventions, but they may play a major role in determining whether the direct interventions will be effective. For example, pretraining older adults in relaxation techniques can improve the effectiveness of mnemonic strategies taught after the relaxation training (Hill, Sheikh, & Yesavage, 1988). Supportive interventions have received very little attention in the memory improvement literature, perhaps explaining part of the failure of many memory improvement interventions. Thus broadly speaking, memory improvement includes any direct or supportive intervention designed to enhance completion of those aspects of a task that normally depend on memory.

The Who of Memory Improvement

The contributors to this book addressed a wide diversity of memory problems and contexts in which memory improvement takes place. They also addressed a wide diversity of subjects, such that there was very little overlap among the chapters in the types of people whose memory was the object of improvement. From the ubiquitous college student to the preschooler to the demented elderly, practically no group is free from attempts at memory improvement. This is not surprising, given the critical role that memory plays in almost all of our daily tasks, but it is important to consider the differences among these groups when developing memory interventions and theories to guide those interventions. What applies to one group of people may or may not apply to others. As shown in Table 12.1, I have roughly separated the subjects of memory intervention studies into three rather fuzzy categories: nonimpaired individuals, individuals with remediable problems, and severely impaired individuals.

The first category includes people who can be considered at least normal, if not above average, in their memory performance prior to any attempts at memory improvement. For example, the development of expertise begins from an adequate baseline of memory performance, as does the situation of college students trying to increase the amount they remember from lectures and texts or the business person hoping to improve memory for the names of clients. For this group, we would not be seeking pharmacologic techniques to improve memory, and in general, we would not have to be concerned with very large negative effects of emotional state, health problems, or medications. This group would benefit from training in various strategies, including classic mnemonics, appropriate use of practice, focusing attention on relevant stimuli, and organizing external memory aids. Perhaps more so than the other two categories, individuals in this group might benefit from metamemory information, such as how and why different memory strategies work, how the physical and social environment affect memory, and so forth.

Table 12.1. Categories of Subjects of Memory Improvement Interventions.

Non-impaired
- Developing expertise
- Improving academic skills
- Improving on-the-job memory skills
- Improvement memory in normal adults

Remediable problems
- Memory loss in later adulthood
- Impairment due to health problems and/or medications
- Impairment due to depression and/or anxiety
- Learning delays
- Impairment due to Attention Deficit Disorder

Severe impairment
- Amnesia
- Brain injury
- Dementing disease
- Profound retardation

For the most part, memory improvement efforts with subjects from this first category include techniques that are taught by others or learned from reading books, and so forth, but that are then initiated by the subject. This differs from many of the techniques used with subjects in the latter two categories, particularly category 3, in which an individual other than the subject might have control over the presentation and use of memory aids. In addition to techniques that are self-applied and those that are applied by others, some techniques are built into the learning situation. Examples of this are the use of multiple study and testing sessions in curricula, which can increase retention of the subject matter over extremely long periods of time (Bahrick & Hall, 1991) and the very effective technique of spacing repetitions (Landauer & Bjork, 1978; Payne & Wenger, this volume). Such curriculum-generated practice effects may be particularly useful with children who are too young to understand the benefit of self-initiated practice.

It's possible that the types of individuals who fall into this first category may be the best prospects for finding techniques of memory improvement that generalize from the immediate training situation to other, related situations. The individuals in this group are essentially normal in memory performance (at least relative to their age peers) prior to engaging in memory improvement activities. Even people with exceptional memories generally demonstrate normal memory performance in areas other than their speciality (Ceci, DeSimone, & Johnson, this volume; Ericsson & Chase, 1982; Frieman, Thompson, & Vogl, 1990). Starting from an adequate baseline of cognitive functioning, generalization might be more likely with these types of subjects.

The issue of generalization of a memory improvement technique was directly addressed by Ericsson and Polson (1988) in their study of a waiter with exceptional memory for dinner orders. They found that the waiter was able to generalize his skill to the memorization of materials with category structures comparable to dinner orders but was not able to generalize to materials that did not have comparable structure. Their findings suggest that when tasks share comparable structure, the learner can apply comparable retrieval processes. When the structure changes, the previously relevant underlying mechanism loses its relevance, and generalization is less likely. Attempts to produce generalization in memory improvement subjects will probably require both shared underlying mechanisms and the subject's understanding of the potential for applying a technique to more than one situation. This latter requirement is most likely to be found in subjects in the first category, who have no a priori memory impairment that might preclude this understanding.

The second category includes people who are experiencing some actual memory impairment due to age, health problems, emotional state, learning disabilities, and so forth. For this group, the goal of memory improvement interventions may be to return the individual, as closely as possible, to premorbid levels of memory performance or to improve performance to the approximate level of nonimpaired cohorts. This goal may be far from attainable with current memory improvement technology, but the fact that some changes do occur with intervention suggests that these problems are at least partially remediable.

One characteristic of the individuals in category 2 that has important implications for theory is that they differ in the locus of their memory problems and the extent to which that locus is amenable to change. With individuals for whom the cause of the problem cannot be changed, memory improvement is designed to augment and enhance remaining skills, rather than reverse the cause. For example, aging cannot be reversed, and many drugs that impair cognition are needed by some patients to sustain life. Memory improvement techniques for these people are designed to remediate a memory problem, not to remediate the cause of that problem.

For others in this category, memory impairment is linked to a treatable condition, such as depression or anxiety, and improvement in the condition is expected to result in improvement of the memory impairment (Raskind, 1984). For these cases, memory improvement techniques are supplemental to treatment of the mood state. Unfortunately, controlled studies of the effects of treatment for depression and anxiety on changes in cognitive performance are lacking. Important areas of needed research, along with controlled treatment studies, include whether memory improvement is feasible prior to treating the mood impairment (Watts, MacLeod, & Morris, 1988) and if so, whether it influences the treatment outcome.

Others in the second category may be experiencing memory impairment due to health problems such as diabetes and hypertension, in which the disease can be controlled, but this control apparently does not totally reverse the associated cognitive problems (Elias, Schultz, Robbins, & Elias, 1989; Hertzog, Schaie, & Gribbin, 1978; Madden & Blumenthal, 1989; Perlmuter et al., 1984). In these situations, control of the medical problem is necessary for any effective memory improvement program, but it is not sufficient. Cognitive interventions for these individuals should supplement the medical treatment of the memory-impairing condition.

Memory improvement efforts with subjects from category 2 should pay particular attention to some of the supportive interventions that can affect memory performance. As Best (this volume) points out, remembering frequently occurs in a social context. Quite often we are required to remember something in the presence of others and perhaps under their scrutiny as well. For subjects who experience some memory loss or intellectual impairment, such as depressed patients, learning-delayed children, or older adults, self-evaluation and perceived evaluation by others may be critical factors in memory performance. These individuals are likely to be more self-conscious of their poor performance than individuals from category 1. Social variables may have direct effects on memory, as when the subject relies on others to do the remembering rather than risk forgetting, and also interactive effects. The use of external aids that can be seen or heard by others, such as pocket notebooks or timers, may not be acceptable to subjects with negative perceptions of how their memory performance is evaluated by those around them. Despite the fact that external aids can be extremely effective, their negative social connotations may preclude their use. Preliminary to any attempts at memory improvement interventions, there should be an evaluation of the subject's attitudes and beliefs so that the intervention can address both the actual memory problems and the attitudes towards those problems.

Our theories might also take into consideration whether subjects in the second category benefit differentially from external and internal memory aids, relative to subjects in the first category. For example, studies have indicated that older adults may rely on external aids to a greater degree than do younger adults (Jackson, Bogers, & Kerstholt, 1988; McEvoy, 1988), but I am unaware of any studies that have looked at the relative efficacy of the different types of aids when used by the elderly. It might be assumed that their greater reliance on external aids reflects a decrease in the effectiveness of internal aids. However, given Brigham and Pressley's (1988) data suggesting that older adults' selection of memory strategies does not correspond well to prior successes and failures with those strategies, it's possible that their preference for one type of aid over the other is determined by factors other than effectiveness. Similarly, therapists working with mood-impaired subjects may reject potential learning strategies based on beliefs about the capabilities of depressed individuals, rather than on actual data. Hertel (this volume, Hertel & Rude, 1991) described an interesting finding: that depressed subjects benefit from a more demanding cognitive task, provided that it is structured to maintain a focus on the task materials. This finding runs counter to the widely held belief that depressed individuals cannot process complex information and suggests that our theories of mood disturbance and memory may need some modifying.

The third category of subjects represents those who are seriously memory impaired, either with specific, focal memory losses, or more global dementing illnesses. For the most part, the memory impairment seen in these individuals is not readily reversed, although there is usually some recovery of function for a period of time in brain-injured patients. Frequently the problems in this third category are superimposed on the less severe impairments represented in the second category. Thus, most demented patients are also elderly, and clinical depression and/or anxiety is a common cooccurrence of dementia (Reifler, Larson, & Hanley, 1982; Reifler, Larson, Teri, & Poulsen, 1986). Substance-abusing young men are overrepresented among the population of head-injured patients, and many cases of stroke-related brain insult and amnesia are coupled with problems of hypertension, and so forth.

For subjects with extremely compromised cognitive systems, we should be much more aware of possible interactive effects of variables that have only slight effects on Category 1 and 2 subjects. To illustrate this point, consider one demented woman with whom we recently worked (McEvoy & Schonfeld, 1989). Mrs. E. was a widow diagnosed with Alzheimer's Disease. She had three adult children in the area, and she alternated living in each one's home on an approximately weekly basis. All three children complained that she "hid" her dirty underwear in various places throughout the houses. After an analysis of the problem, three matching hampers were purchased and placed in identical locations in Mrs. E.'s bedroom in each house. With some prompting and a sign stating "Mom's dirty clothes" taped to each hamper, she eventually learned to use the hampers and stopped hiding her underwear. Several months later, one of the daughters moved the hamper in her home to the bathroom. Almost immediately, Mrs. E. began hiding her dirty underwear again. Interestingly, although the hamper was moved in only one house, the previously successful external memory aid failed in all three houses. In Mrs. E.'s case a seemingly minor environmental change in an external memory aid, moving the hamper from one room to another, rendered the aid useless. This does not often happen with individuals who do not have serious cognitive impairment. When my portable timer buzzes to remind me to take the cake out of the oven, it is just as effective regardless of whether I am in the kitchen, the den, or the back yard.

Many other variables that have minimal effects on more intact subjects may have large effects on the severely impaired. Alzheimer's patients sometimes suffer from "sundowning," an increase in confusion and disorientation in the early evening (Evans, 1987), which might be thought of as an exaggerated time-of-day effect. Anxiety and frustration affect almost anyone faced with a seemingly unsolvable cognitive task, but the harmful effects appear to be greater for brain-injured, profoundly retarded and demented patients. Thus our theories of memory improvement might include a mechanism that weights the influence of environmental, social, and emotional variables as a function of degree of impairment of the subject.

Most of the attempts at memory improvement with individuals in the third category include the use of external aids, structuring of social and physical environments, and pharmacological interventions. Memory performance for these individuals is also more likely to be affected by the presence of another individual who has a caregiving role. Serving as "collateral memories," caregivers can be the most frequently used memory aid for severely impaired individuals. Internal learning strategies and mnemonics are used less frequently and appear to be useful primarily with patients who have very specific, as opposed to global, memory impairment (Wilson, 1984). Use of these intellectually demanding memory aids probably necessitates a more intact cognitive system than is the case for many seriously impaired individuals (Hill, Yesavage, Sheikh, & Friedman, 1989) or extensive training and prompting of the technique (Schacter, Rich, & Stampp, 1985). The one internal device that is seeing a lot of application, particularly with brain-injured patients, is attention training. In theory, attention training is a precursor to other forms of memory improvement and sets the stage for better encoding and retrieval. Unfortunately, as Plude (this volume) points out, we are still awaiting data on the effectiveness of this approach, which has such intuitive appeal.

Finally, it should be pointed out that there is one very large group of individuals who seem to defy categorization in the above scheme. As Best (this volume) noted, young children have characteristics of all three categories. When presented with a memory task that is age appropriate, their performance is relatively normal and probably no more affected by physical, environmental, emotional, or social variables than any other subject in Category 1. However, normal memory performance for young children is far below that of older children on a large variety of tasks, and in particular, their metamemory and self-initiation of strategy use is lacking. In this respect, they more strongly resemble some of the subjects in Category 2 (Conca, 1989). The fact that their memory performance can be enhanced, at least within their "zone of proximal development" (Vygotsky, 1978), is also similar to subjects in the second category. However, for age-inappropriate tasks (those outside the zone of proximal development), young children are more like Category 3 subjects and may have to depend largely on the collateral memory of caregivers. Memory improvement theories may not be able to classify children because of their ongoing maturation, but our theories should provide a broad enough set of functional relationships that memory enhancement can be understood at each stage of development.

Memory Improvement in Context

One of the themes throughout this volume is that memory improvement does not occur in a vacuum. Because the use of memory skills occurs within a context that has social, environmental, biological and emotional components, successful memory improvement is likely to be context dependent. Several years ago, Jenkins eloquently described a contextualist approach to understanding memory performance when he introduced his tetrahedral model (1979). In his model, he identified four sets of variables that can have both direct and interactive effects on memory. His approach has been borrowed and modified countless times since then to understand various aspects of cognitive performance and development. The papers presented in this volume suggest that the tetrahedral model, which was developed to address memory performance, can be applied to memory improvement with very little modification. Table 12.2 represents possible classifications for the four points of a tetrahedron as it might be applied to memory improvement, with all due respect to Professor Jenkins.

The four classes of variables that can affect memory improvement efforts are subject characteristics, orientation of the subject to the memory task, the nature of the task, and the environment in which the subject is attempting to improve memory performance. An important quality of the tetrahedron is that each of these classes of variables can have direct effects on memory improvement and interactive effects. The chapters in this volume have summarized many of the direct and interactive effects of the variables in the tetrahedron, and many more can be found in the literature on memory improvement. The important next step that we must take in developing memory improvement theory is sorting out the effects, and in particular the interactions, in order to improve the focus of our intervention efforts. The question then becomes, which variables matter in the present context and which variables do not?

Many of the variables that we study in relation to memory performance and improvement are likely to be more influential in some situations than in others. By assigning weights to variables, we can focus on those that have the greatest influence in the context in which we are studying memory improvement and disregard those that are known to have little influence in that context. However, we need an a priori framework in which to consider possible variables and their weights. In the previous section of this chapter, I suggested a classification by subject characteristics. Within this classification, I suggested that some internal factors, such as mnemonic strategies, elaborative practice, and metamemory, may have a greater influence on more cognitively intact subjects and may be of less use with the most impaired subjects. External factors, such as the physical and social context, and external memory aids, may have a greater influence on the more impaired individual. This classification approach takes one point in the tetrahedron (*subject variables*) as a starting place and looks for a pattern of interactions with variables from the other points. Another researcher might take *task variables* as the starting place, group them into categories, and look at the pattern of interactions between groups of tasks and the other variables. This approach would be consistent with one of the most enduring modes of study used throughout the history of memory research.

Table 12.2. Variables that can Affect Memory Improvement Efforts.

Subject	*Orientation*
Developmental stage	Attention
Emotional state	Metamemory
Medical condition	Strategies
Expertise	Practice
Dementia	.
.	.
.	.
.	
Memory Task	Environment
Prospective	External aids
Facts	Social context
Motor skill	Caregiver
Implicit	Physical context
.	Time of day
.	.
.	.
	.

One advantage of a contextual approach to memory improvement theory is that variables can have both a direct effect on memory and/or an indirect effect through other variables. Herrmann and Searleman (1990) incorporate both direct and indirect effects in their multimodal approach. For example, they suggest that physical and social manipulations affect memory indirectly through the sensory and response systems. Likewise, we have seen that metamemory affects performance indirectly through strategy selection, criterion setting, and so forth. Time of day may have its primary effect on memory indirectly, through changes in attention, and aging and negative mood state may affect recall through changes in processing resources.

The indirect effects on memory are important to theory, because they suggest one means by which we can weight the influence of variables. To the extent that variable *A* has an indirect effect on recall through variable *B*, we will see effects of *A* only on tasks in which *B* has a significant role. Implicit memory tasks, in which allocation of processing resources to specific learning strategies has negligible effects (Jacoby & Dallas, 1981), should be less affected by aging, negative mood state, and metamemory than are explicit memory tasks. Although of these three, only aging (and to a lesser degree depression) has been studied extensively with respect to implicit memory tasks, it appears that this type of remembering is only slightly affected by aging (Howard, 1988; Hultsch, Masson, & Small, 1991; Light & Singh, 1987). Other variables do affect implicit learning and memory, such as repetitious practice with a physically similar stimulus (Lewicki, Czyzewska, & Hoffman, 1987). To the extent that repetitious practice influences recall through reinstating a physical context, we might expect to see improvement in implicit memory even among subjects who normally show much less improvement in explicit memory, such as those with amnesia, dementia, and learning disabilities.

The contextualist approach to understanding memory improvement is useful for thinking about the many variables that affect memory, but to develop a predictive model, we need to go beyond cataloging the direct and interactive effects of those variables. A preliminary step toward developing such a model might be to treat subject-task combinations as the core elements that define a given memory improvement situation, then assigning weights to the orientation and environment variables as they apply to that situation. Based upon what we know about the underlying mechanisms of the memory task in question, variables can be given large or small weights, depending on the role they play in that task. Thus classic mnemonic strategies would receive a large weighting if the task were remembering the names of several recently met individuals but a small weighting if the task were remembering how to make a sandwich. The variables might also be given valences, depending upon whether the subject is affected by (or capable of utilizing) that variable. Thus, mnemonic strategies would have a positive valence for a mnemonist, a neutral or slightly positive valence for a nonimpaired, healthy child or adult, and a negative valence for a severely brain-injured or demented individual. The combination of weights and valences would describe the predicted effect of that variable in the given subject-task situation. Variables with small weights would have little effect on the task, regardless of the direction of their valence.

Variables with larger weights would enhance performance for groups of subjects having positive valences on that variable and produce poor performance for subjects with negative valences.

One goal of this type of theory would be to categorize tasks and subjects in such a way that all the elements within a category are affected similarly by a given set of variables. Assuming that many tasks share some of their component processes and that subgroups of subjects share similar cognitive strengths and impairments, the large number of possible interactions between subjects, tasks, and other variables might be reduced to a workable set. Of course, at this point, we are far from realizing this goal. We need a great deal of knowledge about our memory tasks, subject characteristics, and learning environment--knowledge that comes to us both from laboratory research and clinical studies. The usefulness of a contextualist approach comes from suggesting which variables might be of interest in a given situation and which might not and in interpreting findings that reflect the operation of multiple determinants of recall. Although we are a long way from a predictive model of memory improvement, progress in this area has already been of interest and use to clinicians and other researchers.

Endnote 1

Preparation of this chapter was supported by National Institute of Mental Health Grant MH 45207.

References

Bahrick, H.P., & Hall, L.K. (1991). Lifetime maintenance of high school mathematics content. *Journal of Experimental Psychology: General*, *120*, 20-33.

Benedict, R., & Harris, A.E. (1989). Remediation of attention deficits in chronic schizophrenia patients: A preliminary study. *British Journal of Clinical Psychology*, *28*, 187-188.

Ben-Yishay, Y., Piasetsky, E.B., & Rattok, J. (1987). A systematic method for ameliorating disorders in basic attention. In M.J. Meier, A.L. Benton, & L. Diller (Eds.), *Neuropsychological rehabilitation* (pp. 165-181). New York: Guilford.

Best, D.L., & Ornstein, P.A. (1986). Children's generation and communication of mnemonic organizational strategies. *Developmental Psychology*, *22*, 845-853.

Borkowski, J.G., Milstead, M., & Hale, C. (1988). Components of children's metamemory: Implications for strategy generalization. In F.E. Weinert & M. Perlmutter (Eds.), *Memory development: Universal changes and individual differences* (pp. 73-100). Hillsdale, NJ: Erlbaum.

Bower, G.H., & Cohen, P.R. (1982). Emotional influences in memory and thinking: Data and theory. In M.S. Clarke & S.T. Fiske (Eds.), *Affect and cognition: The Seventeenth Annual Carnegie Symposium on Cognition* (pp. 291-331). Hillsdale, NJ: Erlbaum.

Brigham, M.C., & Pressley, M. (1988). Cognitive monitoring and strategy choice in younger and older adults. *Psychology and Aging*, *3*, 249-257.

Butler, R.W., & Namerow, N.S. (1988). Cognitive retraining in brain-injury rehabilitation: A critical review. *Journal of Neurologic Rehabilitation*, *2*, 97-101.

Cavanaugh, J.C., Grady, J.G., & Perlmutter, M. (1983). Forgetting and use of memory aids in 20 to 70 year olds everyday life. *International Journal of Aging and Human Development*, *17*, 113-122.

Ceci, S.J., & Bronfenbrenner, U. (1985). Don't forget to take the cupcakes out of the oven: Prospective memory, strategic time-monitoring, and context. *Child Development*, *56*, 152-164.

Cerella, J. (1990). Aging and information processing rate. In J.E. Birren & K.W. Schaie (Eds.), *Handbook of the psychology of aging* (3rd. ed., pp. 201-221). New York: Van Nostrand Reinhold.

Cermak, L.S. (1976). *Improving your memory*. New York: McGraw-Hill.

Conca, L. (1989). Strategy choice by LD children with good and poor naming ability in a naturalistic memory situation. *Learning Disability Quarterly*, *12*, 97-106.

Craik, F.I.M. (1986). A functional account of age differences in memory. In F. Klix & H. Hagendorf (Eds.), *Human memory and cognitive capabilities: Mechanisms and performances* (pp. 409-422). Amsterdam: Elsevier.

Curran, H., Sakulsriprong, M., & Lader, M. (1988). Antidepressants and human memory: An investigation of four drugs with different sedative and anticholinergic profiles. *Psychopharmacology*, *95*, 520-527.

Curran, H., Shine, P., & Lader, M. (1986). Effects of repeated doses of fluvoxamine, mianserin and placebo on memory and measures of sedation. *Psychopharmacology*, *89*, 360-363.

Davis, Z.T. (1987). The effect of time-of-day of instruction on eighth-grade students' English and mathematics achievement. *High School Journal*, *71*, 78-80.

Dobbs, A.R., & Rule, B.G. (1987). Prospective memory and self-reports of memory abilities in older adults. *Canadian Journal of Psychology*, *41*, 209-222.

Einstein, G.O., & McDaniel, M.A. (1990). Normal aging and prospective memory. *Journal of Experimental Psychology: Learning, Memory, and Cognition*, *16*, 717-726.

Elias, M.F., Schultz, N.R., Jr., Robbins, M.A., & Elias, P.K. (1989). A longitudinal study of neuropsychological performance by hypertensives and normotensives: A third measurement point. *Journal of Gerontology*, *44*, P25-P28.

Ericsson, K.A., & Chase, W.P. (1982). Exceptional memory. *American Scientist*, *70*, 607-615.

Ericsson, K.A., & Polson, P.G. (1988). An experimental analysis of the mechanisms of a memory skill. *Journal of Experimental Psychology: Learning, Memory, and Cognition*, *14*, 305-316.

Evans, L.K. (1987). Sundown syndrome in institutionalized elderly. *Journal of the American Gerontological Society*, *35*, 101-108.

Fisk, A.D., & Schneider, W. (1984). Memory as a function of attention, level of processing, and automatization. *Journal of Experimental Psychology: Learning, Memory, and Cognition*, *10*, 181-197.

Frieman, J., Thompson, C.P., & Vogl, R.J. (1990, November). *Exceptional performance in skilled memory: Data and demonstration*. Paper presented at the meeting of the Psychonomic Society, New Orleans.

Giambra, L.M., & Quilter, R.E. (1988). Sustained attention in adulthood: A unique, large-sample, longitudinal and multicohort analysis using the Mackworth Clock-Test. *Psychology and Aging*, *3*, 75-83.

Greenberg, M.S., & Beck, A.T. (1989). Depression versus anxiety: A test of the content-specificity hypothesis. *Journal of Abnormal Psychology*, *98*, 9-13.

Gruneberg, M.M., Morris, P.E., & Sykes, R.N. (Eds.). (1978). *Practical aspects of memory*. London: Academic Press.

Gruneberg, M.M., Morris, P.E., & Sykes, R.N. (Eds.). (1988). *Practical aspects of memory: Current research and issues*. Chichester: Wiley.

Hasher, L., & Zacks, R.T. (1979). Automatic and effortful processes in memory. *Journal of Experimental Psychology: General*, *108*, 356-388.

Herrmann, D.J., & Searleman, A. (1990). The new multimodal approach to memory improvement. In G.H. Bower (Ed.), *Advances in learning and motivation* (Vol. 26, pp. 175-205). New York: Academic Press.

Hertel, P.T., & Hardin, T.S. (1990). Remembering with and without awareness in a depressed mood: Evidence for deficits in initiative. *Journal of Experimental Psychology: General*, *119*, 45-59.

Hertel, P.T., & Rude, S.S. (1991). Depressive deficits in memory: Focusing attention improves subsequent recall. *Journal of Experimental Psychology: General*, *120*, 301-312.

Hertzog, C., Schaie, K.W., & Gribbin, K. (1978). Cardiovascular disease and changes in intellectual functioning from middle to old age. *Journal of Gerontology*, *33*, 872-883.

Hill, R.D., Sheikh, J.I., & Yesavage, J.A. (1988). Pretraining enhances mnemonic training in elderly adults. *Experimental Aging Research*, *14*, 207-211.

Hill, R.D., Yesavage, J.A., Sheikh, J., & Friedman, L. (1989). Mental status as a predictor of response to memory training in older adults. *Educational Gerontology*, *15*, 633-639.

Howard, D.V. (1988). Implicit and explicit assessment of cognitive aging. In M.L. Howe & C.J. Brainerd (Eds.), *Cognitive development in adulthood:*

Progress in cognitive development research (pp. 3-37). New York: Springer-Verlag.

Hultsch, D.F., Masson, M.E.J., & Small, B.J. (1991). Adult age differences in direct and indirect tests of memory. *Journal of Gerontology, 46*, P22-P30.

Humphreys, M.S., & Revelle, W. (1984). Personality, motivation, and performance: A theory of the relationship between individual differences and information processing. *Psychological Review, 91*, 153-184.

Ingram, R.E., Kendall, P.C., Smith, T.W., Donnell, C., & Ronan, K. (1987). Cognitive specificity in emotional distress. *Journal of Personality and Social Psychology, 53*, 734-742.

Intons-Peterson, M.J., & Fournier, J. (1986). External and internal memory aids: When and how often do we use them? *Journal of Experimental Psychology: General, 115*, 267-280.

Jackson, J.L., Bogers, H., & Kerstholt, J. (1988). Do memory aids aid the elderly in their day to day remembering? In M.M. Gruneberg, P.E. Morris, & R.N. Sykes (Eds.), *Practical aspects of memory: Current research and issues: Vol. 2. Clinical and educational implications* (pp.137-142). Chichester: Wiley.

Jacoby, L.L., & Dallas, M. (1981). On the relationship between autobiographical memory and perceptual learning. *Journal of Experimental Psychology: General, 110*, 306-340.

Jenkins, J.J. (1979). Four points to remember: A tetrahedral model of memory experiments. In L.S. Cermak & F.I.M. Craik (Eds.), *Levels of processing in human memory* (pp. 429-446). Hillsdale, NJ: Erlbaum.

Landauer, T.K., & Bjork, R.A. (1978). Optimum rehearsal patterns and name learning. In M.M. Gruneberg, P.E. Morris, & R.N. Sykes (Eds.), *Practical aspects of memory* (pp. 625-632). New York: Academic Press.

Leirer, V.O., Morrow, D.G., Pariante, G.M., & Sheikh, J.I. (1988). Elders' nonadherence, its assessment, and computer assisted instruction for medication recall training. *Journal of the American Geriatrics Society, 36*, 877-884.

Lewicki, P., Czyzewska, M., & Hoffman, H. (1987). Unconscious acquisition of complex procedural knowledge. *Journal of Experimental Psychology: Learning, Memory, and Cognition, 13*, 523-530.

Light, L.L., & Singh, A. (1987). Implicit and explicit memory in young and older adults. *Journal of Experimental Psychology: Learning, Memory, and Cognition, 13*, 531-541.

Loftus, E. (1980). *Memory: Surprising new insights into how we remember and why we forget*. Reading, MA: Addison-Wesley.

Madden, D.J., & Blumenthal, J.A. (1989). Slowing of memory-search performance in men with mild hypertension. *Health Psychology, 8*, 131-142.

Matthews, G., Jones, D.M., & Chamberlain, A.G. (1989). Interactive effects of extraversion and arousal on attentional task performance: Multiple resources or encoding processes? *Journal of Personality and Social Psychology, 56*, 629-639.

McEvoy, C.L. (1988, April). *Teaching everyday memory skills for older adults*. Paper presented at the meeting of the Eastern Psychological Association, Buffalo, NY.
McEvoy, C.L., & Moon, J.R. (1988). Assessment and treatment of everyday memory problems in the elderly. In M.M. Gruneberg, P.E. Morris, & R.N. Sykes (Eds.), *Practical aspects of memory: Current research and issues*, (Vol. 2, pp. 155-160). Chichester: Wiley.
McEvoy, C.L., & Schonfeld, L. (1989). Family treatment in Alzheimer's Disease. *Clinical Gerontologist, 9*, 58-61.
Meacham, J.A., & Leiman, B. (1982). Remembering to perform future actions. In U. Neisser (Ed.), *Memory observed: Remembering in natural contexts* (pp. 327-336). San Francisco: Freeman.
Park, D.C., Smith, A.D., & Cavanaugh, J.C. (1990). Metamemories of memory researchers. *Memory & Cognition, 18*, 321-327.
Perlmuter, L.C., Hakami, M.K., Hodgson-Harrington, C., Ginsberg, J., Katz, J., Singer, D.E., & Nathan, D.M. (1984). Decreased cognitive function in aging non-insulin-dependent diabetic patients. *American Journal of Medicine, 77*, 1043-1048.
Petros, T.V., Beckwith, B.E., & Anderson, M. (1990). Individual differences in the effects of time of day and passage difficulty on prose memory in adults. *British Journal of Psychology, 81*, 63-72.
Plude, D.J. (1990). Aging, feature integration, and visual selective attention. In J.E. Enns (Ed.), *The development of attention: Research and theory* (pp. 467-487). Amsterdam: Elsevier.
Poon, L.W. (1980). A systems approach for the assessment and treatment of memory problems. In J.M. Ferguson & C.B. Taylor (Eds.), The comprehensive handbook of behavior medicine (Vol. 1, pp. 191-212). New York: Spectrum.
Raskind, M. (1984). Electroconvulsive therapy in the elderly. *Journal of the American Geriatrics Society, 32*, 177-178.
Reason, J. (1984). Lapses of attention in everyday life. In R. Parasuraman & D.R. Davies (Eds.), *Varieties of attention* (pp. 515-549). New York: Academic Press.
Reifler, B.V., Larson, E., & Hanley, R. (1982). Coexistence of cognitive impairment and depression in geriatric outpatients. *American Journal of Psychiatry, 139*, 623-626.
Reifler, B.V., Larson, E., Teri, L., & Poulsen, M. (1986). Alzheimer's disease and depression. *Journal of the American Geriatrics Society, 34*, 858-859.
Satlin, A., & Cole, J.O. (1988). Psychopharmacologic interventions. In L.F. Jarvik & C.H. Winograd (Eds.), *Treatments for the Alzheimer patient: The long haul* (pp. 59-79). New York: Springer-Verlag.
Schacter, D.L., Rich, S.A., Stampp, M.S. (1985). Remediation of memory disorders: Experimental evaluation of the spaced-retrieval technique. *Journal of Clinical and Experimental Neuropsychology, 7*, 79-96.

Scogin, F., Storandt, M., & Lott, L. (1985). Memory-skills training, memory complaints, and depression in older adults. *Journal of Gerontology*, *40*, 562-568.

Siegfried, K., & O'Connolly, M. (1986). Cognitive and psychomotor effects of different antidepressants on the treatment of old age depression. *International Clinical Psychopharmacology*, *1*, 231-243.

Sohlberg, M.M., & Mateer, C.A. (1987). Effectiveness of an attention-training program. *Journal of Clinical and Experimental Neuropsychology*, *9*, 117-130.

Stankov, L. (1988). Aging, attention, and intelligence. *Psychology and Aging*, *3*, 59-74.

Thomas-Robe, K. (1990). *Anxiety and depression: A study of cognitive specificity*. Unpublished doctoral dissertation, University of South Florida, Tampa, FL.

Vygotsky, L.S. (1978). *Mind in society: The development of higher psychological processes* (M. Cole, V. John-Steiner, S. Scribner, & E. Souberman, Eds. & Trans.). Cambridge, MA: Harvard University Press.

Watts, F.N., MacLeod, A.K., & Morris, L. (1988). A remedial strategy for memory and concentration problems in depressed patients. *Cognitive Therapy and Research*, *12*, 185-193.

Wenk, G.L. (1989). An hypothesis on the role of glucose in the mechanism of action of cognitive enhancers. *Psychopharmacology*, *99*, 431-438.

West, R. (1985). *Memory fitness over 40*. Gainesville, FL: Triad.

Willis, S.L. (1990). Introduction to the special section on cognitive training in later adulthood. *Developmental Psychology*, *26*, 875-878.

Willis, S.L., & Nesselroade, C.S. (1990). Long-term effects of fluid ability training in old-old age. *Developmental Psychology*, *26*, 905-910.

Wilson, B. (1984). Memory therapy in practice. In B.A. Wilson & N. Moffat (Eds.), *Clinical management of memory problems*. Rockville, MD: Aspen.

Wilson, B. (1987). *Rehabilitation of memory*. New York: Guilford.

Zarit, S.H., Cole, K.D., & Guider, R.L. (1981). Memory training strategies and subjective complaints of memory in the aged. *The Gerontologist*, *21*, 158-164.

Memory in Life, Lab, and Clinic: Implications for Memory Theory

Rose T. Zacks and Lynn Hasher

Basic and applied research on memory should and can inform each other to their mutual benefit much in the same way that laboratory and nonlaboratory studies can (see Bahrick, 1991; Tulving, 1991). Nonetheless, it is a challenge to integrate the wide-ranging contents of the presentations of this conference and to formulate implications for memory theory. Each paper contributed some interesting and unique findings and conceptual points, not all of which can be assimilated. With respect to memory theory, there were a number of themes that cut across several to most of the presentations. We begin with a consideration of those themes.

Themes of the Conference

Dissatisfaction with Past Interaction Between Basic and Applied Memory Research

In one way or another, several conference contributors expressed the view that the standard memory theories of the last 20 to 25 years provide, at best, an incomplete blueprint for designing effective memory improvement strategies. For example, Weingartner and Herrmann (this volume) pointed to the "fragmented or dissociated nature" of basic memory research and to the existence of several distinct "subcultures" of memory research, each with its own methods, findings, and concepts. These subcultures will need to be integrated into a unified framework, they argue, if basic research is to provide useful guidelines for application.

Gruneberg (this volume), Herrmann and Searleman (this volume) and Pressley and El-Dinary (this volume) had a somewhat different concern. They noted with dismay that basic memory researchers have given low priority to memory improvement either as a proper goal of their work or as an arena in which to test the generality of their findings or their theories. For example, Herrmann and Searleman note that since Ebbinghaus, memory researchers have shown little interest in applied issues. From their point of view, the result has been a basic research endeavor that is insensitive to the problems and findings of clinical application. As basic memory researchers, we agree that there has been more separation between basic and applied work on memory than is desirable. Because of this separation, basic researchers have lost opportunities to use the memory clinic as a proving ground for theories and as a field station for the identification of phenomena that may lead to new theoretical insights. However, we should not exaggerate the degree of separation. For example, there is a tradition in Great Britain (e.g., in the work of Baddeley and Broadbent; see also Wilson & Moffat, 1984) of research that bridges the basic-applied gap, and even in North America, there are some notable exceptions to the typical situation. Included among North American basic researchers who have done serious applied work are McEvoy (e.g., this volume), Duke and colleagues (e.g., Duke, Haley, & Bergquist, in press; Duke, Weathers, Caldwell, & Novack, in press), Schacter and Tulving (e.g., Glisky, Schacter, & Tulving, 1986).

The Situational Specificity of Memory Improvement Strategies

A second theme was the conclusion that memory improvement strategies are, in general, "situationally specific". That is, there is frequently poor generalization of any improvement in performance from the training tasks to other tasks tested in the memory clinic or to analogues of the training tasks encountered in everyday situations. Just about every presenter at the conference mentioned situational specificity in one way or another. For example, Herrmann and Searleman (this volume) summarized the discouraging transfer results when people are trained to use one or more of the classical mnemonics such as the method of loci or the peg-word method. Although some instances of situational specificity may reflect metamemory deficiencies, including a lack of knowledge of the potential usefulness of a trained memory strategy or a belief that one is unable to use the mnemonic effectively (Hertzog, this volume), other instances (probably the majority) seem to require a different explanation. For example, a metamemory account of the pattern of memory abilities of Ceci, DeSimone, and Johnson's (this volume) subject, Bubbles P., seems unlikely. Bubbles P. has a truly exceptional memory for numbers but performs at an average level with non-numerical memory materials. He reports no special strategies or monitoring techniques that could account for this differential in performance.

As Payne and Wenger (this volume) make clear, the issue of the specificity of memory-training effects is not a new one for psychology. In fact, it was an important topic of study in the early part of this century, when considerable effort was expended investigating the doctrine of "formal discipline," which proposed that practice would lead to the development of general mental skills. More than 60 years ago, Thorndike (1906) concluded that "several decades" of research had provided little evidence of practice-induced development of general mental skills. Instead, he suggested that positive transfer was largely item and task specific, a view that is in accordance with the results of more recent work on memory improvement.

In addition to the suggestion that specific knowledge (or associations, in Thorndike's time) but not general strategies can transfer from one memory task to another, the conference presenters mentioned two sorts of reasons for the situational specificity of memory improvement strategies. One of these (see Ceci et al., this volume; Herrmann & Searleman, this volume; Weingartner & Herrmann, this volume) is the idea that the memory system itself is not unitary--that it consists of a number of different modules for which different improvement strategies are required. The other proposed source of situational specificity, the embeddedness of memory, stands out as the third overarching theme of this conference and is discussed below.

The Embeddedness of Memory Functions

One of the major contributions of this conference has been to point out in various ways and with considerable force that memory is embedded in a larger cognitive system and in the personal, social, and emotional context in which individuals live. In other words, the claim is that the functioning of the memory system must be considered in relation to a large variety of other cognitive and noncognitive factors. Like memory specificity, just about everyone at the conference stressed this point, and examples of relevant observations can be found in most of the papers. We will mention only a few persuasive examples. One is the discussion by Hertel (this volume) of the complex interplay among emotional state, attentional allocation, and memory performance. Other examples are Best's (this volume) and Hertzog's (this volume) very similar analyses of the profound effects that an individual's perception of his or her memory ability (an aspect of the self-concept) can have on memory performance. The data clearly show that individuals who believe they have poor memories for their age group or for a particular type of information may fail to initiate the kind of effortful processing required for good memory.

These three major themes are, of course, interrelated: There is a strong possibility that memory's embeddedness is a factor in findings of situational specificity. For example, the failure of a face-name recall mnemonic to generalize beyond the training situation may well be due to embedding factors (e.g., social anxiety, cognitive overload, etc.), interfering with the use of this mnemonic in many of the situations (e.g., large parties, job interviews) in which new names need to be learned. It can also be conjectured that applied researchers' dissatisfaction with basic memory theories stems from the weakness of such theories in handling the situational specificity and embeddedness characteristics of applied data. Conversely, it may well be these very characteristics that led basic memory researchers to ignore applied outcomes. That is, from the point of view of a basic memory researcher, whose goal is a nomothetic description of memory, there may be little utility to findings that have minimal generality and that are strongly influenced by factors from outside the memory system.

Reflections on These Themes

The discussion that follows centers on three major claims that jointly summarize our thoughts on the current status of the interplay between basic and applied research as well as our guesses about future prospects: (a) Effective memory improvement strategies *do* already incorporate major findings and concepts of basic memory research, (b) there are some potentially valuable findings and concepts of basic memory research that have not as yet been fully incorporated into memory improvement work, and (c) in part as a response to findings of the memory clinic, general memory theory is changing in a direction that may ultimately increase its applied usefulness.

Basic Memory Research Is Used in Applied Settings

It is clear to us that despite some statements about the irrelevance of basic memory research to the applied setting, memory clinicians make at least tacit (and often explicit) use of major findings and conceptualizations from the experimental laboratory. For example, it would be a rare intervention that did not aim for meaningful (Craik & Lockhart, 1972) and organized (Tulving, 1968) processing of to-be-remembered information. Similarly, the notions that short-term memory has a limited capacity and that chunking of information can help to functionally expand that capacity (Miller, 1956) are likely to be honored, where relevant, by any designer of a memory improvement strategy. So, although currently basic memory theories are not seen as providing complete recipes for memory improvement strategies, they nonetheless have an impact at a more general level. That is, the influence of these theories is at the level of the "folk wisdom" about memory that both basic and applied researchers share. In a few instances, as in the memory rehabilitation interventions designed by Duke and Haley et al. (in press) and Duke and Weathers et al. (in press), the influence is more direct and detailed.

Underused Contributions of Basic Memory Research

We begin our discussion of untapped contributions of basic memory research with a consideration of the products of an earlier (precognitive) era in the study of memory: the verbal learning era. One reason for suggesting a reconsideration of the verbal learning literature is that it focussed on issues of direct relevance to the design of memory improvement strategies, namely, the dynamics of learning, transfer, and forgetting. As noted by Payne and Wenger (this volume; also, Hintzman, in press), the cognitive revolution initiated a shift in memory research away from such concerns and towards the description of static memory structures. An example here is the very large body of research on semantic memory models, fostered in part by widespread acceptance of Tulving's (1972) distinction between episodic and semantic memory. Basic research might better serve the goal of memory improvement if there was a return to the emphases of the verbal learning era. Such a return may have already begun. Hintzman, for example, argues that the currently popular connectionist (or parallel distributed processing, PDP) approach represents a "radical effort" to refocus attention on the learning process.

In the meantime, what kinds of things can we (applied *and* basic researchers) learn from the verbal learning work? Because verbal learners believed that associative strength was *the* major determiner of the memorability of prior experience, much of what we have to learn from their effort relates to the factors controlling associative strength. Building on the British Empiricist tradition, they saw three classes of variables--recency of experience, frequency of repetition, and similarity among items--as the major determiners of associative strength. The in-depth study of these variables yielded a large body of replicable and (within the confines of verbal learning paradigms) highly generalizable findings. This body of data has, we think, been insufficiently explored in terms of implications for memory improvement strategies. For example, a major proportion of the work on similarity had the goal of elucidating item-specific transfer effects. This work might suggest how to better achieve the goal of positive transfer from previous learning.

A more obvious example is the impact of distribution of practice, which verbal learners studied as part of their exploration of how repetition affects associative strength. As reviewed by Payne and Wenger (this volume), the finding that spaced repetitions yield better retention than massed repetitions is a very general one. In a very recent demonstration of this result, Kausler, Wiley, and Phillips (1990) showed that spacing of repetitions benefitted both younger and older adults' memory for repeated actions. The use of spaced, as contrasted to massed repetitions, does not seem to have been widely incorporated into memory amelioration strategies, though given its power to increase recall, it should be.

Another point relates to a contrast between the verbal learning and cognitive approaches in their views on the conditions necessary for good memory encoding. If the tenor of Plude's (this volume) contribution to this conference can be taken as representative (and we think it can), the information-processing approach has assumed that memory acquisition is closely tied to consciously initiated, controlled processing. By contrast, the verbal learners have assumed a somewhat more passive organism, and in doing so, have put relatively more emphasis on the effects of mere exposure or repetition. To a degree at least, the verbal learning view makes sense to us, because much of what we learn in everyday life is acquired unintentionally. This is not to deny that deliberate learning strategies can have major effects on memory but rather to suggest that they perhaps have been given too much weight in the post-verbal-learning era. In line with this claim, we note that there has been a recent resurgence of interest in "implicit learning." This work by Reber (e.g., 1989), Lewicki (e.g., Lewicki, Hill, & Bizot, 1988), and others suggests that much complex and abstract information about the world may be acquired in the absence of deliberate, voluntary attempts to learn. Furthermore, such implicit learning has been shown to be present in young children to the same degree as it is in college students and has been shown to be relatively preserved in older adults and in other people who have deficits in explicit learning (see Reber, in press). Given the pervasiveness of implicit learning, it would seem promising to explore memory improvement strategies that tap into the products of such learning. As far as we know, this possibility has not been systematically explored.

Potential but unrecognized contributions of basic memory research to applied memory work relate not only to the acquisition of information (our emphasis so far) but also to retrieval. The verbal-learning literature could be gleaned for suggestions as to how to improve retrieval (e.g., consideration of the effects of similarity among potential memory targets on retrieval interference might be of interest), but it is probably time to consider newer work.

One of the major contributions of recent memory research has been to increase our understanding of the factors influencing retrieval and the interaction between encoding and retrieval mechanisms. (Some of these issues were discussed at this conference by Intons-Peterson and Newsome, this volume, and Payne and Wenger, this volume.) Memory retrieval, like memory encoding, can occur nonintentionally. Whereas until recently, cognitive theory has ignored nonintentional encoding, the same cannot be said of nonintentional retrieval. Two frequently studied phenomena, in which nonintentional retrieval is thought to play a major role, are semantic priming and "implicit" (Schacter, 1987) or "indirect" (Johnson & Hasher, 1987) memory. In relation to semantic priming effects, most accounts (e.g., Neely, 1977, 1991; Posner & Snyder, 1975) of how a prime facilitates access to semantically related targets involve the concept of *automatic* (i.e., stimulus driven and nonintentional) spreading activation. Similarly, the benefits from prior exposure that are seen on indirect memory tasks, such as fragment completion or perceptual recognition, seem to be largely dependent on nonintentional retrieval of the prior event (Schacter, 1987). It is interesting then that semantic priming effects comparable to those shown by normals are found in individuals who have moderate to even severe deficits on typical explicit memory tasks, including the elderly (Burke, White, & Diaz, 1987; Howard, 1988) and, under some circumstances, amnesics (Graf, Squire, & Mandler, 1984). The same thing can be said of performance on various indirect memory tasks (e.g., Light & Singh, 1987; Nebes, 1989). An example of what can be accomplished with applied strategies that capitalize on such preserved memory abilities is found in Glisky et al.'s (1986) work. With their "vanishing cue" procedure, which seems to rely heavily on nonintentional retrieval, they were able to teach amnesics the rudiments of how to operate a microcomputer. More attempts along these lines might be fruitful.

Another set of issues relates to both nonintentional and intentional retrieval. As Tulving (e.g., Tulving & Pearlstone, 1966) made clear some time ago, the memories that are retrievable ("accessible") at any one time only very partially exhaust the memories that are present ("available") in the memory store. One demonstration of this is the fact that the provision of appropriate recall cues can greatly enhance recall over that obtained without such cues (Tulving & Pearlstone). (By appropriate cues, we mean ones consistent with the way the information was originally encoded [cf. Tulving and Thompson's, 1973, "encoding specificity" principle].) Indeed, the importance of retrieval cues for good memory performance cannot be overestimated: As has been forcefully argued by Duke and Haley et al. (in press), the encoding of effective memory cues may be the single most important means of improving memory.

Because environmental cues are among those that affect retrieval (e.g., Godden & Baddeley, 1975), constancy of the environment may be important to the probability that an earlier learning experience can be retrieved (cf. McEvoy, this volume). Social cues are also important, as Best (this volume) forcefully documented in describing one of the findings obtained in a study in which sixth grade children were able to clearly articulate a meaning-based organizational strategy when teaching younger children how to play a memory game. At the same time, they were unable to describe that strategy to an adult (Best & Ornstein, 1986).

Other considerations apply only to intentional retrieval situations. One is the finding (reviewed by Payne & Wenger, this volume) that memory performance improves with repeated attempts at recalling a set of target memories. Based on the memory-enhancing effects of repeated retrieval attempts and of additional cues, memory clinicians could suggest to their clients that successful recall frequently requires several attempts and that such attempts are especially likely to produce the desired memory if, in the process, additional cues are self-generated. To aid in the cue generation process, clients could be instructed in the use of the procedures included in the "cognitive interview" method developed by Geiselman, Fisher, MacKinnon, and Holland (1985).

Finally, we note that basic memory researchers are increasingly interested in the *interactions* among encoding operations, learning materials, and demands of the retrieval task or environment. One important notion here is that of "transfer-appropriate processing" (Morris, Bransford, & Franks, 1977); this is the idea that performance is not merely a function of the encoding operations or the retrieval environment but of the compatibility between the two.

Another relevant line of work (e.g., Einstein & Hunt, 1980; Hunt & Einstein, 1981) begins with the assumption that materials and processing operations vary in the degree to which they foster the encoding of individual item versus relational information. In addition, because the parameters of the memory test (e.g., recall vs. recognition, length of the retention interval) determine the relative importance of these two types of information for good performance, predictions of memory performance will have to take into account the particulars of the memory test, as well as those of the materials and the encoding activities. Recently, these ideas have been systematized as the "material-appropriate processing" framework (e.g., Einstein, McDaniel, Owen, & Cote', 1990). Again, we believe that this work will soon provide, if it does not already, some useful hints for structuring memory improvement procedures.

Theory Developments

Despite the newly rediscovered value of issues and data from the verbal learning tradition, there were, of course, major shortcomings of this view. Among these, we note a few with special relevance to application of laboratory findings to clinical problems. The verbal learning approach assumed that the study of college undergraduates would illuminate a universal set of laws that characterize the human's unitary learning system. As many papers (e.g., Best, this volume; Ceci et al., this volume; Hertzog, this volume) at this conference demonstrated, there is much to be learned from subjects who are not college students. An adequate general model should recognize both developmental and individual differences in memory.

As many papers (e.g., Herrmann & Searleman, this volume; Weingartner & Herrmann, this volume) at this conference also demonstrated, the assumption of a unitary memory system is extremely problematic: With few exceptions (which possibly include the benefits of spaced over massed practice), general laws of memory are not easily discernable. Perhaps in response to this, the majority of the theories that arose after the demise of the verbal learning perspective proposed that there are different memory functions with distinguishable properties: that is, that memory functioning could not be characterized by a single set of general laws. The shift to a nonunitary view is clearest for those models that propose memory *modules* or *subsystems*, each with its own functional characteristics. However, at least to some degree, a similar point is made by the so-called *processing* views that tie variability in memory functioning to differences in processing, especially during encoding.

The earliest popular example of the subsystem approach is the Atkinson and Shiffrin (1968) model with its multiple memory stores. A few years later, Tulving (1972) forcefully argued that the long-term memory of the Atkinson and Shiffrin formulation includes two distinguishable subsystems: episodic and semantic memory. The episodic-semantic memory distinction has, in turn, undergone a series of modifications and elaborations, culminating perhaps in Squire's (1987) model, which proposes six or more different subsystems of long-term memory. Similarly, Baddeley (1986) has proposed that short-term (or for him, working) memory comprises three distinct subsystems.

The original processing view was that of Craik and Lockhart (1972). They focussed on processing differences and their consequences for memory, arguing that the properties of a memory trace (including its durability, accessibility, etc.) are not primarily a function of the memory store in which the memory resides but instead, of the kind of processing that led to the establishment of the memory trace in the first place. In particular, memorability was tied to the type of rehearsal used (maintenance vs. elaborative) and to the level of processing engaged in (structural, phonological, or semantic).

Like the subsystem approach, the processing approach has not remained constant since its inception. Concepts such as elaboration, distinctiveness, and transfer-appropriate processing have broadened and complicated Craik and Lockhart's original formulation (1972; see Lockhart & Craik, 1990). Additionally, our own (Hasher & Zacks, 1979) description of encoding processes as varying along an automatic to effortful continuum of capacity demands can also be seen as a processing approach. (We note that this framework explicitly addressed the effects of such differences among groups of individuals differing in age and mood state. For us, this was an acknowledgement of the embeddedness of memory in a larger cognitive [e.g., the role of attentional factors] and personal [e.g., the role of mood] context.)

We cannot say that applied memory results, specifically the demonstrations of situational specificity and memory embeddedness, were the primary impetus for most of these developments in memory theory, but we think they were part of that impetus, especially among British psychologists like Baddeley and Broadbent. In addition, Hirst, Schacter, Tulving, and other basic researchers who have studied amnesia (e.g., see Glisky & Schacter, 1986; Hirst & Volpe, 1988) are all attuned to applied memory issues. Regardless of the source of memory theory's evolution, it is clear from this conference that from the point of view of applied memory work, further evolution is needed.

One promising form of such evolution is a view that combines subsystem and processing approaches--in our minds, a sensible idea because each approach makes valid claims and each has limitations. An example of a combined approach is Johnson's (1983; Johnson & Hirst, in press) Multiple-Entry Memory or MEM model. This model includes both multiple memory systems and multiple modes of processing within each. It also begins to take account of the embeddedness of memory and attempts to describe how motivational, emotional, and attitudinal factors interact with more purely cognitive ones in influencing memory trace formation, maintenance, and retrieval.

In our work (e.g., Hasher & Zacks, 1988), we continue to be concerned about embedding memory in a larger cognitive context and about broadening the range of groups whose performance we hope to account for. Additionally, we attempt to include in our analysis some aspects of the personal situations of the individuals under study. Before turning to a description of our framework and some of our recent findings, we address a major theoretical orientation that we have so far ignored. That theoretical orientation is represented by Jenkins' (1979) tetrahedral model of memory. The major claim of such a view is that an adequate account of memory must be highly contextualized, that is, it must simultaneously consider the effects of variables relating to subjects, materials, orienting tasks, and criterial tasks, and their interactions. The influence of this type of view was most clearly seen in McEvoy's (this volume) presentation, but a close cousin is Herrmann and Searleman's (this volume) multimodal model. It is easy to see why the Jenkins' view might be popular with memory improvement researchers. It readily incorporates findings of situational specificity and memory embeddedness. In fact, Jenkins himself predicted (1979, p. 430) that a contextualist view would be popular with memory researchers.

We have a mixed reaction to such views. On the positive side, we believe that ultimately a complete theory will have to speak to the range of variables Jenkins (1979) identified. However, in accepting a contextualist view, we think there is a danger of concluding that it is hopeless to search for broader generalizations: for findings and concepts that have validity across different populations, circumstances, and memory tasks. Additionally, although the tetrahedral model and others like it may serve as "useful heuristics" (Jenkins' description, 1979 p. 431) for memory research, they are, in general, incomplete as mechanistic accounts of memory. For the most part, they have as yet to be fleshed out so as to provide specific predictions for new findings and detailed accounts of existing data. One example of the kind of development we see as moving in the right direction can be found in McEvoy's (this volume) presentation. In particular, we refer to her suggestion that it becomes increasingly important to consider emotional and contextual factors in designing memory improvement strategies, as the degree of memory impairment of the target population increases. Systematic development along such lines can be fruitful but will require a formidable effort.

New Trends in Memory Theory: An Example

Our view of cognitive functioning (Hasher & Zacks, 1988) embeds memory in a series of events that link attention, working memory, retrieval processes and goals. Taken together, these influence a wide array of behaviors, including language comprehension, language production, and decision making.

Attentional processes, we argue, include both activation and suppression processes and, together with goals and aspects of the stimulus array, they determine what gains access to working memory. The role of suppression is particularly important, because it operates to prevent the processing of stimuli and thoughts that are not central to an individual's current goals. In particular, suppression operates at encoding to prevent access to working memory and/or to reduce time in working memory. It operates at retrieval to prevent the exploration of non-goal-path linkages.

To evaluate this model, we have concentrated on the consequences of diminished suppression mechanisms--as, we have argued, may well be the case in aging. (We note that Gernsbacher, 1990, has made a similar argument for low verbal ability young adults). We (Hasher, Stoltzfus, Zacks, & Rypma, 1991) and others (McDowd & Oseas-Kreger, 1991; Tipper, 1991) have reported substantial and consistent evidence that the attentional mechanism variously called inhibition, suppression, or negative priming, is indeed impaired in old age.

If suppression is dysfunctional, more information that is only marginally relevant--or even irrelevant--to the goal path (say of comprehending this presentation or paper) will be able to enter working memory. Indeed, there is now evidence that older adults permit richer access to working memory. For example, Ellen Stoltzfus, in a dissertation project in progress at Duke, has found evidence that both young and older adults show priming (or activation) for the expected ending: such as supplying "baby" to the high cloze sentence, "The famous stork brought him a _____." Only older adults show facilitation for a word related to the high cloze ending, here "child." Apparently, defective suppression mechanisms permit greater access to working memory by information that is beyond the narrow range appropriate for sentences such as those used here.

Another set of experiments used a different procedure, reading in the face of distraction, to explore the ability of older adults to ignore distraction (Connelly, Hasher, & Zacks, 1991). In one of the experiments in this project, younger and older adults read aloud a brief paragraph printed in italics that, in the experimental conditions, was interleaved with extraneous text in another font. The extraneous text was either meaningfully related to the target text or was irrelevant to the target. In either event, it was to be ignored. Older adults were differentially slowed in their reading, relative to younger adults, by the presence of any distraction. For younger adults, text-related and unrelated distraction was equally disruptive. For older adults, related distraction was still more disruptive to their reading than was unrelated distraction. Inefficient suppression appears to create problems, in part by permitting more information to gain access to working memory, perhaps particularly so if that information is at least marginally related to target information. Elsewhere, there is the suggestion that older adults also fail to quickly dismiss ideas that are activated by irrelevant information (e.g., Hamm & Hasher, 1992; Hartman & Hasher, 1991).

In addition to heightened distractibility, what are the consequences of diminished suppression? A major one will most certainly be increased retrieval problems. These will be, in part, the consequence of the enrichment of working memory permitted by weakened suppression mechanisms. This is because events linked by simultaneous occupancy of working memory retain those links, and any memory search initiated for a target may well also activate its associated relevant and irrelevant connections. The more thoughts activated by a retrieval cue, the slower and more inaccurate retrieval will be (these effects are known variously as the "fan" effect or as competition at retrieval). We (Gerard, Zacks, Hasher, & Radvansky, 1991) have recently shown a far greater fan effect for older adults than for youngers.

This slowing of retrieval will also create problems for language comprehension and speech production--insofar as the social contexts in which language occurs are time limited. Both activities require relatively quick access to antecedent information as well as an ability to maintain a topical focus. At their extremes, retrieval problems while speaking will result in meandering and repetition of familiar themes--since access to other information will be momentarily blocked.

Thus, a mechanism of attention appears to have a major role to play in determining memory, language comprehension, and language production. Of course, these problems will impact on other domains that depend on retrieval and topically focussed processing such as problem solving and decision making.

We and others have tried to integrate memory into its larger cognitive context. Cognition, in turn, is embedded in a social world that has expectations of behavior, and constraints as well. These too must ultimately be integrated into a thoughtful picture of human cognition (see Best, this volume; Hertzog, this volume).

What implications does our model have for memory impairment? These we have not yet specified, and we expect that others may see the consequences more clearly than us. Some consequences--and any remediation--will depend on the degree to which suppression is under an individual's control. Logan (1989) has argued eloquently that even the most automatic processes are under partial control by a subject. For example, the degree of Stroop interference in the standard color-naming version of that task will vary as a function of the proportion of congruent items (ones in which the to-be-named hue and the color word are the same) versus incongruent items.

Research on the degree of control of suppression is underway. In the meanwhile, it seems clear that the functioning of individuals with diminished suppression can be aided by a variety of adjustments to their environments. Since many mental activities are stimulus driven, reductions in environmental distractions should prove helpful. (Reductions from thought distraction will be tied to the issue of the degree to which suppression is under voluntary control.) Since retrieval problems can be expected to be profound, ideas or objects that need to be accessed should either be directly visible or nearly so, as is true, for example, when labels are used to indicate the contents of drawers and cabinets. Filing drawers or closet doors, because they visually hide their contents, may actually be impediments to people with diminished suppression.

Furthermore, the physical environment needs to be consistent from day to day. The problem of retrieving your car when you do not park in the same place each day will be greatly magnified for individuals with diminished suppression mechanisms. We have in mind here the clever solution generated by McEvoy (this volume) to the problems of an elderly Alzheimer's patient who moved among her children's houses.

Other applications await both research and the expertise of those more familiar with the everyday problems of people seeking remediation. In sum, we are in substantial agreement with those who see that the problems of cognitive psychology can only be solved by rich, varied, and interconnected approaches (e.g., Bahrick, 1991; Tulving, 1991). We applaud this conference, because we concur with its goals--that of sharing the richness of the empirical data base and the process of theory development in memory, whether those contributions come from the laboratory, life, the clinic, or from another academic discipline.

Summary

In closing, we reiterate what we take as the major contributions this conference offers to mainstream cognitive psychology: New efforts at the classical questions of the acquisition, transfer, and retention of information are to be desired. Memory occurs in a social, personal, and cognitive context and these should be part of the concerns of mainstream cognition. Theories need to be more inclusive of the variability among people; they should be informed by data from subjects of a wider range of ages, abilities, and states than is often the case. These efforts would ensure greater interaction among laboratory, life, and clinic.

Endnotes 1

Preparation of this chapter and our research described therein were supported by National Institute on Aging Grant 2RO1 AG04306.

References

Atkinson, R.C., & Shiffrin, R.M. (1968). Human memory: A proposed system and its control processes. In K.W. Spence & J.T. Spence (Eds.), *The psychology of learning and motivation: Advances in research and theory* (Vol. 2, pp. 89-95). New York: Academic Press.

Baddeley, A.D. (1986). *Working memory*. New York: Oxford University Press.

Bahrick, H.P. (1991). A speedy recovery from bankruptcy for ecological memory research. *American Psychologist, 46*, 76-77.

Best, D.L., & Ornstein, P.A. (1986). Children's generation and communication of mnemonic organizational strategies. *Developmental Psychology, 22*, 845-853.

Burke, D.M., White, H., & Diaz, D.L. (1987). Semantic priming in young and older adults: Evidence for age constancy in automatic and attentional processes. *Journal of Experimental Psychology: Human Perception and Performance, 13*, 79-88.

Connelly, S.L., Hasher, L., & Zacks, R.T. (1991). Age and reading: The impact of distraction. *Psychology and Aging, 6*, 533-541.

Craik, F.I.M., & Lockhart, R.S. (1972). Levels of processing: A framework for memory research. *Journal of Verbal Learning and Verbal Behavior, 11*, 671-684.

Duke, L.W., Haley, W.E., & Bergquist, T.F. (in press). Cognitive-behavioral interventions for age-related memory impairment. In P.A. Wisocki (Ed.), *Handbook of clinical behavior therapy with the elderly client*. New York: Plenum.

Duke, L.W., Weathers, S.L., Caldwell, S.G., & Novack, T.A. (in press). Cognitive rehabilitation after head trauma: Toward an integrated cognitive/behavioral perspective on intervention. In C.J. Long, L.K. Ross, & M.G. Mutchnick (Eds.), *Head trauma: Acute care to recovery*. New York: Plenum.

Einstein, G.O., & Hunt, R.R. (1980). Levels of processing and organization: Additive effects of individual-item and relational processing. *Journal of Experimental Psychology: Learning, Memory, and Cognition, 6*, 588-598.

Einstein, G.O, McDaniel, M.A., Owen, P.D., & Cote', N.C. (1990). Encoding and recall of texts: The importance of material appropriate processing. *Journal of Memory and Language, 29*, 566-581.

Geiselman, R.E., Fisher, R.P., MacKinnon, D.P., & Holland, H. (1985). Eyewitness memory enhancement in the police interview: Cognitive retrieval mnemonics versus hypnosis. *Journal of Applied Psychology, 70*, 401-412.

Gerard, L., Zacks, R.T., Hasher, L., & Radvansky, G.A. (1991). Age deficits in retrieval: The fan effect. *Journal of Gerontology, 46*, 131-136.

Gernsbacher, M.A. (1990). *Language mechanisms as structure building*. Hillsdale, NJ: Erlbaum.

Glisky, E.L., & Schacter, D.L. (1986). Remediation of organic memory

disorders: Current status and future prospects. *Journal of Head Trauma Rehabilitation*, *1*, 54-63.
Glisky, E.L., Schacter, D.L., & Tulving, E. (1986). Computer learning by memory-impaired patients: Acquisition and retention of complex knowledge. *Neuropsychologica*, *24*, 313-328.
Godden, D.R., & Baddeley, A.D. (1975). Context-dependent memory in two natural environments: On land and under water. *British Journal of Psychology*, *66*, 325-332.
Graf, P., Squire, L.R., & Mandler, G. (1984). The information that amnesic patients don't forget. *Journal of Experimental Psychology: Learning, Memory, and Cognition*, *10*, 164-178.
Hamm, V.P., & Hasher, L. (1992). Age and the availability of inferences. *Psychology and Aging*, *7*, 56-64.
Hartman, M., & Hasher, L. (1991). Aging and suppression: Memory for previously relevant information. *Psychology and Aging*, *6*, 587-594.
Hasher, L., Stoltzfus, E.R., Zacks, R.T., & Rypma, B. (1991). Age and inhibition. *Journal of Experimental Psychology: Learning, Memory, and Cognition*, *17*, 163-169.
Hasher, L., & Zacks, R.T. (1979). Automatic and effortful processes in memory. *Journal of Experimental Psychology: General*, *108*, 356-388.
Hasher, L., & Zacks, R.T. (1988). Working memory, comprehension, and aging: A review and new view. In G.H. Bower (Ed.), *The psychology of learning and motivation* (Vol. 22, pp. 193-225). New York: Academic Press.
Hintzman, D.L. (in press). 25 years of learning and memory: Was the cognitive revolution a mistake? In D.E. Meyer & S. Kornblum (Eds.), *Attention and performance XIV*. Hillsdale, NJ: Erlbaum.
Hirst, W., & Volpe, B.T. (1988). Memory strategies with brain damage. *Brain and Cognition*, *8*, 379-408.
Howard, D.V. (1988). Aging and memory activation: The priming of semantic and episodic memories. In L.L. Light & D.M. Burke (Eds.), *Language, memory, and aging* (pp. 77-79). New York: Cambridge University Press.
Hunt, R.R., & Einstein, G.O. (1981). Relational and item-specific information in memory. *Journal of Verbal Learning and Verbal Behavior*, *20*, 497-514.
Jenkins, J.J. (1979). Four points to remember: A tetrahedral model of memory experiments. In L.S. Cermak & F.I.M. Craik (Eds.), *Levels of processing in human memory* (pp. 429-446). Hillsdale, NJ: Erlbaum.
Johnson, M.K. (1983). A multiple-entry, modular memory system. In G.H. Bower (Ed.), *The psychology of learning and motivation* (Vol. 17, pp. 81-123). New York: Academic Press.
Johnson, M.K., & Hasher, L. (1987). Human learning and memory. *Annual Review of Psychology*, *38*, 631-668.
Johnson, M.K., & Hirst, W. (in press). Processing subsystems of memory. In R.G. Lister & H.J. Weingartner (Eds.), *Perspectives in cognitive neuroscience*. New York: Oxford University Press.
Kausler, D.H., Wiley, J.G., & Phillips, P.L. (1990). Adult age differences in

memory for massed and distributed repeated actions. *Psychology and Aging, 5*, 530-534.

Lewicki, P., Hill, T., & Bizot, E. (1988). Acquisition of procedural knowledge about a pattern of stimuli that cannot be articulated. *Cognitive Psychology, 20*, 24-37.

Light, L.L., & Singh, A. (1987). Implicit and explicit memory in young and older adults. *Journal of Experimental Psychology: Learning, Memory and Cognition, 13*, 531-541.

Lockhart, R.S., & Craik, F.I.M. (1990). Levels of processing: A retrospective commentary on a framework for memory research. *Canadian Journal of Psychology, 44*, 87-112.

Logan, G.D. (1989). Automaticity and cognitive control. In J.S. Uleman & J.A. Bargh (Eds.), *Unintended thought* (pp. 52-74). New York: Guilford.

McDowd, J.M., & Oseas-Kreger, D.M. (1991). Aging, inhibitory processes and negative priming. *Journal of Gerontology, 46*, P340-P345.

Miller, G.A. (1956). The magical number seven plus or minus two: Some limits on our capacity for processing information. *Psychological Review, 63*, 81-97.

Morris, C.D., Bransford, J.D., & Franks, J.J. (1977). Levels of processing versus transfer appropriate processing. *Journal of Verbal Learning and Verbal Behavior, 16*, 519-533.

Nebes, R.D. (1989). Semantic memory in Alzheimer's disease. *Psychological Bulletin, 106*, 377-394.

Neely, J.H. (1977). Semantic priming and retrieval from lexical memory: Roles of inhibitionless spreading activation and limited-capacity attention. *Journal of Experimental Psychology: General, 106*, 226-254.

Neely, J.H. (1991). Semantic priming effects in visual word recognition: A selective review of current findings and theories. In D. Besner & G. Humphreys (Eds.), *Basic processes in reading: Visual word recognition*. Hillsdale, NJ: Erlbaum.

Posner, M.I., & Snyder, C.R.R. (1975). Attention and cognitive control. In R. Solso (Ed.), *Information processing and cognition: The Loyola Symposium* (pp. 55-85). Potomac MD: Erlbaum.

Reber, A.S. (1989). Implicit learning and tacit knowledge. *Journal of Experimental Psychology: General, 118*, 219-235.

Reber, A.S. (in press). An evolutionary context for the cognitive unconscious. *Philosophical Psychology*.

Schacter, D.L. (1987). Implicit memory: History and current status. *Journal of Experimental Psychology: Learning, Memory, and Cognition, 13*, 501-518.

Squire, L.R. (1987). *Memory and brain*. New York: Oxford University Press.

Thorndike, E.L. (1906). *Principles of teaching*. New York: A.G. Seiler.

Tipper, S.P. (1991). *Less attentional selectivity as a result of declining inhibition in older adults*. Manuscript submitted for publication.

Tulving, E. (1968). Theoretical issues in free recall. In T.R. Dixon & D.L. Horton (Eds.), *Verbal behavior and general behavior theory* (pp. 2-36).

Englewood Cliffs, NJ: Prentice Hall.
Tulving, E. (1972). Episodic and semantic memory. In E. Tulving & W. Donaldson (Eds.), *Organization of memory* (pp. 381-403). New York: Academic Press.
Tulving, E. (1991). Memory research is not a zero-sum game. *American Psychologist*, *46*, 41-42.
Tulving, E., & Pearlstone, Z. (1966). Availability versus accessibility of information in memory for words. *Journal of Verbal Learning and Verbal Behavior*, *5*, 381-391.
Tulving, E., & Thompson, D.M . (1973). Encoding specificity and retrieval processes in episodic memory. *Psychological Review*, *80*, 352-373.
Wilson, B., & Moffat, N. (Eds.). (1984). *Clinical management of memory problems*. Rockville, MD: Aspen Systems.

Author Index

Subject Index

MIX
Papier aus verantwortungsvollen Quellen
Paper from responsible sources
FSC® C105338

If you have any concerns about our products,
you can contact us on
ProductSafety@springernature.com

In case Publisher is established outside the EU,
the EU authorized representative is:
Springer Nature Customer Service Center GmbH
Europaplatz 3, 69115 Heidelberg, Germany

Printed by Libri Plureos GmbH
in Hamburg, Germany